MEDICAL EMERGENCIES

CONTEMPORARY ISSUES IN SMALL ANIMAL PRACTICE VOLUME 1

Editorial Advisory Board

Forthcoming Volumes in the Series

Vol. 2 Infectious Diseases
Fredric W. Scott, D.V.M., Ph.D., Guest Editor
Vol. 3 Surgical Emergencies
Ronald M. Bright, D.V.M., Guest Editor
Vol. 4 Disorders of Exotic Animals
Elliott R. Jacobson, D.V.M., Ph.D. and
George V. Kollias, Jr., D.V.M., Ph.D.,
Guest Editors
Vol. 5 Neurological Disorders
Joe N. Kornegay, D.V.M., Ph.D., Guest Editor
Vol. 6 Nephrology and Urology
Edward B. Breitschwerdt, D.V.M., Guest Editor
Vol. 7 Dermatology
Gene Nesbitt, D.V.M., Guest Editor
Vol. 8 Oncology
Neil T. Gorman, B.V.Sc., Ph.D., Guest Editor

MEDICAL EMERGENCIES

Edited by

Robert G. Sherding, D.V.M.

Associate Professor of Veterinary Clinical Sciences
Head, Small Animal Internal Medicine Section
College of Veterinary Medicine
The Ohio State University
Columbus, Ohio

Churchill Livingstone
New York, Edinburgh, London, and Melbourne   1985

Acquisitions editor: *Gene C. Kearn*
Copy editor: *Kim Loretucci*
Production editor: *Fred L. Kantrowitz*
Production supervisor: *Joe Sita*
Compositor: *Maryland Composition Company, Inc.*
Printer/Binder: *The Maple-Vail Book Manufacturing Group*

© Churchill Livingstone Inc. 1985

Distributed in the United Kingdom by Churchill Livingstone,
Robert Stevenson House, 1-3 Baxter's Place, Leith Walk,
Edinburgh EH1 3AF and by associated companies, branches
and representatives throughout the world.

First published 1985

Printed in U.S.A.

ISBN 0-443-08333-9

9 8 7 6 5 4 3 2 1

Library of Congress Cataloging in Publication Data
Main entry under title:

Medical emergencies.

   (Contemporary issues in small animal practice ; v. 1)
   Includes bibliographies and index.
   1. Veterinary emergencies.   I. Sherding, Robert G.
II. Series.   [DNLM: 1. Emergencies—veterinary.
W1 C0769MRW v.1 / SF 911 M489]
SF914.3.M43   1985   636.089′6025   84-19893
ISBN 0-443-08333-9

Manufactured in the United States of America

This book is dedicated to my children, Cameron and Heather

Contributors

Timothy A. Allen, D.V.M. Associate Professor of Veterinary Clinical Sciences, College of Veterinary Medicine and Biomedical Sciences, Colorado State University, Fort Collins, Colorado

Debra S. Barrett, D.V.M. Resident in Toxicology, Comparative Toxicology Laboratories, Kansas State University, Manhattan, Kansas

John Bonagura, D.V.M., M.S. Associate Professor of Veterinary Clinical Sciences, College of Veterinary Medicine, The Ohio State University, Columbus, Ohio

Janice M. Bright, D.V.M., M.S. Research Fellow, Department of Physiological Sciences, College of Veterinary Medicine, University of Florida, Gainesville, Florida

Dennis J. Chew, D.V.M. Associate Professor of Veterinary Clinical Sciences, College of Veterinary Medicine, The Ohio State University, Columbus, Ohio

Stephen P. DiBartola, D.V.M. Assistant Professor of Veterinary Clinical Sciences, College of Veterinary Medicine, The Ohio State University, Columbus, Ohio

William Fenner, D.V.M. Associate Professor of Veterinary Clinical Sciences, College of Veterinary Medicine, The Ohio State University, Columbus, Ohio

Richard B. Ford, D.V.M., M.S. Associate Professor of Internal Medicine, Department of Companion Animal and Special Species Medicine, North Carolina State University School of Veterinary Medicine, Raleigh, North Carolina

Steve C. Haskins, D.V.M., M.S. Associate Professor of Anesthesiology and Critical Care, Department of Surgery, School of Veterinary Medicine, University of California, Davis, California

Susan Johnson, D.V.M., M.S. Assistant Professor of Veterinary Clinical Sciences, College of Veterinary Medicine, The Ohio State University, Columbus, Ohio

William Muir, D.V.M., Ph.D. Professor and Chairman, Department of Veterinary Clinical Sciences, College of Veterinary Medicine, The Ohio State University, Columbus, Ohio

Frederick W. Oehme, D.V.M., Ph.D. Professor of Toxicology, Medicine and Physiology, Director, Comparative Toxicology Laboratories, Kansas State University, Manhattan, Kansas

Michael Schaer, D.V.M. Associate Professor of Medical Sciences, Chief, Small Animal Medicine Service, Head, Small Animal Hospital, College of Veterinary Medicine, University of Florida, Gainesville, Florida

Robert G. Sherding, D.V.M. Associate Professor of Veterinary Clinical Sciences, Head, Small Animal Internal Medicine Section, College of Veterinary Medicine, The Ohio State University, Columbus, Ohio

Carol M. Szymanski, D.V.M. Assistant Professor of Veterinary Clinical Sciences, College of Veterinary Medicine, The Ohio State University, Columbus, Ohio

Todd R. Tams, D.V.M. Clinical Assistant Professor of Medicine, Angell Memorial Animal Hospital, Tufts University School of Veterinary Medicine, Boston, Massachusetts

Preface

The veterinarian who is called upon to diagnose and treat medical emergencies must be prepared to meet the challenge of serious, life-threatening conditions involving all disciplines and body systems. In an emergency situation, swift life-and-death decisions must be made based on limited patient information, and a course of action must be implemented within minutes—sometimes even seconds. The margin for error is narrow and delay can mean catastrophe.

Emergency medicine is gradually becoming a recognized clinical specialty within veterinary practice. A major evolution in the initial diagnosis and treatment of critically ill animals is currently taking place with the widespread emergence of specialized emergency/critical care facilities in many communities. These modern, specialized facilities are staffed with specially trained personnel and equipped with emergency drugs, special instruments, resuscitative equipment, and sophisticated life-support systems. Overall, these developments have promoted improved standards of emergency care for animals.

Medical Emergencies is intended to provide a clinically useful, state-of-the-art reference and guide for the practicing veterinarian who must manage medical emergency situations. We have tried to bring together in one book information that will be helpful to both the general-practice veterinarian who must periodically treat critically ill animals and the veterinarian who practices exclusively in an emergency clinic. Emphasis has been placed on the emergency conditions and situations most frequently encountered.

An introductory chapter offers an overview of emergency care. Most of the rest of the book is organized by body system, and there are additional chapters on fluid, electrolyte, and acid-base disturbances; toxicologic emergencies; environmental injuries; and life-threatening sepsis. Although the book is organized by body system, it should be emphasized that multiple organ failure is the rule rather than the exception in emergency situations. Thus, the clinician will often be required to integrate the information from several chapters in the emergency care of a single patient. Each chapter discusses background pathophysiology, clinical signs, recognition, diagnosis, and management of the various emergency conditions. A basic understanding of pathophysiology is essential since therapy of a life-threatening condition, perhaps more than in other situations, is based on physiologic criteria and principles.

Emergency medicine is by nature multidisciplinary. A distinguished group of experts, skilled and knowledgeable in a variety of clinical specialties, have contributed to this book. The editor thanks these authors for their dedication to the development of a quality medical emergency reference.

Robert G. Sherding, D.V.M.

Contents

1 | Overview of Emergency and Intensive Care

Steve C. Haskins

It is impossible to precisely define the nature of an emergency because in its broadest scope it is entirely in the eyes of the beholder (Table 1-1). The designation "emergency" generally implies that the situation must be taken care of now and that it cannot wait until such time as it is convenient to do so. The "emergency" vaccination because the family is leaving for Canada at 6 o'clock in the morning or the "emergency" ovariohysterectomy because the surgeon is going on sabbatical are emergencies of the truest sense to these individuals. These situations would hardly be considered as such by the casual observer who can usually be overhead muttering something about a lack of organization. Emergencies of ignorance are perhaps more tolerable than emergencies of convenience. A pet vomited twice between 1 and 2 o'clock in the morning, and the owner has no idea as to whether the pet is suffering or is in danger of dying. The owner seeks out the expert advice of a veterinarian, who usually mumbles something about pet owners who cannot apply the same common sense, patience, and thoughtful neglect to their pets that they do to their children. Although attending to their presumably genuine concerns is somewhat of a nuisance, it does provide a useful service to the client: The consultation has relieved their concern. They will be able to sleep easy, knowing that the veterinarian is now morally and legally liable for any unforseen, untoward happenings.

CLASSIFICATION OF EMERGENCIES

Emergencies having medical significance are divided into three categories. Each is determined primarily by the extent of the systemic involvement of the disease process(es) and the patient's ability to compensate.

Table 1-1. Classification of Emergencies

Emergencies of convenience
Emergencies of ignorance
Noncritically ill critical patients
Subseriously ill critical patients
Immediate life-threatening crises
Cardiac arrest

The noncritically ill critical patient is mildly involved with the disease process and seems to be compensating well: The patient with a contused lung and a small, nonprogressive pneumothorax; the patient receiving continuous chest drainage or fluid administration; or the patient with the healing fractured spine. Although these are potential candidates for major catastrophes, they are at that moment stable. These are not especially high-level nursing care problems, but they nevertheless require diligent attention if an uneventful convalescence is to be achieved. Waiting, watching, and periodic corrections here and there underlie a successful endeavor.

The subseriously ill critical patient is one who is moderately involved with a systemic disease process. These are diseases which cause some embarrassment but which at the time are not likely to cause the patient's demise: a diaphragmatic hernia sustained a few hours previously, severe dehydration from a week of vomiting secondary to a gastrointestinal foreign body, pyometra, a prolapsed intervertebral disc, a badly fractured long bone. These patients often present a considerable therapeutic dilemma. Should surgical repair be attempted in a critical patient in the middle of the night when support personnel are less available? Is early surgical repair in the best interest of the patient? Will the patient's condition improve with time and/or therapy so that he will be a better surgical risk, or will his condition deteriorate if surgery is delayed? Definitive cures of all illnesses need not be rendered in the emergency room; stabilization of those aspects of the illness which are potentially life-threatening, however, must be. Critically ill patients must be stabilized as much as possible before any surgical or diagnostic intervention. Many times stabilization therapy converts a subseriously ill critical patient into a noncritically ill critical patient. Once homeostasis compatible with long-term survival has been achieved, definitive corrective procedures can be completed in a carefully planned and orderly manner. A disease is defined as a subserious illness if the patient is so unstable that the veterinarian feels compelled to remain in constant attendance. If a disease is serious enough to elicit the question of whether it is an emergency, it is probably serious enough to be categorized as at least a subserious illness.

Severe involvement with virtually any disease process may be a serious threat to the life of the patient. Hypovolemic or septic shock, decompensated heart or pulmonary failure, end-stage renal or hepatic disease, severe hypoglycemia or fluid and electrolyte disorders, head trauma, heat stroke, dystocia, and gastric torsion represent major homeostatic instabilities. Rapid, effective

Table 1-2. Guidelines for Categorizing the Seriousness of the Illness

Parameter	Noncritically Ill Critical Patient	Subseriously Ill Critical Patient	Life-Threatening Crisis
Bradycardia	Heart rate in normal range	<60/min	<40/min
Tachycardia	Heart rate in normal range	>180/min	>250/min (?)
Ventricular arrhythmias	Occasional	Frequent (>several/min), ventricular rhythm <160/min	Increasingly frequent, multifocal ventricular tachycardia (>180/min)
Hypovolemia	No clinically apparent compensatory changes	Of sufficient magnitude to cause compensatory changes and a lowering of blood pressure	Of sufficient magnitude to cause severe hypotension and mental obtundation
Hypotension	Blood pressure in normal range	60–80 mm Hg (mean)	<60 mm Hg (mean)
Dehydration	Barely decreased skin turgor (5–6%)	Moderately decreased skin turgor (7–9%)	Severely decreased skin turgor (>10%)
Upper airway obstruction	Stertorous breathing but no change in respiratory pattern	Stertorous breathing, long slow inspiratory efforts, no cyanosis	Stertorous breathing, long slow inspiratory efforts with intercostal retraction, "dyspnea," and cyanosis
Pleural filling defect or pulmonary parenchymal disease	No change in respiratory pattern, nonprogressive	Some increased breathing effort	Severely increased breathing effort, progressive disease, cyanosis

This table represents some general categorizations representing the author's best approximation to give the reader some guidelines in decision-making processes about the seriousness of the disease process. No part should be quoted or referenced as having any basis in fact. All abnormalities should be correlated with all other historical, physical, physiological, and laboratory findings before any decisions are made regarding the importance of any individual parameter or the overall status of the patient.

[a] The physiological consequence of an electrolyte imbalance depends to a large extent on the rate of development of the imbalance.

intervention is of paramount importance. A disease may be defined as life-threatening if, as the term implies, the patient would not be expected to survive its immediate manifestations.

How does one decide just how sick a patient is and which category of emergency or critical illness he represents? It is a decision based on general guidelines (which are presented throughout this chapter and this book), experience, intuition, and common sense (Table 1-2). There is not, unfortunately, a well-established clear-cut perimeter of health beyond which the patient becomes obviously critically ill or life-threatened.

The necessary therapy is initially provided to alleviate the crisis, regardless of the time or the inconvenience, and then the patient is monitored to make sure he remains stable until he recovers or until definitive therapy can be rendered. When one is not sure if the disease is life-threatening, the patient is monitored carefully until it can be determined whether it is or is not. If it is decided that a condition is not a life-threatening problem, it is always advisable to monitor the patient frequently enough to make sure that it does not become one. Long-term (overnight) forecasting about the nature and progress of a crit-

Table 1-2. (*continued*)

Parameter	Non critically Ill Critical Patient	Subseriously Ill Critical Patient	Life-Threatening Crisis
CNS-induced hypoventilation	Hypoventilation or bradypnea not clinically apparent; minute volume >150 ml/kg/min; $Paco_2$ <45 mm Hg	Hypoventilation or bradypnea clinically apparent; minute volume 100–150 ml/kg/min; $Paco_2$ 45–60 mm Hg	Severe hypoventilation or bradypnea; minute volume <100 ml/kg/min; $Paco_2$ >60 mm Hg
Hypoxemia	No change in respiratory pattern; Pao_2 >80 mm Hg	Some increased breathing effort; Pao_2 60–80 mm Hg	Marked increased breathing effort; Pao_2 <60 mm Hg; cyanosis
CNS disease	Some dementia or disorientation; all cranial nerves normal	Depression, lethargy; all cranial nerves normal	Stupor, coma; cranial nerves abnormal
Hypothermia	>34°C (94°F)	29–34°C (85–94°F)	<29°C (85°F)
Hyperthermia	<40°C (104°F)	40–41°C (104–106°F)	>41°C (106°F)
Hypokalemia[a]	No apparent clinical signs; >3.0 mEq/L	Evidence of skeletal and smooth muscle weakness; 2.0–3.0 mEq/L	Evidence of ECG alterations and/or ventricular ectopic beats; <2.0 mEq/L
Hyperkalemia[a]	No apparent clinical signs; <6.0 mEq/L	Mild ECG alterations; 6.0–8.0 mEq/L	Marked ECG alterations; >8.0 mEq/L
Hyponatremia[a], hypoosmolality[a]	No apparent clinical signs; <135 mEq/L; <280 mOsm/kg	Some mental obtundation; <125 mEq/L; <260 mOsm/kg	Severe mental obtundation; <115 mEq/L; <240 mOsm/kg
Hypernatremia[a], hyperosmolality[a]	No apparent clinical signs; >155 mEq/L; >320 mOsm/kg	Some mental obtundation; >165 mEq/L; >340 mOsm/kg	Severe mental obtundation; >175 mEq/L; >360 mOsm/kg
Anemia	>20%	15–20%	<15%
Polycythemia	<60%	60–70%	>70%
Hypoproteinemia	>3.5 g/dl	2.5–3.5 g/dl	<2.5 g/dl
Hyperproteinemia	<10 g/dl	10–14 g/dl	>14 g/dl
Hypoglycemia	>60 mg/dl	40–60 mg/dl	<40 mg/dl
Uremia	Mildly elevated BUN (<50 mg/dl); stable	Moderately elevated BUN (50–100 mg/dl); stable; no mental obtundation	Severely elevated BUN (>100 mg/dl); progressive mental depression; vomiting

ically ill patient is not necessary. Adequate monitoring is the key, and with the advent of emergency night-time veterinary facilities it can be a reality.

What should be monitored? As many parameters as possible should be monitored. The more that is known about the patient, the better one is able to accurately assess the patient's response to the disease and to the therapy. All findings and observations should be recorded. Trends are much more meaningful than individual values and much more accurate than memory.

How often should the patient be monitored? Each parameter is monitored as often as is necessary to ensure that it is normal, stable, or at least improving. The more unstable the parameter, the more often it should be evaluated. If at any time there is reason to believe that a parameter has changed since the last evaluation, it is remeasured.

How long should it be monitored? Monitoring frequency may decrease as the patient convalesces, but there are only two reasons to stop monitoring: recovery and death.

Cardiac arrest is presented as a distinct emergency category. It is one step beyond a life-threatening crisis; it is a "12" on an emergency scale of "1 to 10," it is the grandfather of all emergencies. Its prevention is the reason that books are written on the treatment of life-threatening crises; it is much easier to prevent than to treat. Early recognition and aggressive therapy is of paramount importance (Ch. 2). Careful preplanning is a necessary precursor to a successful resuscitation endeavor. A management protocol and drug dosages should be established and posted in plain view in the animal care facility.[9] All personnel in the hospital should be trained to be a functional part of the resuscitation team. Necessary equipment and supplies should be readily available and in working order at all times.

ORGANIZATION OF AN EMERGENCY/INTENSIVE CARE UNIT

There are several important components to an effective emergency and critical care endeavor. Each should be as fully developed as possible and all should be as well-coordinated as possible.

Software

The knowledge of what to look for in the history, physical examination, laboratory analyses, and physiological measurements, as well as how to interpret the findings and return them to normal, are of course basic to the endeavor. It is important to know the normal and to be able to recognize, characterize, and quantitate the abnormal and its effects on the patient. It is important to know patterns of disease and to develop problem lists of possible causes for all abnormalities. Perhaps most important is common sense or the ability to apply the knowledge to a wide variety of clinical circumstances, many of which the clinician may never have encountered before.

Knowledge, without the technical expertise to implement it, is of little value. One should be sufficiently familiar with each diagnostic or monitoring procedure or therapeutic technique that it can be utilized in a variety of circumstances so as to provide repeatable information and reliable results. Because new procedures and techniques are plagued with technical misadventures, they should first be learned on noncritical patients in nonstressful situations.

Emergency medicine and especially intensive care tend to be prolonged, intense projects requiring a team of knowledgeable and technically competent personnel. Each member of the team must be prepared, alert, and diligently attentive to the task at hand. Each must be able to work independently, think creatively, and yet follow instructions precisely. The management of critically ill patients may consume a substantial portion of a person's time. The cost of such an intense, sometimes prolonged endeavor may be high.

Hardware

Diagnostic equipment increases the accuracy of the initial evaluation of the patient; monitoring equipment enhances the effectiveness of surveillance of the patient's response to therapy; and therapeutic equipment facilitates administration of the appropriate treatment. Equipment is not a substitute for frequent patient observation and reevaluation; it merely extends and expands basic clinical skills and allows more meaningful, more interesting, and more effective use of the veterinarian's time (Table 1-3).

Expendable supplies (e.g., catheters, fluids, drugs, paper, and soap) are inevitably utilized to a greater extent in the management of critically ill patients because of the depth of involvement of monitoring and treatment procedures (Table 1-3).

A wide variety of drugs are necessary to accommodate a diverse array of critical care and emergency situations (Table 1-3). The user should know the relative indications, preferred technique of administration, and appropriate precautions and dangers for each drug.

Little is accomplished without an accurate written record of observations and treatments. Because there is such a wide variation in normal values, individual numbers are much more meaningful when they are compared to a series of previous measurements. It is important to keep track of trends during treatment. Future reference to treatment records may be required for medical or legal purposes.

The absolutely essential hardware item to the practice of intensive care is money. The cost of such care is inevitably high: the time commitment for the academic and technical preparation, the time commitment for the patient care endeavor, the quantity and quality of the personnel, the purchase of equipment, the upkeep and repairs on the equipment, and the purchase of expendable supplies and drugs. A wide variety of software and hardware must be on hand so as to be prepared for most of the emergencies that may be encountered. It is not economically feasible, however, to have all of the personnel, equipment, and inventory on hand and no cases to pay for them. An emergency which can be rapidly resolved is usually affordable. Abnormalities which are not easily stabilized require careful and sometimes prolonged postacute care and observation in order to ensure an uneventful recovery. Such cases are unquestionably more common than is the availability of the financial backing.

The need for centralized critical care facilities is readily apparent. The advent of emergency practices where professional supervision is available during the "off" hours is a beginning. Shuttling the patients between the daytime and the off-time practice is a technical problem that, for the most part, seems to have been worked out by delegating this responsibility to the owner. If the patient is stable, this practice is quite acceptable. If the patient is not stable, a more qualified ambulance service probably should be arranged.

An emergency practice should be equipped as well as, if not better than, a regular daytime practice (Table 1-3). The emergency practice serves a concentrated population of emergency and critically ill patients. A diverse array

Table 1-3. Equipment, Supplies, and Drugs Which May Be of Use in the Emergency and Intensive Care Setting

I. Equipment
  A. Highest priority
    1. Means of providing oxygen
    2. Means of providing positive-pressure ventilation
    3. Assortment of endotracheal tubes
    4. Sterile surgical instruments and towels
    5. Surgical lights
    6. Assortment of stomach tubes and stomach pumps
    7. Electrocardiograph
    8. Anesthetic machine
    9. Hematocrit tubes and centrifuge
    10. Refractometer
    11. Microscope
    12. Spectrophotometer
    13. Defibrillator with small and large external and internal paddles
    14. Suction apparatus and catheters
    15. Chemistry strips for blood glucose and urea nitrogen
    16. Ophthalmoscope
    17. Face masks
    18. Coagulation testing method
    19. Blood pressure measuring equipment
    20. Radiographic equipment
    21. Laryngoscope and assortment of blades
    22. Circulating warm water blanket or infrared heat lamp
  B. Desirable
    1. Tracheostomy tubes
    2. Harleco total CO_2 apparatus or Oxford titrator
    3. Blood gas analyzer
    4. Flame photometer
    5. Osmometer
    6. Fluid infusion pump
    7. Nebulizer (ultrasonic)
II. Supplies
  A. Highest priority
    1. Full assortment of peripheral and jugular venous catheters
      a. Outside-the-needle catheters for peripheral veins, 2.5 inch 18 and 20 gauge
      b. Outside-the-needle catheters for small peripheral veins, 1.0 and 0.75 inch 22 and 24 gauge
      c. Outside-the-needle catheters for temporary chest or abdominal drains, tracheal catheters, jugular veins, or femoral arteries or veins (5.5 inch 14 or 16 gauge)
      d. Inside-the-needle catheters for jugular veins or tracheal catheters, 8 and 12 inch 17, 19, and 21 gauge
    2. Wide selection of fluids
      a. Lactated Ringer's (or equivalent solution)
      b. Saline
      c. Dextrose in water 5%
      d. Maintenance solution
      e. High- and low-molecular-weight dextran
      f. Source of whole blood (A-negative) and plasma
      g. Mannitol
    3. Wide selection of concentrates
      a. Sodium bicarbonate
      b. Potassium chloride
      c. Dextrose in water 50%
      d. Heparin
    4. Administration sets—regular and pediatric (blood filter sets)
    5. Extension sets, three-way stopcocks, and catheter caps
    6. Chest drain cannulas
    7. Urinary catheters

Table 1-3. (*continued*)

    8. Closed urine collection bags
    9. Tape, cotton, gauze, and other bandaging materials
    10. Fleece pads for cage padding
    11. Sandbags for positioning
  B. Desirable
    1. Water-trap chest drain system
    2. Calibrated burette for accurate fluid administration
III. Drugs
  A. Highest priority
    1. Epinephrine
    2. Sodium bicarbonate
    3. Atropine
    4. Blood pressure stimulant (choose one)
      a. Mephentermine
      b. Dopamine
      c. Dobutamine
      d. Ephedrine
    5. Vasoconstrictor (choose one)
      a. Phenylephrine
      b. Norepinephrine
    6. Cardiotonics (several)
      a. Calcium
      b. Digitalis
      c. Isoproterenol
      d. Blood pressure stimulant
      e. Glucagon
    7. Antiarrhythmic agents (several)
      a. Lidocaine
      b. Procainamide
      c. Quinidine
      d. Beta-receptor blocking agent (propranolol)
    8. Tranquilizers, sedatives
      a. Meperidine
      b. Acepromazine
    9. Anesthetics for cardiovascularly debilitated patients
      a. Oxymorphone and diazepam
      b. Ketamine and diazepam
    10. Any other anesthetic of choice for other patients
    11. Analeptics
      a. Narcotic reversing agent (naloxone)
      b. Doxapram
    12. Glucocorticoids (either)
      a. Dexamethasone phosphate
      b. Prednisolone succinate
    13. Diuretics (all)
      a. Furosemide
      b. Mannitol, dextrose
      c. Dopamine
    14. Antipyretic
      a. Dipyrone
      b. Antiprostaglandins
    15. Antiemetics
      a. Thorazine
      b. Prochlorperazine
    16. Antitoxins
      a. Activated charcoal
      b. Pralidoxime (for organophosphates)
      c. Edathamil Calcium-Disodium (CaEDTA) (for lead)
      d. Dimercaprol (for arsenic)
      e. Atropine (for organophosphates)

Table 1-3. (*continued*)

f. Sodium nitrite and sodium thiosulfate (for cyanide)
g. Sodium bicarbonate and vinegar (for neutralization of acids and alkalis, respectively)
h. Apomorphine
i. Kaolin-pectate
j. Vitamin K
17. Broad-spectrum antibiotics
B. Desirable
  1. Antihistamine (diphenhydramine)
  2. Aminophylline
  3. Vasodilator
    a. Nitroprusside
    b. Nitroglycerin
    c. Phentolamine
    d. Clonidine
    e. Prazosin
  4. Neuromuscular blocking agent and reversing agent

of diagnostic, monitoring, and therapeutic equipment, supplies, and drugs should be readily available and in working order. An underequipped, undersupplied, understaffed, or underknowledged emergency practice may provide relief from emergency calls for area veterinarians, but it provides limited service to its clients.

A successful emergency and intensive care endeavor requires at least:

1. Veterinary supervision
2. Animal health technician support
3. Knowledge
4. Common sense
5. Technical ability
6. Equipment
7. Expendable supplies
8. Patients
9. Money
10. Records

Lack of any one item severely undermines the efforts and effectiveness of all other aspects of the operation.

INITIAL EVALUATION AND THERAPY OF AN EMERGENCY

When the patient is first presented, the presence of any life-threatening emergency should be determined. Is the heart still beating? If not, cardiopulmonary resuscitation should be instituted (Ch. 2). Is the heartbeat regular? If not, an electrocardiographic (ECG) diagnosis is obtained and the condition treated accordingly (Ch. 2). Is there an adequate pulse? If not, is it due to heart failure or hypovolemia (Ch. 2)? Is the patient breathing? If not, he should be intubated and ventilated. Is the patient breathing adequately and with minimal effort? If not, why not (Ch. 3)? Is the patient convulsing? If so, anticonvulsant therapy should be instituted (Ch. 9). Is there profuse external hemorrhage? If so, it must be stopped. What is the patient's temperature?

Once effective intervention for all life-threatening emergencies has been instituted, a more thorough history, physical examination, and plan for diagnostic procedures and laboratory analyses can be contemplated. The owners should be asked for a brief version of their story. Specific but nonleading questions may help ferret out additional useful information. The pattern of the history and the presenting signs help to differentiate between the likely diseases and to guide further diagnostic endeavors and laboratory analyses. Lists of differential diagnoses help guide the work-up and reduce the likelihood of missed diagnoses. As the diagnostic work-up evolves and the underlying problem becomes more apparent, the provisional hypothesis, prognosis, treatment protocol, and expected costs can be discussed with the owner.

Evaluation and Initial Therapy of the Cardiovascular System

Is the heart still beating? Is it still regular? Is the pulse still acceptable? What is the heart rate? The normal heart rate varies between 80 and 160 beats per minute (bpm). Slow or fast heart rates or rapid changes in a previously stable heart rate should be investigated (Ch. 2). Very slow or fast heart rates or irregular heart rates should be characterized electrocardiographically and treated when necessary (Ch. 2). If the bradycardia, tachycardia, or arrhythmia is not life-threatening, only the underlying disease process need be corrected. If the bradycardia is severe, a beta-receptor stimulating sympathomimetic drug is administered (epinephrine, dopamine, mephentermine, dobutamine, isoproterenol). The heart rate should be maintained above 60 bpm unless blood pressure, cardiac output, or mixed venous oxygen content can be measured and adequate tissue perfusion ensured. No maximum heart rate has been established; however, if pulse quality, blood pressure, cardiac output, or mixed venous oxygen content reflect inadequate cardiac output, attempts should be made to slow the heart (infusion of any beta-receptor stimulant stopped, propranolol administered to block sympathetic tone, carotid sinus pressure applied, or perhaps narcotics or neostigmine administered to increase vagal tone or digitalis given to slow atrioventricular conduction). Ventricular arrhythmias that are rapid (> 180 bpm), multifocal, or worsening in severity should be treated (lidocaine, procainamide, lidocaine plus procainamide, propranolol, verapamil, bretylium). See Chapter 2 for a detailed discussion of therapy of cardiac emergencies.

Is the patient dehydrated or hypovolemic? Is there historical or physical evidence of a disease which is compatible with whole blood, plasma, or fluid loss (blunt trauma, big dog/little dog encounter, penetrating injury, bone fracture, hydrothorax, ascites, gastrointestinal losses, lack of food and water intake, polyuric renal disease, etc.)? Gastrointestinal, renal, and third space fluid losses typically have high sodium levels (60–120 mEq/L) and moderate potassium levels (5–25 mEq/L). Dehydrated patients are always hypovolemic. Dehydrated and hypovolemic patients should receive a bolus of fluids. A large-bore catheter should be aseptically placed in a peripheral or jugular vein. The initial replacement fluid should be approximately isotonic and isoelectric [sodium 130–155 mEq/L, potassium 5 mEq/L, bicarbonate-like anion (lactate, acetate, gluconate) about 24 mEq/L]. For specific circumstances there may be an indication to increase or decrease the sodium, potassium, and/or bicarbonate concentrations.[8] Whole blood or plasma infusion may be indicated to maintain the packed cell volume above 20% and the total protein above 3.5 g/dl. Fluids should be administered in a volume that is sufficient to eliminate the signs of dehydration, hypovolemia, and peripheral vasoconstriction and to restore arterial blood pressure and central venous pressure to acceptable levels (Table 1-4). The volume administered may range from 10 to 90 ml/kg or more. See Chapter 4 for a detailed discussion of fluid therapy.

Is there evidence of peripheral vasoconstriction? Peripheral vasoconstriction is most often a compensatory response to hypovolemia, although it may be caused by any stress which increases sympathetic tone. Vasoconstriction impairs visceral tissue perfusion and should not be allowed to persist. Usually correction of the underlying disease process is sufficient to alleviate it. Specific vasodilator therapy may be useful under some circumstances, e.g., during therapy for hypovolemic or septic shock or congestive heart failure (glucocorticosteroids, phenothiazine tranquilizers, morphine, nitroprusside, nitroglycerin, phentolamine, clonidine, prazosin). The continuous measurement of arterial blood pressure is beneficial during the use of potent vasodilators to avoid excessive hypotension.

Is the patient hypotensive? Blood pressure should be measured if possible.[9] Hypotension may be suspected if: (1) there is a history or physical evidence of fluid loss or heart failure; (2) the heart rate is very slow, fast, or irregular; or (3) there is excessive vasodilation (Ch. 2; Tables 2-1 and 2-2). Blood pressure is important to cerebral and coronary perfusion and must be preserved at all cost. If the patient seems to be in danger of dying from hypotension and the heart is beating regularly and fast, an alpha-receptor stimulating agent (phenylephrine or norepinephrine) should be administered; if the heart is slow and weak, an alpha- and beta-receptor stimulating agent (epinephrine or dopamine) should be given. These temporary maneuvers may be necessary to keep the patient alive long enough to allow introduction of an intravenous catheter and administration of a suitable dose of fluids, to digitalize the heart, or to stabilize the underlying disease process.

Central venous pressure and pulmonary arterial wedge pressure measurements reflect the ability of the right and left heart, respectively, to accommodate the venous return. Measurement of central venous pressure may aid in the evaluation of the effectiveness of therapy in right heart failure or may help delineate the endpoint of fluid therapy when very large volumes are administered in the treatment of such conditions as hypovolemic or septic shock. Meas-

Table 1-4. Important Considerations in Replacement Fluid Therapy

Applicable Measurement and Desired Level	Fluids of Choice If Measured Parameter Is Outside the Desired Level
Volume Central venous pressure: 2–10 cm H_2O Arterial blood pressure: 80–120 mm Hg (mean) Pulse quality: strong Capillary refill time: <1 sec Mucous membrane color: pink Normal skin turgor	1. Crystalloid sodium replacement solution (lactated Ringer's or equivalent solution) 2. Colloid expander (dextran, plasma) 3. Whole blood
Oxygen-carrying capacity Packed cell volume: >20% Hemoglobin: >7 g/dl	1. Whole blood
Colloid oncotic pressure Total plasma protein: >3.5 g/dl	1. Colloid expander (plasma, dextran) 2. Whole blood
Electrolytes Sodium: 135–155 mEq/L	1. Lactated Ringer's if sodium concentration is in normal range 2. Lactated Ringer's plus 5% dextrose in water if sodium >155 mEq/L 3. Saline (plus potassium and bicarbonate) if sodium <135 mEq/L
Potassium: 3.5–5.5 mEq/L	1. For bolus dosages of fluids, potassium concentration should be 5 mEq/L 2. For a slower repair of dehydration, potassium concentrtion should be 20 mEq/L 3. Omit all potassium if patient is hyperkalemic 4. Potassium 40, 60, or 80 mEq/L if plasma concentration is 3.0–3.5, 2.5–3.0, or <2.5, respectively
Bicarbonate: 18–28 mEq/L	1. Administer a fluid with a bicarbonate concentration of about 24 mEq/L if patient has no acid-base disturbance 2. Add 1–5 mEq/kg if patient has metabolic acidosis 3. Use saline without bicarbonate if patient has metabolic alkalosis

urement of pulmonary capillary wedge pressure may aid in the evaluation of the effectiveness of therapy in left heart failure or in the control of capillary hydrostatic pressure in pulmonary edema.

The clinical measurement of cardiac output by thermal-indicator dilution techniques is currently possible. The measurement of cardiac output and its response to disease, cardiotonics, fluid loading, and treatment of the underlying disease would be very helpful in maximizing the effectiveness of the therapeutic endeavor.

If the mucous membrane color is pale, is it due to peripheral vasoconstriction or anemia?

Is there any evidence of acute or chronic heart failure (Ch. 2)? If so, a cardiotonic, e.g., a beta-receptor agonist catecholamine (mephentermine, dobutamine, dopamine, or isoproterenol), calcium, or digoxin, should be administered. Reducing venous return and preload by administering venodilators or diuretics, positive-pressure ventilation, or phlebotomy may also be helpful. Reducing arterial blood pressure and afterload by administering arteriolar vasodilators may be helpful. Propranolol may be useful in the treatment of hypertrophic cardiomyopathy.

Evaluation and Initial Therapy of the Respiratory System

Is the animal breathing? If not, it should be intubated and positive-pressure ventilated until the underlying disease process is corrected to a sufficient degree that it can spontaneously maintain its own respiratory requirements (Ch. 3; Table 3-4).

The airway should be secured with an endotracheal tube. Although commercial endotracheal tubes are the safest, any hollow tube made of any material may be used in the emergency situation. Although dogs and cats can be ventilated with a face mask or by blowing through their nose while holding the mouth closed, there is a great tendency to inflate the esophagus and stomach instead of the lungs. This can be minimized by gently pressing upward on the larynx (not the trachea) and occluding the esophagus during the application of positive pressure to the airway. Artificial ventilation is usually accomplished by manual compression of a rebreathing bag or a mechanical ventilator. In the absence of these, a T-tube attached to a pressurized gas source or air compressor,[12] mouth-to-tube, large syringe, or an ordinary tire pump can be used. Pulmonary resuscitation is discussed in Chapter 3.

What is the breathing rate? Rate alone has little meaning without reference to the nature of the ventilatory effort and the volume. A change in rate, however, may signify a change in the status of an underlying disease process.

What is the character of the ventilatory effort? Is it weak and slow as might be expected in central nervous system (CNS) or neuromuscular disease? Is it slow and deep as might be expected with partial airway obstruction, or is it fast and shallow as might be expected with pleural space or parenchymal lung disease or abdominal distention? Is it fast and deep as might be expected with nonrespiratory causes of hyperventilation or mechanical apparatus-related hypoxemia or hypercapnia? Is it irregular as might be expected in brainstem disease? Is the patient breathing adequately and with minimal effort? If not, the cause should be determined and treated accordingly (Ch. 3). The extent of the involvement with the disease process should be assessed at the beginning and then at regular intervals thereafter by evaluating as many parameters as are available.

Hypoxemic animals are difficult to manage because of their tendency to react adversely to diagnostic or therapeutic stresses. Preliminary insufflation of oxygen through an intratracheal catheter (Ch. 3; Fig. 3-1) can be lifesaving and reduces the hazards associated with diagnostic examination, restraint procedures, and the administration of sedative or anesthetic drugs.

Is the integrity of the thoracic wall intact? An open hole in the chest wall should be occluded immediately. A chest tube should be introduced at the same time and air rapidly aspirated with a high-flow suction unit, a simple water faucet Venturi T-tube, or a large syringe. The patient should then be anesthetized, intubated, and the opening surgically repaired. Damage to intrathoracic organs should be evaluated at the time of surgery. Fractured ribs may require surgical repair if they are displaced. If not, cage rest and analgesic support is indicated. Thoracic puncture wounds from any cause associated with thoracic complications, e.g., pneumothorax or hemothorax, warrant thoracotomy. The underlying damage can be surprisingly extensive. Thoracic injuries are discussed in Chapter 3.

Is there auscultatory evidence of an upper or lower airway obstruction? Symptomatic relief of a partial, non-life-threatening upper or lower airway obstruction can many times be accomplished if the patient can be made to breath in a less vigorous fashion by the administration of a small dose of tranquilizer or sedative. Careful monitoring is necessary during the onset of action of the drug to ensure that excessive respiratory depression does not develop. Insufflation of oxygen may be necessary.

If the obstruction is severe and an immediate danger to the life of the patient, more definitive therapy should be instituted (Ch. 3). Examination of the pharynx and larynx may reveal a removable foreign body or a nonremovable lesion that can be bypassed by endotracheal intubation or tracheostomy. Endotracheal intubation may require general anesthesia. If the larynx is difficult to visualize, a small-diameter, stiff urinary catheter can be inserted to serve as a guide for the endotracheal tube. If the larynx is impossible to visualize or intubate, a tracheostomy is performed. Emergency tracheostomies are plagued with technical complications, and careful attention must be given to aseptic surgical technique and accurate surgical dissection of the tissues. If the obstruction occurs subsequent to endotracheal intubation, the cuff is deflated and the tube repositioned or replaced. If the severe obstruction is intrathoracic, oxygen insufflation, general anesthesia, endotracheal intubation, and positive-pressure ventilation are palliative and provide the time necessary for a complete investigation and repair of the underlying problem (Ch. 3). Young puppies play with small objects and occasionally inhale them. If this is a possibility, the dog is lifted by the hind legs and shaken. Several brisk compressions should be applied around the circumference of the abdomen (taking care to avoid the ribs and liver). This forced "cough" may cause the object to be expelled.

If the obstruction is thought to be due to severe diffuse bronchospam, a potent beta-stimulating bronchodilator (epinephrine, dopamine, dobutamine, albuterol, or terbutaline) is administered intravenously, intramuscularly, or subcutaneously. If the bronchospasm is not life-threatening, aminophylline or nebulization of beta$_2$-stimulants may be indicated. This is discussed further in Chapter 3.

Are there regional, unilateral, or bilateral decreases in the amplitude of the lung and/or heart sounds, and percussion evidence of a decreased or increased resonance? A diagnostic thoracentesis (with an intravenous catheter system) is performed at a high and a low point on the thoracic wall if a pleural space filling disease is expected. If air or fluid is obtained, as much as possible should be removed and the fluid saved for cytologic examination and culture and sensitivity. Chyle, transudates, and exudates are usually slow to reaccumulate. Hemothorax or pneumothorax due to blunt trauma may or may not reaccumulate. Rapid reaccumulation of any fluid is an indication for placement of an indwelling chest drain (Ch. 3). If auscultation, percussion, and abdominal palpation indicate a diaphragmatic hernia and the respiratory distress is severe, one can try to shake the viscera back into the abdomen. An emergency laparotomy and manual retrieval of the viscera may be necessary. Surgical intervention is usually required for repair of a diaphragmatic hernia, internal wounds due to big dog/little dog encounters, projectile injuries, penetrating injuries from sharp objects, or displaced rib fractures.

Is there auscultatory, radiographic, or blood gas evidence of parenchymal lung disease? The major emphasis of symptomatic support of diffuse infiltrative pulmonary parenchymal disease is the prevention of hypoxemia until the underlying disease process can be identified and effectively treated (Ch. 3). When a dyspneic, hypoxemic patient is first presented, it is convention to start treatment with oxygen. If inspired oxygen concentrations up to 60% fail to provide symptomatic relief, the concentration is temporarily increased to 100% and positive airway pressure is then instituted as described in Chapter 3. A patient should not be allowed to breath oxygen in concentrations above 80% for more than about 12–24 hr. If the patient is breathing well (as determined by clinical estimation or by a Paco$_2$ of less than 40 mm Hg) and yet is hypoxemic, continuous positive pressure may be applied during spontaneous breathing. If the patient is not breathing well, intermittent positive-pressure ventilation should be instituted with quantities of positive end-expiratory pressure sufficient to keep the patient well oxygenated with minimal depression of venous return, cardiac output, and arterial blood pressure.

Once the immediate life-threatening status of the pulmonary parenchymal disease has been ameliorated, the nature of the infiltrate is evaluated and the patient treated in an appropriate manner. The protein content of any pulmonary edema fluid can be compared with that of plasma to help determine the nature of the underlying abnormality. Exudates are cytologically characterized and cultured. Physical therapeutic techniques (postural drainage, chest percussion or vibration, nebulization, and perhaps tracheal suctioning) are used to mobilize and facilitate removal of airway secretions.

Evaluation and Initial Therapy of the CNS

Is the patient convulsing (Ch. 9)? If so, glucose 0.5–1.0 g/kg is administered intravenously. If hypocalcemia is suspected, 2 ml of 10% calcium chloride is administered slowly intravenously (IV) (for an average sized dog). If the seizures do not cease, diazepam (0.25 mg/kg IV) is given. Diazepam may be repeated two to four times if the seizure activity does not stop within a few minutes after administration. If the diazepam controls the seizure, it should be readministered as often as is necessary to achieve continued control. If repeated doses of diazepam do not terminate the seizures, the patient can be lightly anesthetized with pentobarbital (2 mg/kg at 2-min intervals to effect, up to 25 mg/kg). Continued seizure control is maintained with phenobarbital (2 mg/kg/dose to effect). A detailed discussion of seizure management can be found in Chapter 9.

Seizures must be terminated as soon as possible for reasons discussed in Chapter 9. Seizuring patients ventilate poorly and are hypoxemic and hypercapnic. They are in danger of vomiting and aspiration as well as hyperthermia. The patient should be evaluated for these abnormalities during and after the seizure. Is there any physical or historical evidence of poisoning (Ch. 11)? Samples of blood, urine, vomitus, feces, and possibly cerebrospinal fluid (CSF) are taken and saved for laboratory analysis.

Is the patient comatose or severely depressed (Ch. 9)? Is there historical, physical, or laboratory evidence of poisoning, visceral organ failure, or metabolic disorder? Is there evidence of blunt trauma to the head? Is there diffuse cerebral or brainstem dysfunction (Ch. 9)? Cerebral injuries, which cause patients to progress from demented to stuporous to comatose, and brainstem injuries (which produce coma at the outset) are associated with a poor prognosis. A thorough neurologic examination and careful evaluation of pupillary reflexes are performed according to the guidelines in Chapter 9.

Are there any irregularities in the breathing cycle? A Cheyne-Stokes breathing pattern is evidence of diencephalic involvement and carries a guarded prognosis. Central neurogenic hyperventilation is indicative of lower midbrain/pons involvement apneustic breathing indicates caudal pons damage; cluster, ataxic, and Biot's breathing indicate medullary injury; and agonal gasps and apnea indicate severe respiratory center dysfunction. All indicate severe brainstem disease and a poor prognosis.

Decerebrate rigidity or flaccid paralysis indicate midbrain to medullary injury, respectively, and warrant a poor prognosis. Decerebrate rigidity must be differentiated from decerebellate rigidity and Schiff-Sherrington syndrome (Ch. 9).

Is there evidence of depressed skull fracture? Such fractures must be decompressed as soon as possible after CNS dehydration therapy has begun. If elevated intracranial pressure or CNS edema are thought to be present, CNS dehydration therapy is instituted as described in Chapter 9, including fluid restriction, hyperosmotic agents (mannitol, glucose), glucocorticosteroids (dexamethasone), hyperventilation (to reduce CO_2 and cerebral blood flow), elevation of the head, and prevention of hypotension or hypoxemia. Dimethylsulfoxide may have some beneficial effects: diuresis, reduction of edema, and minimization of further mechanical brain damage (1–2 g/kg IV of a 40% solution).

The progression of the CNS signs should be noted. Surgical decompression may be indicated if the patient's signs deteriorate in spite of aggressive medical therapy or if there is a depressed skull fracture.

Fluid overloading should be avoided in patients with CNS injury. CNS autoregulation of local blood flow and the blood-brain barrier may not be intact, and this increases the susceptibility to cerebral edema.

Is there evidence of spinal cord disease: paresis or paralysis of any of the limbs? If so, the vertebral column should be stabilized. CNS dehydration therapy should be initiated and the severity and progression of the disease process evaluated. Surgical decompression may be indicated if the patient's signs deteriorate or if onset of the disability has been within the last few hours and the cord damage is not too severe, as evidenced by the retention of deep pain sensation. Spinal cord injury is discussed in Chapter 9.

Evaluation and Initial Therapy of Abdominal Disease

Is there abdominal pain with palpation (Table 1-5)? If the problem had an acute onset, what was the patient doing just before the onset? Are bowel sounds normal (as in diseases which do not involve the gastrointestinal tract), increased (as in gastroenteritis or acute bowel obstruction), or decreased (as in any diffuse peritonitis)? The presence of bowel sounds per se does not preclude serious gastrointestinal involvement and their absence does not prove it. Is there vomiting or diarrhea (Ch. 7); what is its character (color, consistency, abnormal constituents)? Is there evidence of abdominal wall blunt trauma or penetrating injury? Penetrating wounds due to high-speed projectiles or associated with abdominal pain, peritonitis, or free abdominal air warrant a diagnostic laparotomy. Abdominal paracentesis or peritoneal lavage may help establish a diagnosis or delineate the need for surgery.[4] What is the radiographic appearance of the abdomen?

Is there abdominal distention (Table 1-6)? If so, is there increased or decreased resonance upon percussion? If the distention is due to fluid, what is the nature of the fluid (paracentesis)? If the distention is due to air, is it a gastric

Table 1-5. Causes of Abdominal Pain

A. Acute pain associated with trauma
    1. Ruptured kidney, liver, spleen, urinary bladder, ureter, pancreas, or hollow viscera
    2. Renal contusion
B. Acute onset pain which may or may not be associated with vomiting or diarrhea
    1. Gastrointestinal obstruction
       a. Foreign body
       b. Volvulus
       c. Intussusception
       d. Strangulated hernia
    2. Gastroenteritis
    3. Pancreatitis
    4. Hepatitis
    5. Torsion of a retained testicle
    6. Passage of a gallstone or kidney stone
    7. Urethral obstruction and bladder distension
    8. Prostatitis
    9. Nephritis
    10. Cholecystitis
    11. Metritis
C. Insidious onset of pain
    1. Ischemia and necrosis of a segment of bowel
    2. Bile peritonitis
    3. Urine peritonitis
    4. Septic peritonitis
       a. Intestinal perforation
       b. Penetrating injuries
D. Nonabdominal lesions which may cause abdominal splinting upon palpation
    1. Spinal trauma, disk disease
    2. Abdominal muscle or skin injuries
    3. Lumbar muscles
    4. Pancreatitis in cats
    5. Fractured pelvis or femur
    6. Polyarthritis, osteomyelitis

dilation or torsion? If the abdominal distention is severe and is interfering with breathing or venous return, it must be decompressed as soon as possible. Is an emergency laparotomy necessary?[2] The management of abdominal emergencies is discussed in Chapter 7.

Evaluation of Other Organ Systems

Orthopedic injuries must be identified, thoroughly decontaminated if compound, and at least temporarily stabilized if necessary. Is there any vascular or nerve injury associated with the fracture? Fractures around the CNS or peripheral nervous system may require early surgical decompression or stabilization. Luxations are easiest to replace immediately after they occur.

Are there any ocular emergencies, e.g., proptosis, corneal abrasions, ulcers, or lacerations, globe lacerations, glaucoma, intraocular foreign bodies, hyphema, retinal hemorrhage or detachment (Ch. 10)? Can the eye and vision be saved? Conjunctival exudate or chemical irritants are removed by irrigation and topical cycloplegics, and antibiotics are applied as necessary. General anes-

Table 1-6. Causes of Abdominal Distention

A. Free fluid
  1. Transudate
    a. Congestive heart failure
    b. Cirrhosis
    c. Hypoproteinemia
    d. Lymphangiectasis
    e. Neoplasia
  2. Exudate
    a. Intestinal perforation
    b. Urine peritonitis
    c. Bile peritonitis
    d. Penetrating wounds
    e. Ruptured pyometra or abscess
    f. Feline infectious peritonitis
  3. Blood
    a. Major organ trauma
    b. Neoplasia
    c. Bleeding disorders
    d. Splenic torsion
B. Air
  1. Gastric dilation or torsion
  2. Free air—perforated intestine
  3. Intestinal obstruction
C. Visceral organ
  1. Pregnancy
  2. Pyometra
D. Miscellaneous
  1. Pendulous abdomen associated with Cushing's disease
  2. Neoplasia

thesia, when necessary for surgical repair of proptosis or severe corneal ulceration and lacerations, is induced without excitement as sudden changes in intraocular pressure may cause expulsion of intraocular contents and loss of the eye.

Is there intraocular evidence of severe systemic disease, e.g., polycythemia, anemia, hyperviscosity, hypertension, uremia, coagulopathies, diabetes, lipemia, or an infectious disease?[11]

Skin lacerations are thoroughly cleaned and sutured if advisable. Puncture wounds are thoroughly investigated for any associated internal damage.

Is there any physical evidence of hemorrhage, hematoma, or petechiae; of pale, injected, bluish, or icteric discoloration to the mucous membranes; of central or peripheral hypo- or hyperthermia, or cold or heat injury; of cutaneous electrical, thermal, or caustic injury?

It is very helpful to be able to measure a few of the important blood components which are commonly abnormal in emergency and critically ill patients: packed cell volume, total plasma protein, glucose, urea nitrogen, plasma bicarbonate or total CO_2, alanine aminotransferase (GPT), gamma glutamyltransferase or alkaline phosphatase, total white blood cell count and differential, estimation of platelet numbers on a blood smear, and coagulation screening. Blood pH and gas analysis, electrolytes (sodium, potassium, and chloride), and osmolality are often helpful, but blood samples may have to be sent to an outside laboratory for analysis.

ANESTHETIC CONCERNS IN CRITICALLY ILL PATIENTS

It is often necessary to administer general anesthesia to a critically ill patient in order to effectively diagnose or manage the emergency situation. The sicker the patient, the more likely it is that he will succumb to the anesthetic procedure.

The clinician should obtain a thorough understanding of the extent of involvement of the disease process(es) via the history, physical examination, and various diagnostic procedures and laboratory analyses. It should be determined whether the patient ate within the last 8–12 hr. Patients with food in their stomachs are likely to vomit during induction or recovery. If it is suspected that there is food in the stomach, the general anesthetic should be postponed, the patient made to vomit before induction if he is not depressed (apomorphine 0.04 mg/kg), or an endotracheal tube introduced as early as possible after induction and maintained in place as long as possible during recovery. It is advisable to correct as many of the underlying disturbances as much as possible before anesthetic induction, or even to delay the surgical intervention until the patient is more stabilized.

The veterinarian should prevent perioperative stresses which are additive to the stress of the primary disease and which may not be well tolerated by the patient (excitement, inadequate or inappropriate fluid administration, hypoxia, hypercapnia, hyperthermia, hypothermia, etc.).

The seriousness of any organ dysfunction is assessed with regard to anesthetic drug selection, monitoring, and support. Cardiovascular disease usually represents the greatest immediate risk to the patient and therefore is usually the concern of highest priority. Respiratory disease is second, and CNS and visceral organ functions are third. Anesthetic drugs with pharmacologic characteristics best suited to the physiological abnormalities of the patient are selected. Narcotics alone, narcotics and diazepam or neuromuscular blocking agent combinations, or a ketamine-diazepam combination best support blood pressure in cardiovascular-compromised patients. Rapid induction (ultrashort barbiturate or ketamine), endotracheal intubation, and positive-pressure ventilation best support most respiratory diseases (except closed pneumothorax). An anesthetic technique with which the clinician is familiar should be selected.

Because there is no way to predict how an individual patient will respond to any chosen anesthetic protocol, monitoring the physiological response of the patient to the anesthetic drugs and the state of general anesthesia is of paramount importance. The emphasis of the monitoring is placed on the cardiovascular and pulmonary systems and any of the other organ systems which are compromised. Continuous audible and automatic monitors (e.g., heart sound amplifiers, Doppler blood flow detectors, respiratory monitors, and electrocardiographs) are ideal. They supplement, but do not replace, the frequent evaluation of the vital signs by trained observers. Both the depth of anesthesia and the physiological status of the patient are monitored and recorded. Any change from previous measurements are noted.

Intraoperative support of organ function must be as effective as possible to minimize any further deterioration. All abnormalities in organ function detected during the operative period are corrected. Support of cardiovascular and circulatory function may depend on crystalloid, colloid, or whole blood administration in appropriate volumes; central venous and arterial blood pressure measurement; cardiotonic and vasoactive drugs; antiarrhythmic drugs; glucocorticosteroids; concentrated electrolyte solutions; and/or various anesthetic combinations. Respiratory function may be supported by oxygen, positive-pressure ventilation, positive end-expiratory pressure, tracheal aspiration, chest drainage, and tracheostomy. Fluid loading, urinary bladder catheterization, natriuretic or osmotic diuretic agents, or dopamine may be necessary to support renal function. Fluid restriction, hyperventilation, hyperosmotic agents, corticosteroids, glucose, and prevention of hypoxemia and hypotension may be necessary to support CNS function. Monitoring and support procedures should be continued well into the postoperative period.

Although there may be minor surgical procedures, there is no such thing as a minor general anesthetic. The state of general anesthesia imposes a tremendous stress on a patient. The risk is high, particularly in critically ill patients. Undesirable events can be rapid in onset and serious in nature. Emergency personnel should be prepared for the worst, yet hope for the best.

EXTENDED MANAGEMENT

The transition from initial emergency care to extended intensive care is gradual and often imperceptible. There is a tendency to relax once the initial lifesaving measures have been successfully completed. However, further care is often required in the hours and days following the initial crises to ensure that the patient does not destabilize. The vigil is ongoing and should be sufficiently in-depth and repetitive to provide an uneventful convalescence. The intensity of the postcrisis monitoring and support depends on the degree of instability of the patient.

The most important component of an intensive care endeavor is the quality of the basic nursing care. The nurse must evaluate the patient frequently enough to develop a sense of whether the patient is improving. The patient must be well padded so as to prevent decubital ulcers, and immobile patients are repositioned at regular intervals to minimize decubiti, hypostatic congestion of the lung, and pneumonia. Critically ill patients are highly susceptible to systemic infection. The patient and his environment must be clean of debris, secretions, and exudates at all times. All indwelling catheters are cleaned and disinfected at regular intervals, and all administered fluids and drugs must be sterile. In addition, there must be a high level of personal hygiene among those individuals working with the patient to prevent contamination and cross-contamination between patients.

Indwelling Vascular Catheters

Indwelling vascular catheters expose the patient to local and systemic infections. Their use is indicated for lifesaving fluid administration, but they must not be utilized any longer than absolutely necessary. Appropriate aseptic safeguards during the insertion and maintenance of an indwelling catheter decrease the risk of untoward mechanical or infectious complications. Catheters that were inserted during emergency resuscitation, under less than ideal circumstances, must be replaced as soon as possible after the patient is stabilized.

Insertion of Indwelling Vascular Catheters. Catheters may be percutaneously placed in awake patients in the cephalic vein, lateral and medial saphenous veins, jugular vein, femoral vein, ear veins in some breeds, abdominal veins in some patients, femoral artery, and dorsal metatarsal artery. In anesthetized patients, they can be placed in the sublingual vein and artery and brachial artery. The carotid artery is available via cutdown. Peripheral veins are used for short-term isotonic fluid administrations, and central veins are used if long-term or hypertonic fluid administration is intended. Percutaneous insertions are preferred because they are associated with a lower infection rate compared to cutdown insertions. However, a cutdown should be used when the vessel is small and/or difficult to catheterize percutaneously or if multiple percutaneous attempts have failed.

Catheter-inside-the-needle systems are easy to insert in a sterile manner, but the needle makes a larger hole in the vessel than is filled by the indwelling catheter, which can result in early postinsertion hemorrhage. For this reason these catheters are not used for arterial catheterization. The needle is generally much larger than the catheter and sometimes is too large for the intended vein even though the catheter per se would fit nicely. The length of the catheter available in this format is longer than that with catheter-outside-the-needle systems. Catheter-outside-the-needle systems are more difficult to insert in a sterile manner because the catheter is exposed; however, they are not generally as likely to cause postinsertion hemorrhage.

An area over the vessel is clipped. The area should be sufficiently large that the catheter is not accidentally contaminated by unprepared areas during the insertion. The skin is prepared with antiseptic solutions in a manner similar to that used for any surgical procedure. Tincture of iodine 1–2% is the antiseptic solution of choice, but chlorhexidine, iodophors, and 70% alcohol can also be used. Benzalkonium-like compounds and hexachlorophene are not recommended.[6] Sterile drapes are used if it is necessary or helpful to extend the surgical field beyond the margins of the prepared area.

The hands are washed well, but it is not necessary to wear sterile gloves if neither the catheter nor the skin puncture site is to be touched during insertion. Sterile gloves are worn if it is necessary to manipulate the catheter or the skin puncture site, or if a cutdown procedure is intended.

Proper positioning of the vessel greatly facilitates catheter insertion. Excessive movement of the vessel during the catheterization procedure is to be avoided. Vessels are most effectively immobilized by stretching them between two points of traction. If the vessel rolls laterally or wrinkles longitudinally, insufficient traction has been applied. On the other hand, excessive traction may collapse the vessel. Digital pressure against the side of the vessel usually collapses it, rather than effectively immobilizing it and is therefore best avoided. Immobilization of a peripheral vein is accomplished by stretching the skin between the hand or tourniquet that occludes the vein proximally at the elbow or stifle and the hand that holds the limb distally. Extension of the limb and flexion of the carpus or extension of the tarsus increases the stretching of the skin and the immobilization of the vein. The jugular vein is stretched by pressing into the thoracic inlet and extending the head.

It may be helpful to make a relief incision in the skin to minimize skin–catheter resistance and to help prevent tearing of the end of the catheter. This is easily accomplished by puncturing the skin with a regular hypodermic needle and then widening the hole by sawing back and forth with the cutting edge of the bevel of the needle.

The catheter is first inserted subcutaneously. There should be minimal skin–catheter interaction. The catheter and needle tip (bevel upward) are placed on top of the vessel and aligned as closely as possible to the longitudinal axis of the vessel (to minimize the incidence of penetration of the deep wall of the vessel). The catheter is then inserted into the vessel with a sharp, almost stabbing motion. It may be necessary to initially approach the vein from a steeper angle in order to secure the superficial wall of the vessel by the needle tip. Sometimes it is possible to feel first the tip of the needle and then the shoulder of the catheter tip pop into the lumen of the vessel. At other times the relative position of the vessel lumen and the needle tip must be "visualized" and estimated. It is usually not a good idea to attempt to insert the needle and catheter unit far into the vessel because of its tendency to puncture the deep wall. The needle and catheter tip must be inserted far enough to be entirely through the superficial wall and into the lumen, and yet must not have penetrated the deep wall. The insertion is completed by gently sliding and rotating the catheter into the vessel to its full length.

Failure to successfully advance the catheter even though blood was aspirated through the needle may be due to several errors: (1) The needle or catheter tip may have been only partially through the superficial wall of the vessel. Then when the catheter was inserted it caught on the vessel wall. This may bend or tear the catheter tip or tear the vessel wall. (2) The bevel of the needle may be partially through the deep wall of the vessel. (3) Movement of either the vessel or the needle between the time blood was aspirated and the time the catheter was inserted may cause the needle and/or catheter tip to no longer be entirely within the lumen of the vessel. (4) A tear or barb on the catheter tip may catch on the vessel wall and impair smooth introduction. (5) If the catheter was not inserted along the longitudinal axis of the vessel, the end of the catheter may catch on the wall of the vessel or may puncture it. (6)

Because vessels do not course in a straight line, the catheter may catch at a bend in the vessel. If this happens, it is usually helpful to change the position of the limb. All conceivable positions should be tested. It may be helpful to forcefully inject saline through the catheter at the time of insertion. (7) Internal thrombosis of the vein from previous catheterizations may prevent advancement of the catheter within the lumen. (8) The catheter may be too large for the vessel. Most vessels constrict after they have been manipulated for a while and become too small to catheterize. This is particularly common in cutdown procedures. Rapid insertion and minimal manipulation of the vessel is an important goal. The catheter can be lubricated to facilitate insertion.

Once the catheter is in place, the needle-stylet is removed, the catheter is capped with an infusion plug, and the system is flushed with heparinized saline (1,000 units of heparin per 250–500 ml of saline). The catheter is fixed at the skin puncture site to prevent it from sliding in and out, which can predispose to the introduction of infectious agents and enhance mechanical trauma to the vessel intima. On a limb, fixation may be accomplished by taping around the circumference of the catheter and then taping the catheter to the leg. On flat body surfaces, e.g., the neck or femoral fossa, it is better to suture the catheter in place. This may be accomplished by placing a snug skin suture close to the puncture site on one side of the catheter and then tying around the circumference of the catheter (tight enough to just barely indent it but not to occlude it); a snug skin suture is then placed on the opposite side of the catheter. All three ties are done as a continuous suture.

An antibiotic-antifungal ointment is placed on the skin puncture site and the site wrapped occlusively. The catheter must be sufficiently bound by the wrap that accidental extraction of the catheter is avoided. It may be necessary to prevent the animal from chewing or pulling the catheter out by using an Elizabethan collar or a specialized bandaging material (e.g., aluminum or steel). Finally, the name of the person who inserted the catheter and the date is recorded in the medical record and directly on the bandage.

Maintenance of the Indwelling Catheter and Infusion Apparatus. Indwelling catheters must be redressed and inspected every 1–2 days and all soiled bandage material discarded. The puncture site is cleaned with antiseptic solutions and fresh antibiotic-antifungal ointment and the occlusive wrap reapplied.

The skin puncture site and vessel is inspected at each redressing. There is normally a very small ring of inflammation at the puncture site. Excess inflammation, diffuse tissue swelling, expulsion of exudate from the puncture site upon palpation, and tenderness or pain upon palpation are indications of untoward effects from the indwelling catheter. Cellulitis is characterized by warm, erythematous, and tender skin around the insertion site. Phlebitis, which may be caused by mechanical, chemical, or infectious irritation of the vein, is recognized as warm, erythematous skin overlying a tender, indurated vessel. Purulent thrombophlebitis is heralded by all of the signs of simple phlebitis plus exudate, which may drain or be expressed. It also may drain internally resulting in a severe septicemia. Thrombotic occlusion of the vessel is recognized by severe hardening ("ropiness") of the vessel. It is associated with the inability to infuse fluids by gravity and may result in severe subcutaneous fluid accumulation if the fluids are administered with a pump. Thrombosis also generally prevents the withdrawal of blood samples. In occult infection of the IV site,[6] local inflammatory, thrombotic, or exudative signs are minimal or nonexistent. Unexplained fever and leukocytosis may be the only early signs. The diagnosis may be confirmed by culturing the catheter tip.

Infusion fluids and administration tubing must be kept sterile. Connections are not disconnected unless absolutely necessary and then must be done aseptically. All injection caps are cleaned well with an antiseptic solution prior to needle insertion. The fluid bottles and all administration tubing are changed every 1–2 days, and tubing is changed after each blood or colloid infusion. The primary catheter or infusion line should not be used for the collection of blood samples except in emergencies. The fluid bottle must be clearly marked if any drug or concentrate has been added to the bottle, along with the time and date that the bottle was started and the name of the person responsible. In-line filters are not necessary for infection control for routine fluid administration,[6] but they may be necessary for parenteral hyperalimentation solutions.

The catheter must be removed if: (1) there is evidence of cellulitis, phlebitis, thrombosis, purulent thrombophlebitis, or catheter-associated bacteremia or septicemia; (2) the catheter ceases to function properly because of thrombosis or occlusion by clot or kink; (3) the catheter has been in place for 3 days (assuming there is another location to move it to); (4) the patient begins to lick or chew at the bandages; and (5) the use of a catheter is no longer necessary.

Maintenance Fluid Therapy and Nutrition

Once the initial fluid volume and electrolyte disturbances have been corrected the patient is given a maintenance fluid. Maintenance fluids should be low in sodium (40–60 mEq/L) compared to plasma and high in potassium (15–20 mEq/L). Patients receiving replacement solutions for maintenance requirements become hypernatremic if they cannot eliminate the excessive sodium load and hypokalemic if they are not eating. Maintenance solutions are commercially available or may be homemade by mixing 1 part lactated Ringer's (or an equivalent solution) with 1–2 parts 5% dextrose in water (to dilute the sodium concentration) and then supplementing the potassium. The volume of fluids to be administered for maintenance is determined from a chart (Table 1-7). Note that the relationship between body weight and the volume of the maintenance fluids is not linear. A detailed discussion of fluid therapy can be found in Chapter 4.

The patient is weighed daily to ascertain the adequacy of the fluid therapy. A change in body weight from one day to the next is almost entirely related to changes in body water and is a reasonable way to determine if the water volume requirements are being met each day. The volume of all losses is measured or estimated and totaled at the end of the day. Total inputs and outputs do not necessarily need to balance, depending on the initial status of the patient

Table 1-7. Daily Caloric and Water Requirements for Dogs (140 kcal/
day/kg$^{0.73}$)

Body Weight (kg)	Total kcal/day or Water (ml/day)	ml/kg	ml/hr
1	140	140	6
2	232	116	10
3	312	104	13
4	385	96	16
5	453	91	19
6	518	86	22
7	580	83	24
8	639	80	27
9	696	77	29
10	752	75	31
11	806	73	34
12	859	71	36
13	911	70	38
14	961	68	40
15	1,011	67	42
16	1,060	66	44
17	1,108	65	46
18	1,155	64	48
19	1,201	63	50
20	1,247	62	52
25	1,468	59	61
30	1,677	56	70
35	1,876	54	78
40	2,068	52	86
45	2,254	50	94
50	2,434	49	101
60	2,781	46	116
70	3,112	44	130
80	3,431	43	143
90	3,739	41	156
100	4,038	40	168

and the intent of the fluid therapy plan. Major blood components are monitored at periodic intervals to ensure that their concentrations are restored to and maintained within acceptable limits (Table 1-4).

Critically ill patients are weaned back onto oral nutrition as soon as resolution of the disease process allows. Oral voluntary feeding, oral force-feeding, and indwelling nasogastric, pharyngostomy-gastric, or gastrostomy stomach tubes are techniques that have been used with good results.[3,10] When the oral-gastric route is undesirable or unavailable, jejunostomy[13] or intravenous[12] administration of nutrients may be efficacious. Patients stressed by disease, infection, major trauma, or surgery exhibit hormonal changes that are catabolic in nature and which are responsible for metabolic rates that are much in excess of resting energy expenditure or simple starvation. Early nutritional support decreases catabolic tissue losses, increases wound healing and immunologic competence, and improves patient survival. Extended starvation in stressed patients may result in decreased wound healing which necessitates additional surgery and/or in death secondary to pneumonia or septicemia.

The objective of nutritional support is to provide: (1) the patient's energy requirements; (2) amino acid building blocks for antibodies, white blood cells, platelets, coagulation factors, fibroblasts, and other necessary protein tissue reconstruction; and (3) some of the essential water-soluble vitamins (B-complex), minerals (calcium, phosphorus, zinc, magnesium, manganese), and essential fatty acids (linoleic, linolenic, and arachidonic acids) that would eventually become depleted if they were not supplemented.

An intravenous infusion of a 25–35% dextrose solution is required if the patient's daily energy needs are to be met within a normal daily volume of water. Rampant hyperglycemia can be avoided by weaning the patient onto the high dextrose infusion over a period of 1.5–3 days. Some patients require supplemental insulin. (Weaning the patient off the dextrose infusion is necessary later to avoid withdrawal hypoglycemia.) Dextrose infusion alone may interfere with the normal hormonal response to stress and the necessary mobilization of endogenous amino acids. If partial or total intravenous nutrition is contemplated, it is appropriate to utilize a balanced protein-caloric solution (approximately 6 g of metabolizable amino acid/150 kcal of energy [42 g of dextrose]).

Indwelling Urinary Catheters

Indwelling urinary catheters are occasionally necessary to monitor urine output in order to ensure adequate renal function, an empty urinary bladder, or an unobstructed urethra. Intermittent or indwelling catheters predispose to mechanical and septic cystitis and urethritis and should be used with appropriate caution. Sterile introduction often requires a second person to help position the patient.

Insertion of Indwelling Urinary Catheters. The hair around the prepuce or vulva is clipped and the area washed with a povidone-iodine soap solution. The prepuce or vestibule is flushed with a povidone-iodine solution. The prepuce is retracted and the penis also gently washed with the povidone-iodine solution.

The female urethra is either visualized with the aid of a previously disinfected laryngoscope, otoscope, or vaginal speculum, or is palpated with the finger of a sterile-gloved hand.

A long, soft sterile catheter is used. The catheter should be as thin in caliber as possible to minimize urethral trauma. Human infant feeding tubes work well for indwelling urinary catheters. The catheter is generously lubricated, inserted into the urethra, and advanced until urine can be obtained. Introducing excessive lengths of catheter is to be avoided because it may cause mechanical trauma of the bladder.

The catheter is sutured in place to minimize its sliding in and out, which can predispose to the introduction of infectious agents and cause mechanical trauma to the urethra. A snug suture is placed in the prepuce or vulva on one side of the catheter and then tied around the circumference of the catheter (tight enough to just barely indent the catheter but not so tight as to occlude it); finally, a snug skin suture is placed in the prepuce or vulva on the opposite side of the catheter. All three ties are done as a continuous suture. The catheter is then immediately attached to a closed drainage system.

Maintenance of Indwelling Urinary Catheters and Collection Units. To prevent the migration of infectious agents into the bladder around the urinary catheter, it may be helpful to flush the prepuce or vestibule with a dilute iodine solution three times daily. Hands should always be washed before and after handling the catheter.

To prevent the migration of infectious agents into the bladder through the lumen of the catheter: (1) The collection system must be completely closed and all joints firmly attached or taped to prevent accidental disconnection. (2) The collection system is positioned so that it drains downhill—urine must not be allowed to drain back into the bladder because it may be contaminated. (3) Draining the collection reservoir or needle puncture of the collection tube to obtain a urine sample must be accomplished aseptically. (4) Bubbles must not be allowed to form in the collection tube and rise toward the patient as they may carry infectious agents with them. It may be helpful in this regard to form a coil in the collection tubing so that the bubble rises only as far as the top of the coil. (5) Ten milliliters of 3% hydrogen peroxide or 0.25% acetic acid is put in the collection reservoir to help prevent bacterial growth.

The collection tubing is taped to the hind leg or abdomen to prevent accidental traction on the catheter and suture sites. Enough slack in the tubing is provided to allow the patient a full range of motion of the hind leg.

Irrigation of the catheter with anything is discouraged. Antibiotic flushes have not been shown to prevent urinary infections, only to delay them and select for resistant infections.[6] Flushing obstructed catheters may force contaminated urine and debris into the bladder. Instead, obstructed catheters should be replaced. The indwelling urinary catheter should be removed as early as possible.

If catheterization can be accomplished easily, aseptically, and atraumatically, and continuous urine drainage is not necessary, intermittent bladder catheterization may be preferred as it is associated with a lower morbidity than indwelling catheterization.

Indwelling Tracheal Tubes

Occasionally it becomes necessary to gain access to the airway for an extended period of time for the purpose of providing ventilatory support, bypassing a laryngeal or other upper airway obstructive disorder, or effectively treating a respiratory infection. Indications are discussed further in Chapter 3. Awake animals tolerate orotracheal tubes poorly, and some form of heavy sedation or even a general anesthetic may be necessary to enforce patient acceptance. Indwelling translaryngeal tubes predispose to laryngeal damage in the form of laryngitis, epiglottitis, subglottic edema, and postintubation stenosis. Indwelling tracheostomy tubes are well tolerated by unsedated canine and feline patients with or without continuous ventilatory support. The maintenance of an indwelling tracheostomy tube, however, represents an intensive nursing care endeavor and is not without hazard.

Technique of Tracheostomy.   Insertion of the tracheostomy tube must be a well-controlled surgical procedure. Aseptic technique and careful dissection are necessary to minimize contamination of and damage to the trachea and surrounding tissues. The patient is positioned in exact dorsal recumbency so that the head, neck, and thorax are not rotated in either lateral direction. A longitudinal skin incision is made caudal to the cricoid cartilage, the length of which is two to three times the diameter of the tube to be inserted. The sternohyoid muscles are divided on the midline, and the fascia is completely dissected away from the trachea. The trachea is grasped between tracheal rings and held firmly with thumb forceps or mosquito hemostatic forceps. A longitudinal incision through two to three tracheal rings is made exactly on the ventral midline of the trachea beginning with the second or third tracheal ring. If the incision is not made on the midline or if it is not straight, the tube will not rest comfortably within the lumen of the trachea and undue pressure will be applied to the tracheal wall and epithelium. A small transverse incision at one or both ends of the longitudinal incision may facilitate introduction of the tube. The tube is inserted while continuing to hold the trachea with the forceps.

The majority of the incision (muscle, subcutaneous tissue, and skin) is closed, but an airtight closure around the tube is to be avoided. Air often escapes from the tracheal incision and must be allowed to vent to the outside. If trapped, it may accumulate subcutaneously and migrate into the chest, causing a pneumomediastinum and pneumothorax.

The skin incision is covered with an antibacterial-antifungal ointment and a sterile gauze sponge which has been cut so as to fit comfortably around the tube. The tube is then bandaged securely to the patient's neck in a manner that does not distort the position of the tube within the trachea.

Management of the Indwelling Tracheostomy Tube.   The cuff of the tube must be a high-volume, low-pressure type to minimize cuff-induced tracheal trauma. The cuff is inflated to a minimal occlusive volume that is just sufficient to prevent most of the back-flush of air during positive-pressure inflation of the lungs. Complications of excessive cuff pressure include tracheal inflammation, ischemia, ulceration, granuloma formation, necrosis, hemorrhage, malacia and dilation, fibrosis and stenosis, or tracheoesophageal fistulation. The volume of cuff inflation is recorded. Any subsequent increase in this volume could be attributed to technical error, overinflation of the cuff, a leaky cuff, or tracheomalacia and dilation.

Airway humidity must be provided on a regular basis, either by direct installation of saline at hourly intervals or by nebulization of water at 4- to 6-hr intervals. This is to prevent drying of the mucosa and respiratory secretions. In addition, systemic hydration of the patient must be maintained.

The inner cannula is cleaned and the trachea and tracheostomy tube suctioned approximately every 2 hr or as often as necessary. Suction catheters must be soft and flexible in order to minimize epithelial trauma during suctioning. They must have more than one hole in the tip to prevent excessive attraction of the catheter to the tracheal wall. When this does occur, an epithelial plug is sucked into the hole and is likely to be ripped away when the catheter is withdrawn. A terminal flange on the tip of the catheter adjacent to the holes also helps to prevent this. The catheter must also have as large a lumen as possible to facilitate removal of thick secretions, but its outside diameter should not be larger than 50% of the inside diameter of the smallest portion of the airway through which the catheter is placed. The tracheal suctioning procedure must be aseptic to prevent contamination of the lower respiratory tract. Suction catheters should not be reused unless they have been properly resterilized; however, catheters must not sit in a vat of antiseptic solution between suctionings.

Mobilization of peripheral respiratory secretions to the central airways by postural drainage and percussion just before suctioning may improve the results of the suctioning procedure. If the patient is laterally recumbent, it may be advantageous to percuss and suction while the patient is lying on one side and then to repeat the procedure with the patient lying on the opposite side. Immediately before the suctioning procedure, it is helpful to instill 2–5 ml of saline into the trachea. Supplemental preoxygenation may help prevent suction-induced hypoxemia.

The sterile catheter is gently inserted into the trachea as far as it will advance (without applying suction) with a sterile-gloved hand. Suction is then intermittently applied while the catheter is removed. The negative pressure must not be applied to the airway for more than a total of 10–15 sec to minimize the amount of airway collapse and hypoxemia. The catheter is withdrawn with a rotating, winding motion of the hand. This motion helps minimize the attraction of the tip of the catheter to the tracheal epithelium and maximizes removal of secretions from the entire circumference of the trachea and tube. The suctioning procedure must cease immediately if excessive patient discomfort or restlessness occurs, or if changes in cardiac or respiratory rhythm are noted. The patient is manually hyperinflated after the suctioning procedure to alleviate small airway collapse and hypoxemia, and should breathe an oxygen-enriched mixture for several minutes.

The absence of any aspirated material in intubated patients is indicative of inadequate airway humidification and excessive drying of secretions. The presence of blood in the aspirate is indicative of excessive tracheal damage, and if this occurs the suctioning technique must be altered. Trauma may be secondary to excessive manipulation of the catheter within the trachea or excessive attraction of the catheter to the tracheal wall.

The tracheostomy wound is treated as an open surgical wound on a daily basis. The soiled bandages are removed and all exudate cleaned from the wound; then the antibiotic-antifungal ointment and the light sterile dressing are reapplied. The patient is monitored for the development of lumen occlusion, tube dislodgement, local infection, subcutaneous or intrathoracic emphysema, hemorrhage, or tracheomalacia.

Chest Drainage

An indwelling chest drain is indicated whenever thoracentesis of fluid or air must be repeated frequently because of rapid reaccumulation. Any rigid but soft and pliable tube which is nonirritating to the tissues may be used as an indwelling chest drain. The tube must be sufficiently large to accommodate the passage of cellular debris and fibrin clots, yet small enough to be comfortably passed between the ribs. The tube should have many large holes toward its tip to maximize the opportunity for fluid drainage. If the holes are homemade, they must not be so large as to weaken the wall of the tube, and the edges of the holes should be smooth so that they do not catch on any tissues when the tube is removed. Commercial trocar chest drains, foley or other urinary catheters, gastric feeding tubes, Silastic or polyvinyl chloride tubing, and intravenous catheters have been used as chest drains.

Chest Tube Insertion and Management.   An indwelling chest tube must be inserted carefully and with all the precautions of aseptic surgical technique. Sedation is usually not necessary. The dorsal and caudal quadrant of the thorax is clipped and prepared with antiseptic solutions. Sterile surgical gloves and drapes or towels are utilized. A small volume of 1–2% lidocaine is deposited subcutaneously and a small incision made in the dorsal-caudal quadrant of the thorax (1.5–2 times the diameter of the tube) at approximately the 9th or 10th intercostal space. The skin incision is slid forward (if the tip of the tube is to be placed in the dorsum of the thoracic cavity) or forward and downward (if the tube is to be placed in the ventrum of the thoracic cavity) at least two intercostal spaces. This provides a subcutaneous tunnel between the point of entry of the tube through the skin and the point of entry into the thoracic cavity, which helps prevent leakage of atmospheric air into the chest after the tube is placed.

A midintercostal point is selected for the intercostal puncture and a small volume of 1–2% lidocaine is deposited. If a trocar catheter is being used, the end of the trocar is placed in the palm of one hand. The thumb and index finger of the opposite hand grasps the tube 2–4 cm from the tip of the stylet (depending on the size of the patient). This provides a "stop" so that the stylet is not advanced too far into the thorax. The trocar is plunged into the chest. The tube is then slanted so that it is more or less parallel to the pleural surface. The stylet is kept stationary as the tube is advanced to its proper location in the chest. The stylet is then removed and the tube occluded between the thumb and forefinger until the catheter can be capped.

If forceps are being used to insert a flexible catheter, it may be helpful to make a small relief incision partially through the intercostal musculature. The end of the catheter is occluded before introduction. Once the forceps and tube unit is inserted into the thoracic cavity, the hold of the forceps is released and the tube is advanced further into the pleural space. The forceps is gently removed.

As the stylet or forceps is removed, the skin is allowed to slide back to its normal resting position, and the skin incision is closed around the chest tube. A suture is placed snugly in the skin on one side of the tube and then tied tightly around the tube; finally, it is sutured snugly to the skin on the opposite side of the catheter. The skin incision site is covered with an antibiotic-antifungal ointment and a sterile gauze pad. It is cleaned and redressed daily. A gentle loop is placed in the drainage tube so that any traction placed on it will not pull directly on the sutures or pull the tube out. The tube is loosely bandaged to the patient's thorax.

The chest tube can then be fitted with a self-sealing injection cap or a capped three-way stopcock and periodically drained with a large syringe. The force of aspiration must be very mild as extremely low subatmospheric pressures (-200 to -500 cm H_2O) can be generated with ease. The chest tube may be attached to a homemade or commercial closed-chest drainage system (Ch. 3; Fig. 3-2). The patient with an indwelling chest tube is monitored at regular intervals for: (1) iatrogenic hemothorax, pneumothorax, or subcutaneous emphysema; (2) rate of pleural fluid or air drainage; (3) local or pleural infections or septicemia; and (4) chest tube occlusion.

Corticosteroid Therapy

High dosages of glucocorticosteroids have multiple beneficial effects in hemorrhagic and septic shock, many of which are a result of the stabilization of cellular and organelle membrane integrity (endothelial, platelet, leukocyte, lysosome, intestinal epithelium).[14] They also normalize the sympathetic influence on the vasculature, improve visceral perfusion, and enhance venous return and cardiac output. High dosages of glucorticosteroids are administered to patients suffering moderate to severe hypovolemic, cardiogenic, or septic shock, and severe hypoglycemia, hypoxemia, or hyperthermia. Water-soluble succinate or phosphate esters of dexamethasone, prednisolone, methylprednisolone, or hydrocortisone are administered intravenously. The most effective dose for methylprednisolone was found to be at least 30 mg/kg.[1] Prednisolone is usually considered to be slightly less potent than methylprednisolone. The most effective dose for dexamethasone was found to be at least 15 mg/kg,[15] although the commonly accepted shock dose is 4–6 mg/kg. The potential benefit of administering less than the optimal dose of corticosteroid is unknown but is presumed to be less than that desirable. If the decision is made to give corticosteroids for the treatment of one of the above conditions, the full dosage is administered. The role of corticosteroids in the therapy of shock is discussed in more detail in Chapter 2.

Infection Control

Critically ill patients have an increased susceptibility to infection. This is because they are stressed by their disease process; they have high levels of immunosuppressive endogenous or exogenous corticosteroids; they are subjected to invasive surgical, diagnostic, or therapeutic procedures, as well as indwelling cannulas; they suffer varying degrees of malnutrition; they may be receiving antibiotics which predispose to resistant bacterial or fungal overgrowth; they are often surrounded by other sick, contaminated, and infected patients; they are minimally mobile; and they may have diseases such as diabetes mellitus, hyperadrenocorticism, or uremia which are known to lower an animal's threshold for infection.

Emphasis is placed on nursing care protocols which minimize contamination and infection of critically ill patients: (1) The patient and the immediate vicinity must be clean and antiseptic. (2) All indwelling cannulas must receive regular insertion site care, as discussed previously. (3) All surgical, diagnostic, or therapeutic procedures are completed under strict aseptic conditions utilizing properly sterilized equipment. (4) All fluids administered to the patient must be sterile; all fluids drained from the patient must be collected in sterile containers which are completely closed to the atmosphere. All administration and collection apparatus are changed at regular intervals. (5) All mechanical therapeutic equipment to which the patient is attached must be properly sterilized and changed at regular intervals. (6) Immobile patients are repositioned regularly (every few hours), and convalescing patients are encouraged to ambulate early to minimize the retention of respiratory secretions, which predispose to pneumonia. (7) Personnel must wash their hands well between patients, and soiled clothing changed immediately. (8) Disposable gloves are worn when handling patients with known infections. (9) Patients and their excretions must be isolated from all other patients at all times. (10) Soiled bedding and bandages are placed in designated receptacles and not on the floor or counter. (11) Floors, counters, and kennels must be regularly scrubbed with soap, water, and appropriate antiseptic solutions. (12) Supraphysiological dosages of corticosteroids must not be administered for longer than 48 hr without antibiotic backup.

Antibiotic therapy must not be administered for longer than 48 hr without a culture and sensitivity to verify microorganism susceptibility. Antibiotics should be broad spectrum in nature (or in combination) and must be given in the appropriate dosage.[5] Antibiotics may be a mixed blessing. They may prevent or treat systemic infection by susceptible microorganisms, but they predispose to overgrowth of resistant microorganisms and fungi. Where clinicians draw the line between the benefit and risk of antibiotic therapy is highly variable. It seems reasonable to recommend that antibiotics not be routinely used in emergency or instrumented patients, nor that they be used to take the place of adequate surgical or nursing care technique. However, they should be used in patients who are heavily contaminated or are suspected or known to already be infected.

Psychological Stress of Intensive Care

In our enthusiasm to minimize the pathophysiological stress of the disease process, we attend to the patient in an intensive manner at frequent intervals throughout the day. The patient's normal daily routine is totally upset. He is isolated from familiar surroundings and his owners, and is subjected to a series of examinations, probings, and injections by a variety of strangers who may not take the time to show that they care. The metabolic and pharmacologic obtundation is compounded by the lack of restful sleep. These psychological stresses may lead to mental confusion, lethargy, apathy, disorientation, delirium, exhaustion, restlessness, and aberrant behavior, e g., a reduced tolerance to manipulation or an outward aggressiveness.

The psychological well-being of the intensive care patient warrants as much attention as is given to the physiological disturbances. Intensive care unit (ICU) personnel must take time to talk to the animals, reassuring and befriending them. The patient's mental activity can be mobilized with short walks outdoors and by scheduling regular owner visits. Treatments and monitorings should be scheduled at discrete intervals so that the patient can sleep in between. The lights in the ICU should be turned down at night.

SUGGESTED READING

It is readily apparent that trauma and emergency/intensive care are devoid of disciplinary boundaries. People who deal with these critical patients on a routine basis should be more than casually familiar with a diverse spectrum of diseases and treatments. This book certainly provides the most current thoughts on the matter. Additional sources of information are available for the interested student of critical care:

Amis TC: Manual of Small Animal Respiratory Disease. Churchill Livingstone, New York, 1984

Archibald J. Holt JC, Sokolovsky V: Management of Trauma in Dogs and Cats. American Veterinary Publications, Santa Barbara, CA, 1981

Brasmer TH, Piermattei D: The acutely traumatized small animal patient. In: Major Problems in Veterinary Medicine. W.B. Saunders, Philadelphia, 1984

Crane SW (ed): Symposium on Trauma. Vet Clin North Am, Vol. 10, 1980

Ettinger SJ (ed): Textbook of Veterinary Internal Medicine, Saunders, Philadelphia, 1983

Kirk RW (ed): Current Veterinary Therapy, Vol. 8 (1983) Vol. 7 (1980). W.B. Saunders, Philadelphia

Kirk RW, Bistner SI: Handbook of Veterinary Procedures and Emergency Treatment. Saunders, Philadelphia, 1981

Sattler FP, Knowles RP, Whittick WG (eds): Veterinary Critical Care. Lea & Febiger, Philadelphia, 1981

Schaer M (ed): Symposium on Fluid and Electrolyte Balance. Vet Clin North Am, Vol. 12, 1982

Wingfield WE (ed): Symposium on Emergency Medicine. Vet Clin North Am, Vol. 11, 1981

Zaslow IG (ed): Veterinary Trauma and Critical Care. Lea & Febiger, Philadelphia, 1984

REFERENCES

1. Altura BM: Glucocorticoid-induced protection in circulatory shock: role of reticuloendothelial system function. Proc Soc Exp Biol Med 150:202, 1975

2. Crane SW: Evaluation and management of abdominal trauma in the dog and cat. Vet Clin North Am, 11:655, 1981
3. Crane SW: Placement and maintenance of a temporary feeding tube gastrostomy in the dog and cat. Comp Contin Educ Pract Vet 2:770, 1980
4. Crowe DT: Evaluation of abdominal trauma. Am Anim Hosp Assoc Sci Proc 42:258, 1975
5. Davis LE: Antimicrobial therapy. p. 2. In Kirk RW (ed): Current Veterinary Therapy VII — Small Animal Practice. W. B. Saunders, Philadelphia, 1980
6. Guidelines for prevention of intravenous therapy-related and catheter-associated urinary tract infections and nosocomial pneumonia. In U.S. Department of Health and Human Services (ed): Guidelines for the Prevention and Control of Nosocomial Infections. National Technical Information Service, Springfield, 1900
7. Haskins SC: A flowchart for cardiopulmonary resuscitation. In Slatter D (ed): Textbook of Small Animal Surgery. Inside front cover. Saunders, Philadelphia, (in press)
8. Haskins SC: Fluid and electrolyte therapy, compendium of continuing education for veterinarians. Pract Vet 6:244, 1984
9. Haskins SC: Standards and techniques of equipment utilization. In Sattler FP, Knowles RP, Whittick WG (eds): Veterinary Critical Care. Ch. 3. Lea & Febiger, Philadelphia, 1981
10. Lantz GC: Pharyngostomy tube installation for the administration of nutritional and fluid requirements. Comp Contin Educ Pract Vet 3:135, 1981
11. Martin CL: The eye and systemic disease. p. 593. In Kirk RW (ed): Current Veterinary Therapy VII — Small Animal Practice. W. B. Saunders, Philadelphia, 1980
12. Mullen JL, Crosby LO, Rombeau JL: Symposium on Surgical Nutrition. Surgical Clinics of North America. W. B. Saunders, Philadelphia, 1981, Vol. 61
13. Page CP, Carlton PK, Andrassy RS, et al: Safe, cost-effective postoperative nutrition: defined formula diet via needle-catheter jejunostomy. Am J Surg 138:939, 1979
14. Shatney CH: The use of corticosteroids in the therapy of hemorrhagic shock. In Cowley RA, Trump BF (eds): Pathophysiology of Shock, Anoxia, and Ischemia. Williams & Wilkins, Baltimore, 1982
15. Vargish T, Turner CS, Bond RF: Dose-response relationship in steroid therapy for hemorrhagic shock. Am Surg 43:30, 1977

2 | Cardiovascular Emergencies

William Muir
John Bonagura

The phrase "cardiovascular emergency" implies a disorder of the heart or vascular system which is important enough to require immediate attention. The cardiovascular system demands special attention because, unlike emergency situations involving other organ systems, inadequate, untimely, or inappropriate therapy often results in the immediate death of the animal. The goals of this chapter are to familiarize the reader with the common causes, pathophysiology, and treatment of cardiovascular emergencies including *shock, acute heart failure, pericardial tamponade,* and *cardiac arrhythmias.* A discussion of cardiopulmonary resuscitation with emphasis on therapy is included for completeness.

SHOCK

Categories of Shock

Shock, an acute syndrome characterized by inadequate tissue perfusion, is caused by disturbances in normal cardiovascular function.[7,9] Critical reductions in capillary perfusion result in generalized ischemia, hypoxia, and the inability of the body cell mass to metabolize nutrients normally. If shock is severe or allowed to persist for extended periods of time, cell death and the death of the animal occur. Because shock implies abnormal cardiovascular function, it can be categorized as originating from one of four hemodynamic deficits: hypovolemia, cardiac failure, abnormal distribution of blood, or obstruction to blood flow (Table 2-1).[14] Collectively, these hemodynamic deficits

Table 2-1. Causes of Shock

Major Category	Cause
Hypovolemic shock Exogenous	1. Blood loss caused by hemorrhage 2. Plasma loss caused by thermal or chemical burns and inflammation 3. Fluid and electrolyte loss caused by dehydration, vomiting, diarrhea, renal disease, severe exercise, heat stress, or excessive diuresis
Endogenous	1. Extravasation of fluids, plasma, or blood into a body cavity or tissues (third space losses) caused by trauma, endotoxins, hypoproteinemia, anaphylaxis, or burns
Cardiogenic shock	1. Myocardiac mechanical factors caused by regurgitant or obstructive defects 2. Myopathic defects caused by heritable traits, chemicals, or toxins 3. Cardiac arrhythmias
Distributive shock High resistance	1. Distribution of blood volume and flow to vital organs caused by endotoxins, anesthetic drug overdose, CNS trauma, anaphylaxis
Low resistance	1. Distribution of blood away from vital organs caused by severe infections, abscesses, or arteriovenous fistulas
Obstructive shock	1. Obstruction to blood flow through the heart (pericardial tamponade, neoplasia, embolism), aorta (embolism, aneurysm), vena cava (gastric bloat, heartworm, neoplasia), lungs (embolism, heartworm, positive-pressure ventilation).

can be thought of as resulting in a decrease in the effective circulating blood volume, which is defined as that portion of the extracellular fluid volume that is effectively perfusing tissues.

Hypovolemic Shock.   Depletion of the extracellular fluid volume is the most common cause of a reduction in the effective circulating blood volume encountered in veterinary medicine. Fluid loss from the body occurs during bleeding, vomiting, and diarrhea. Other less common causes of fluid loss are burns, insensible losses from skin and the respiratory tract, and polyuric states.

Volume depletion is also produced by the loss of interstitial and intravascular fluid into a nonexchangeable "third space." Traumatized dogs or cats, for example, can lose as much as 20% of their blood volume into the tissues surrounding a severely traumatized fracture site (e.g., fractured femur). Severe crush injuries, intestinal obstruction, peritonitis, pancreatitis, and clotting defects are additional examples of insults which can result in the acute sequestration of extracellular fluid into body cavities or tissues.

Cardiogenic Shock. Any compromise of the heart's ability to pump blood can potentially result in a decrease in the effective circulating blood volume. Cardiogenic shock is caused by a critical reduction in cardiac output and is produced by significant depression of myocardial contractility, cardiac rate and rhythm disturbances (arrhythmias), and acquired or congenital cardiac disease. Drug overdose (e.g., anesthesia, tranquilization) resulting in severe bradycardia and hypocontractility is a relatively common cause of hypotension and shock.

Distributive Shock. Any major disturbance in the distribution of blood flow to vital organs due to drastic alterations in peripheral vascular tone can result in a decrease in the effective circulating blood volume to those tissues. High-resistance forms of distributive shock are characterized by the vascular sequestration of blood and the redistribution of blood volume and flow to those organs essential to the maintenance of life (i.e., heart, lung, and brain) at the expense of supplying adequate blood flow to the splanchnic viscera, kidney, skeletal muscle, and skin. Bacterial endotoxins and anesthetic drug overdose are causes of high-resistance distributive shock. Low-resistance causes of distributive shock are characterized by blood being shunted (arteriovenous fistulas) away from vital organs and by blood traversing capillary beds without sufficient time to exchange oxygen and nutrients. Septic shock caused by grampositive or gram-negative bacteria is the most common cause of low-resistance distributive shock. The net effect of either high- or low-resistance forms of distributive shock is a reduction in the blood volume that is effectively perfusing body tissues even though the absolute intravascular volume may be normal.

Obstructive Shock. Pathogenic conditions which prevent effective tissue perfusion because of major intravascular or extravascular physical obstruction to blood flow can cause shock. Embolism from various causes (air, trauma) and positive intrathoracic pressure during mechanical or manual ventilation of an anesthetized or unconscious patient can obstruct blood flow, leading to hypotension and shock.

Summarizing: trauma, severe infection, cardiac disease, and major surgical operation are examples of common clinical problems which can result in cardiovascular embarrassment and shock from several causes. Thoracic trauma, for example, could result in hemorrhage into the thoracic cavity (hypovolemic shock) and a marked reduction in the heart's pumping ability due to the development of cardiac arrhythmias (cardiogenic shock). A clear understanding of the various causes for shock and the mechanism(s) whereby they induce a decrease in tissue perfusion is the basis for a rational approach to the design of therapeutic regimens.

Overview of the Pathophysiology of Shock

During health, neural, hormonal, and local tissue factors are responsible for maintenance and regulation of the effective circulating blood volume. The exchange of nutrients, including oxygen, between the vascular compartment and the interstitium and between the interstitium and cells, is essential for normal cellular metabolism. Similarly, the waste products of cellular metabolism, e.g., carbon dioxide and fixed acids (lactic acid), must be removed by the blood and eventually excreted by the lung or kidney if normal cellular metabolism is to be maintained. These vital exchange processes are totally dependent on the normal function of all the organs of the body and adequate blood flow to these organs. The effective circulating blood volume is considered to be decreased even when total blood volume or flow is increased if vital tissues are not being adequately perfused.[4]

The accumulation of cellular waste products due to poor tissue perfusion triggers neuroendocrine and local responses which result in a redistribution of cardiac output and local fluid shifts. If these fluid shifts are successful in removing cellular waste products and supplying adequate nutrients and oxygen, normal cell function returns. Temporary decreases in the effective circulating blood volume, however, can produce a critical series of cellular events that, if uncorrected, threaten the survival of the tissue bed involved and, potentially, the animal's life. Alterations in cellular membrane transport function and permeability are the first changes which occur during shock. Membrane potential becomes less negative because of a loss of intracellular K^+ and an accumulation of intracellular Na^+. There is a reduction in the rate of conversion of pyruvate to acetyl-CoA, leading to an increase in the lactate/pyruvate ratio and intracellular acidosis, and progressive reduction in ATP production. Intracellular concentrations of 3',5'-cyclic AMP decrease, which limits the regulatory effects of various hormones and neurotransmitters on cellular metabolism and vascular tone. Cellular calcium metabolism is compromised, resulting in the accumulation of intracellular free Ca^{2+}, loss of mitochondrial function, and cellular swelling. Hemorrhagic and traumatic shock decrease the tissues' ability to respond to insulin and produce an intracellular deficit in glucose metabolism. These changes in cellular metabolism cause a progressive accumulation of many metabolites, resulting in increased circulating concentrations of free fatty acids and amino acids. Accumulation of these cellular metabolites and waste products combined with hypoxia depresses the reticuloendothelial phagocytic function, which is responsible for metabolizing and removing cellular remnants, bacteria, and circulating toxins.

If the body's responses to these initial ischemia-induced changes in cellular function are inadequate or if therapy is inappropriate, insufficient, or delayed, anaerobic glycolysis supervenes and mitochondrial and endoplasmic reticulum injury continue, resulting in the intracellular accumulation of acid metabolites (lactic acid), Na^+, and Ca^{2+}. Parenchymal and endothelial swelling impede the return of normal blood flow, the utilization of nutrients, and normal diffusional processes. Blood becomes sludged or trapped in capillaries, causing

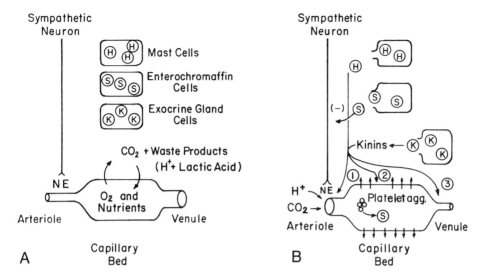

Fig. 2-1. Effects of histamine (H), serotonin (S), and kinins (K) on vascular tone and capillary permeability. During health (A) vascular tone is regulated by the release of norepinephrine (NE) from sympathetic nerve terminals and by local tissue factors (CO_2, H^+). Shock results in (H), (S), and (K) release from various tissue beds causing arteriolar dilation (1), increases in capillary membrane permeability (2), and venular constriction (3). Histamine and serotonin interfere with normal adrenergic neurotransmission ($-$).

further ischemia. Intracellular organelles called lysosomes begin to leak hydrolytic enzymes, which cause cellular autolysis. Lysosomes are found in highest concentration in liver, kidney, and spleen. Their release is believed to be one of the major mechanisms responsible for the degranulation of mast cells (histamine release) and the destruction of neighboring cells, resulting in the release of their toxic waste products. Histamine and serotonin released from platelets and enterochromaffin cells cause decreases in arteriolar tone, increases in venous tone, inhibition of the sympathetic regulation of vascular tone, and increases in capillary membrane permeability. Kinins dilate arterioles, increase capillary membrane permeability, and constrict venules (Fig. 2-1). Various prostaglandins (thromboxane, leukotrienes) inhibit sympathetic nerve activity, increase capillary membrane permeability, induce platelet aggregation, and activate the complement system. The latter two effects and kinin release cause the activation and consumption of the body's clotting factors, resulting in coagulopathy and eventually diffuse bleeding. This syndrome, referred to as disseminated intravascular coagulation (DIC), results in uncontrollable hemorrhage. Other toxic by-products of abnormal protein metabolism which are believed to reach significant plasma concentrations during prolonged cellular ischemia are myocardial depressant factor (MDF) and reticuloendothelial depressant substance (RDS). MDF is the product of an ischemic pancreas and causes negative inotropic effects. RDS is produced in ischemic splanchnic viscera and depresses phagocytic and detoxification processes. The release of significant quantities of lysosomal hydrolases, cellular waste products, and blood sludging are believed to herald irreversible shock, which inevitably leads to death.

Any situation leading to an acute reduction in the effective circulating blood volume triggers a variety of acute hemodynamic and hormonal compensatory and corrective responses aimed at restoring tissue blood flow (Fig. 2-2). The magnitude of these responses is determined by the severity of the decrease in the effective circulating blood volume and those factors responsible for its decrease. The absorption of toxins from a devitalized bowel, for example, can lead to the lysis of mast cells, neutrophils, and platelets, resulting in the release of histamine, serotonin, kinins, and a variety of prostaglandins (thromboxane, leukotrienes) which interfere with vascular control and capillary permeability (Fig. 2-1). In addition to the compensatory and corrective changes which are outlined in Figure 2-2, hypotension or a decrease in blood or plasma volume induces homeostatic restorative fluid shifts from cells to the interstitium, a contraction of capacitance blood vessels in the spleen, liver, and great veins, and a redistribution of blood flow to the brain, heart, and lung. The last of these effects is accomplished at the expense of providing adequate blood flow to the splanchnic viscera, kidney, skeletal muscle, and skin. These internal adjustments in vascular tone, cardiac performance, and the volume of body fluid compartments may be adequate to prevent significant alterations in cellular metabolism until the factors responsible for shock are eliminated or corrected. If the cause of shock is not eliminated, however, and the internal compensatory and corrective changes are inadequate, progressive tissue ischemia and hypoxia occur, resulting in death.

Specific Organ Defects

Heart. Provided that heart failure is not the cause of poor tissue perfusion, cardiac performance is remarkably well maintained and may actually be increased during the initial stages of shock.[5] Decreases in cardiac contractility, cardiac output, and arterial blood pressure, occurring as a result of decreased venous return and increases in peripheral vascular resistance, are initially compensated for by sympathoadrenally induced increases in cardiac contractility and heart rate. Cardiac output may actually increase above preshock levels during low peripheral vascular resistance forms of distributive shock (Table 2-1). The continued loss of blood from damaged vessels, fluid loss from leaky capillaries, and the absorption or release of cardiotoxic substances (H^+, K^+, endotoxin, MDF) eventually reduce cardiac performance regardless of compensatory effects.

Vasculature. The causal factor in most forms of shock (except low-resistance distributive shock) is a progressive decline in cardiac output, resulting in a decrease in arterial blood pressure and a decreased effective circulating blood volume. Blood pressure is initially maintained by sympathetically in-

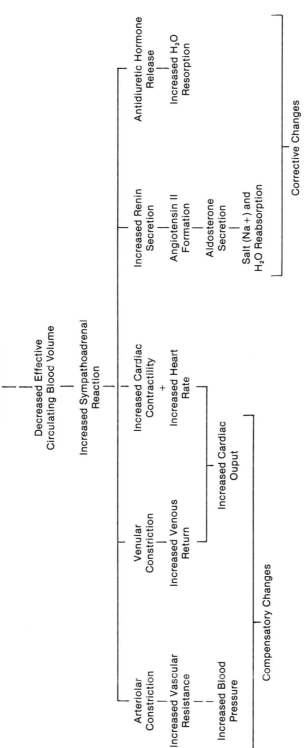

Fig. 2-2. Compensatory and corrective responses to a decrease in the effective circulating blood volume caused by shock.

duced increases in peripheral and pulmonary vascular resistance and marginal increases in venous return caused by reflex venoconstriction. These protective responses ensure a redistribution of blood flow to the brain, heart, and lungs at the expense of other organs, e.g., the splanchnic viscera and kidney. The lower hydrostatic pressure in the latter organs favors the uptake of fluid from the tissues, which helps to maintain blood volume. Continued depression of cardiac output and arterial blood pressure, however, eventually limits tissue oxygen supply which, together with the accumulation of metabolic products (CO_2, H^+, etc.), causes dilation of constricted arterioles. The postcapillary venules remain constricted as venous smooth muscle is relatively insensitive to metabolic changes. These vascular changes increase capillary pressure and permeability. Exudation of fluid into the tissues reduces the circulating blood volume further. Terminally, the capacitance veins dilate, exaggerating vascular pooling and resulting in dramatic decreases in the effective circulating blood volume.

Low-resistance forms of distributive shock (Table 2-1) are characterized by a generalized reduction in peripheral vascular resistance due to opening of arteriovenous shunts or the inability to regulate peripheral vascular tone. These changes result in the redistribution of blood flow away from vital organs (heart, brain) and the rapid accumulation of large volumes of fluid in capacitance vessels and peripheral tissues. Because low-resistance forms of distributive shock generally begin as hypermetabolic disorders, tissue requirements for nutrients and oxygen can exceed supply. Excessive peripheral vascular pooling of blood and the hypermetabolic state can result in sudden deterioration of the effective circulating blood volume and death.

Lung.   Shock-induced increases in sympathoadrenal discharge provoke an initial hyperventilatory state characterized by normal arterial oxygen tension and a low carbon dioxide tension. Decreases in pulmonary blood flow or pressure induce ventilation/perfusion mismatches, an increase in pulmonary shunting of venous blood, and arterial hypoxemia. Compensatory pulmonary arteriolar and venous constriction result in poor pulmonary blood flow, increases in pulmonary capillary hydrostatic pressure, and increases in pulmonary capillary permeability. Hypoxia, accumulation of circulating prostaglandins (thromboxane, leukotrienes), and the absorption of extrapulmonary toxins cause additional increases in pulmonary capillary permeability. Hypoxia and the accumulation of plasma in the pulmonary tissues interfere with pulmonary surfactant production, resulting in alveolar atelectasis and a decrease in lung compliance. The accumulation of proteinaceous fluids in small airways, if severe, can lead to hyaline membrane formation and respiratory failure.

Central Nervous System.   Cerebral blood flow is maintained during the early stages of shock, regardless of cerebral vasoconstriction secondary to hyperventilation and moderate reductions in arterial blood pressure. A mean arterial blood pressure below 55 mm Hg causes blood to be redistributed away from a cerebrum to the medulla in order to maintain vital vegetative functions. Central nervous system (CNS) depression, mental clouding, and unconsciousness may occur if hypotension is severe or lasts for an extended period of time.

Prolonged CNS ischemia and hypoxia can result in a breakdown of the blood-brain barrier, cerebral edema, and death.

Splanchnic Circulation.   Blood flow to the gastrointestinal tract, spleen, and pancreas is dramatically reduced in the initial phases in all forms of shock. Hepatic arterial blood flow is maintained, although portal flow is dramatically reduced. If blood flow is not returned to normal, the sensitive mucosal and submucosal linings of the gastrointestinal tract are damaged, resulting in submucosal edema and eventually hemorrhage. Third space accumulation of fluids into a devitalized intestinal wall can cause substantial decreases in the effective circulating blood volume. Continued splanchnic ischemia results in a breakdown of the gastrointestinal epithelium and the absorption of endotoxins from enteric bacteria. Pancreatic ischemia results in the release of proteolytic enzymes into the intestinal tract, predisposing to hemorrhagic enteritis. If severe, pancreatic ischemia also results in the release of MDF into the systemic circulation.[5] The release of enteric toxins and lysosomal hydrolases into the portal circulation depresses the liver's phagocytic and detoxification properties and triggers the release of other vasoactive substances (histamine, thromboxane). Histamine release causes intense hepatic venoconstriction in dogs, which eventually produces centrilobular hepatocellular swelling, portal hypertension, and intestinal congestion. Increases in portal venous pressure combined with the inability of the nervous system to regulate arteriolar tone results in the pooling of large volumes of blood in the intestinal tract.

Kidney.   The kidney can withstand relatively severe and prolonged periods of reduced blood flow and return to normal function. Severe ischemia, however, causes acute renal tubular necrosis, resulting in the loss of renal concentrating ability and renal failure. Renal blood flow is reduced during the initial phases of all forms of shock which cause hypotension. Renal blood flow is occasionally increased early during low-resistance forms of distributive shock.

Clinical Evaluation of the Patient in Shock

Shock is diagnosed after careful physical examination with emphasis on the cardiovascular system. Examination of the respiratory system and the CNS combined with pertinent laboratory data help to confirm the severity of shock (Table 2-2). Accurate historical details and special procedures (radiographs, abdominal tap) are useful in confirming suspicions. Because a diagnosis of shock is determined by the status of the cardiovascular system, as many indices of cardiac function as possible must be evaluated. Tissue blood flow is dependent on blood volume and cardiac output. Cardiac output is regulated by heart rate, venous return, aortic blood pressure (afterload), and cardiac contractility (Fig. 2-3).

Heart Rate and Rhythm.   A change in heart rate is one of the easiest clinical indicators of cardiovascular compromise to detect but is often difficult to interpret. The heart rate increases in direct proportion to the severity of cardiovascular compromise in an attempt to restore tissue perfusion, blood

Table 2-2. Clinical Characteristics of Early and Late Stages of Shock

Characteristic	Early Stage	Late Stage
Cardiovascular		
Heart rate	Moderately increased	Markedly increased
Heart rhythm	Regular	Regular or irregular
Pulse pressure	Normal	Reduced (weak thready pulse)
Capillary refill time	Minimally prolonged	Markedly prolonged (>3 sec)
Mucous membrane color	Pale pink (injected in septic shock)	White (red or blue in septic shock)
CVP	Minimally reduced	Markedly reduced (<1 cm H_2O)
Arterial blood pressure	Normal or decreased (elevated in septic shock)	Decreased (mean pressure <60 mm Hg)
ECG	Normal	Normal, arrhythmia, S-T segment deviation
Respiratory		
Respiratory rate	Increased	Rapid shallow breathing
Pattern of respiration	Regular	Normal, intermittent dyspneic
Auscultation	Normal	Increased bronchovesicular sounds, crackles
Tidal volume	Increased	Decreased
Arterial oxygen tension	Normal	Normal or decreased
Arterial carbon dioxide	Decreased	Normal or increased
Central nervous system		
Level of consciousness	Alert, anxious, minimally depressed	Depressed, semiconscious, coma
Laboratory evaluation		
Packed cell volume	Normal or increased	Normal or decreased
Total protein	Normal or increased	Decreased
Blood lactate	Normal	Increased
Serum K^+	Normal or decreased	Increased
BUN and creatinine	Normal	Normal or increased
Urine volume and Na^+	Decreased	Markedly decreased
White blood cell count	Increased (left shift)	Decreased (left shift)

pressure, or both. Unfortunately, excitement, pain, fever, hypoxia, CNS trauma, and hypokalemia can result in an elevated heart rate regardless of whether shock is present. Close inspection of the electrocardiogram (ECG) during shock frequently reveals S-T segment depression or elevation suggestive of myocardial ischemia. Extreme tachycardia or bradycardia occur during the late stage of shock due to myocardial ischemia and hypoxemia.

Cardiac arrhythmias are infrequent during the early stage of shock unless cardiac trauma or disease are present. Atrial fibrillation may develop in giant-breed dogs in shock. Ventricular arrhythmias are frequently observed during cardiogenic shock (cardiomyopathy), canine bloat, or following thoracic trauma. A rapid ventricular rate or frequent ventricular extrasystoles reduces arterial blood pressure and cardiac output. Abnormalities in cardiac rhythm are accurately diagnosed by an ECG but can be detected by careful auscultation of the heart and digital palpation of a peripheral artery. Rapid irregular heart sounds of varying intensity, a rapid irregular pulse, and a pulse deficit are

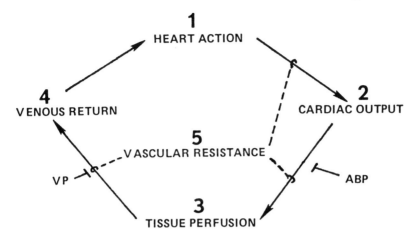

Fig. 2-3.   Overview of circulatory dynamics. Normal heart action (1) pumps sufficient cardiac output (2) to supply the needs of the metabolizing tissues (3). At equilibrium, cardiac output equals venous return (4). Systemic vascular resistance (5) influences heart action by changing the resistance to left ventricular outflow and modulating both arterial blood pressure (ABP) and venous pressure (VP). Mean arterial blood pressure, the product of cardiac output and vascular resistance, falls if either of these parameters is decreased.

indicators of a cardiac arrhythmia. Return of the pulse rate and rhythm to normal after therapy is an excellent prognostic sign.

Arterial Blood Pressure.   The peripheral pulse can be a good indicator of arterial blood pressure. The arterial blood pressure is directly dependent on the cardiac output and indirectly related to the peripheral vascular resistance. Cardiac output is increased by increases in heart rate, venous return, and cardiac contractility; it is decreased by increases in peripheral vascular resistance. A strong regular pulse occurring at a normal rate generally indicates that venous return, cardiac contractility, and peripheral vascular resistance are normal. Rapid pulse rates, a decreased pulse pressure (difference between systolic and diastolic blood pressure), prolonged capillary refill time, and hypothermia are signs of hypovolemia, a reduced perfusion pressure, and poor peripheral blood flow. Prolonged capillary refill time combined with pale or white mucous membranes are an indication of hemorrhage, intense peripheral vasoconstriction, a reduction in arterial blood pressure, and a redistribution of blood flow. During low-resistance forms of distributive shock (septic shock), the mucous membranes may become injected (bright red), although capillary refill time is prolonged. This is a poor prognostic sign indicative of low arterial blood pressure and the loss of the animal's ability to regulate vascular tone.

Blood pressure can be quantitated by direct and indirect techniques. Direct measurement of arterial blood pressure requires arterial (femoral, dorsal metatarsal, radial, brachial) catheterization and is relatively easily accomplished with experience. Direct measurement of arterial blood pressure is used to guide therapy, evaluate arterial pH and blood gases (O_2 and CO_2), and determine prognosis. Fluid-filled catheters are connected to aneroid manometers or pressure transducers for the display of pressure on oscilloscopes (Tektronix, Datascope Corp.). Indirect assessment of arterial blood pressure is not as accurate as direct techniques, particularly during hypotension, but does not require arterial puncture. Several devices employing arterial occluding pressure cuffs (Criticon Corp, Datascope Corp.) or pressure cuffs and ultrasonic crystals which determine blood flow (Parks Electronics) are available.

Central Venous Pressure.   Central venous pressure (CVP) is dependent on cardiac performance, blood volume, and venous vascular tone. Decreases in CVP can be caused by tachycardia, hypovolemia, or decreases in venous vascular tone (increased compliance). Blood loss (>25% blood volume) and low-resistance forms of distributive shock (Table 2-1) commonly produce marked reductions in CVP. Cardiogenic shock may cause an initial increase in CVP due to right heart failure; but as shock progresses and blood pools in the tissues, CVP falls. CVP therefore is a good indicator of absolute or relative hypovolemia and is useful in assessing the adequacy of volume replacement. The CVP is determined by placing a catheter in the jugular vein so that its tip lies within the anterior vena cava. The catheter is connected to a fluid-filled manometer. Zero pressure is considered to be a point at the level of the right atrium. Trends in CVP measurement are more important than single determinations. Changes in the CVP by greater than 2 cm H_2O are considered significant and indicate that fluid administration should be increased (decreased CVP) or decreased (increased CVP). Dyspnea and intermittent positive-pressure ventilation (IPPV) can cause transient but large changes in CVP.

Occasionally, pulmonary capillary wedge pressure (P_{cwp}) is determined by inserting a specialized catheter (balloon-tipped Swan-Ganz catheter) via the jugular vein, out the pulmonary artery, and wedging it into a pulmonary arteriole (Fig. 2-4). The pressure recorded is a reflection of the left atrial pressure. The measurement of P_{cwp} is a useful index of left ventricular output. During pure left-sided heart failure, P_{cwp} is elevated, predisposing the patient to pulmonary edema.

There is a predictable relationship between right (CVP) and left (P_{cwp}) atrial pressures providing there is no obstruction of blood flow through the heart and pure right- or left-sided heart failure are not present. During shock, decreases in right atrial pressure indicate a decrease in left atrial pressure and a reduction in cardiac output. Conversely, increased CVP is indicative of poor forward flow of blood, an elevated left atrial pressure, and a predisposition to pulmonary edema.

Respiratory Function.   Activation of the sympathoadrenal system from any cause (Fig. 2-1) results in increases in respiratory rate. Respiratory rate also increases when fluid begins to accumulate in the lung. Tachypnea may lead to the excessive elimination of carbon dioxide, resulting in mild respiratory alkalosis. If hypoxemia accompanies shock or pulmonary fluid accumulation, respiratory rate and volume are increased, producing significant respiratory alkalosis (Table 2-2). CNS depression or the development of metabolic acidosis

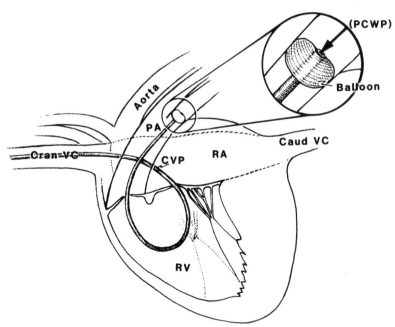

Fig. 2-4. The hemodynamic correlates to right-sided and left-sided congestive heart failure or fluid overload are elevations in right and left atrial pressures, respectively. When balloon-tipped (Swan-Ganz) catheters are used, the balloon can be inflated so that the catheter moves across the tricuspid and pulmonic valves and into the pulmonary artery (PA). When the balloon is fully inflated (**inset**) the end hole port can be used to measure distal pressure in the pulmonary capillaries. This is the pulmonary capillary wedge pressure (P_{cwp}), and it closely approximates the pulmonary venous, left atrial, and left ventricular diastolic pressures. (Reproduced by permission from Bonagura JD: Fluid and electrolyte management of the cardiac patient. p. 501. In Schaer M (ed): Symposium on Fluid and Electrolyte Balance. Veterinary Clinics of North America. W. B. Saunders, Philadelphia, 1982, Vol. 12.)

is observed as shock progresses and results in a decrease in respiratory rate even though the tidal volume may remain normal or is only slightly depressed. Intermittent breathing patterns (Cheyne-Stokes, Biot's) or markedly reduced respiratory rates are an indication of marked cerebral depression, cerebral ischemia, and the retention of significant amounts of carbon dioxide (respiratory acidosis). The return to normal breathing patterns and rates after therapy is a good prognostic sign.

Central Nervous System. CNS activity is usually increased during early stages of shock. Most animals are alert and apprehensive, and they may be aggressive. As shock progresses and cerebral blood flow diminishes, disorientation, depression, and coma occur.

Laboratory Data. A wide variety of laboratory data can be used to monitor the shock patient. The value of these indices in determining prognosis is increased by serial measurements and frequent determination. Red blood cells and total protein are normally limited to the vascular space. A reduction in plasma volume (Table 2-2) causes an increase in both packed cell volume and total protein, suggesting volume depletion. Aggressive fluid therapy with balanced electrolyte solutions reduces both packed cell volume and total protein. Acute hemorrhage, however, may result in little change in the packed cell volume or total protein. Blood cells and particularly protein may leak across damaged capillaries during later stages of shock, reducing both the packed cell volume and total protein. A stable packed cell volume and steadily decreasing total protein are indicative of severe capillary damage with the loss of protein and fluids into the tissue (third space loss). Total protein values below 3.5 g/100 ml predispose to edema formation.

Frequent blood gas and electrolyte determinations help to determine the severity of shock and suggest therapy. During early stages of shock, hyperventilation results in respiratory alkalosis with an intracellular shift of potassium ions (hypokalemia). Sustained reductions in tissue perfusion lead to anaerobic metabolism, metabolic acidosis, a shift of potassium out of cells (hyperkalemia), and the release of intracellular enzymes. Measurements of alanine transaminase (ALT) and alkaline phosphatase (ALP) can detect liver damage; aspartate transaminase (AST) and lactic dehydrogenase (LDH) are indicators of generalized tissue damage; elevated lipase and amylase indicate pancreatic ischemia; and elevated blood urea nitrogen (BUN) and creatinine indicate poor renal blood flow. Low urine sodium concentrations are pathognomonic for volume depletion. Sustained elevations of lactic acid are indicative of continued tissue ischemia and hypoxia, anaerobic metabolism, and a poor long-term prognosis. Similarly, reduced platelets, increased fibrin split products, and prolonged activated coagulation times indicate coagulopathy and severe tissue damage. Finally, early in shock, blood glucose and white blood cell counts are generally elevated because of increased sympathetic tone, insulin resistance, and the mobilization of white blood cells from storage sites. Both blood glucose and white blood cells are dramatically reduced late in shock and suggest a poor prognosis.

Therapy for Shock

Shock therapy has two principal goals: (1) to stabilize the patient; and (2) to compensate for or eliminate the cause of shock.[7,9] When shock is caused by a single factor, e.g., acute hemorrhage, both goals can be accomplished rapidly and simultaneously by fluid replacement. Frequently, however, the cause of shock is uncertain or represents the terminal event in a longstanding disease process. Therapy during the latter situations requires a multifaceted approach oriented toward restoring normal cardiovascular function and stabilizing the patient (Table 2-3). Because shock by definition is a reduction in the effective circulating blood volume leading to inadequate tissue perfusion, patient stabilization is accomplished by providing adequate blood or fluid volume, maintaining proper cardiac function, and ensuring vascular integrity. During the later stages of shock, therapy is often oriented toward minimizing or combating the deleterious effects of anaerobic metabolism and the toxic components of cellular lysis.

Maintenance of Adequate Fluid Volume. Restoring or maintaining adequate fluid volume is the single most important therapy in shock. Regardless of cause, all forms of shock require the administration of fluids to maintain tissue perfusion. Less critical yet important goals of fluid therapy are to restore a normal fluid volume and correct acid-base and electrolyte disturbances. Ideally, proper fluid selection and volume of administration require careful and frequent monitoring of arterial blood pressure, CVP, arterial pH, serum electrolytes, hematocrit, urine output, and the level of consciousness. Polyionic salt solutions, e.g., lactated Ringer's, are desirable for initial fluid replacement when extensive laboratory data are not available or cannot be rapidly obtained. Such fluids contain physiological concentrations of extracellular electrolytes and a potential source of base (lactate, acetate, citrate) which is rapidly metabolized to bicarbonate (HCO_3^-), providing acidosis and perfusion deficits are not severe. Saline is an adequate substitute for lactated Ringer's when fluid is needed to replace a volume deficit due to acute blood loss. The administration of large volumes of saline can lead to hypokalemia and hypoproteinemia. Hypotonic fluids, e.g., 5% dextrose, should be avoided if possible in order to prevent excessive electrolyte dilution, hypoproteinemia, and cellular edema. Although polyionic salt solutions are beneficial in restoring volume and preventing microcirculatory sludging, they must be used cautiously when the plasma protein falls below 3.5 g/dl or the packed cell volume falls below 20%. Plasma expanders (dextran 40 or 70), plasma, or blood are indicated in hypovolemia during protein-losing states, during the acute loss of large volumes of blood, or when large volumes of polyionic solutions result in hypoproteinemia or a reduction in the packed cell volume. The intravenous administration of low (dextran 40) or high (dextran 70) molecular weight dextrans increases plasma volume directly and by drawing fluid into the vascular space. Both solutions reduce platelet and red blood cell aggregation, decrease blood viscosity, and improve microcirculatory blood flow. Although infrequent, the intravenous administration of either solution can cause fever and allergic reactions in susceptible animals. Excessive volumes of dextrans can also produce peripheral and pulmonary edema, and may cause a hemorrhagic diathesis. Plasma is superior to dextran because it does not produce the described untoward reactions and contains proteins which can serve metabolic needs. In addition, plasma albumin supports blood volume and oncotic pressure 10–15 times longer than solutions containing synthetic colloids.

Fresh blood is an ideal replacement fluid in animals who are anemic (hemoglobin < 5 g/dl) or continue to bleed. Transfusion reactions are uncommon in dogs (providing A-negative donors are used) and even less frequent in cats. Blood cross-matching and careful patient observation for hemolysis, hemoglobinuria, fever, vomiting, and jaundice are recommended when donors with unknown blood types are used and multiple transfusions are required. Stored blood can be administered when fresh blood is unavailable. Stored blood contains the same cellular components as fresh blood but, because of the addition

Table 2-3. Therapeutic Management of Problems Associated with Shock

Problem	Treatment	Trade Name or Device	Dosage	Side Effects or Contraindications
Hypovolemia				
Fluid loss	Crystalloid	Lactated Ringer's	50–100 ml/kg/hr IV	Hypervolemia, pulm. edema, hypoproteinemia
Plasma loss	Colloid expander	Gentran 40 (Travenol)	20–40 ml/kg IV	Hypervolemia, pulm. edema, allergic reactions
Blood loss	Whole blood *See* Hypovolemia	—	10–40 ml/kg IV	Hypervolemia, allergic reactions
Hypotension	Calcium chloride	—	1 ml 10% sol./10 kg IV	
	Phenylephrine	Neo-Synephrine (Winthrop)	10–50 µg/kg IV	
	Epinephrine	Adrenaline (Parke Davis)	3–5 µg/kg IV	Hypertension, tachycardia, arrhythmias
	Dopamine	Intropin (Arnar Stone)	3–10 µg/kg/min IV	
	Dobutamine	Dobutrex (Lilly)	3–10 µg/kg/min IV	
Cardiac arrhythmias				
Bradycardia	Atropine	— (Elkins-Sinn)	0.01–0.02 mg/kg IV	Tachycardia
	Glycopyrrolate	Robinul (Robins)	0.005–0.01 mg/kg IV	Tachycardia
Tachycardia	Digoxin	Lanoxin (Burroughs Wellcome)	0.01–0.02 mg/kg IV slowly	Bradycardia, cardiac arrhythmias
	Propranolol	Inderal (Ayerst)	0.05–0.01 mg/kg IV	Bradycardia, cardiac failure
Atrial arrhythmias	Quinidine	Quinidine gluconate (Lilly)	4–8 mg/kg/10 min IV	Hypotension
Ventricular arrhythmias	Lidocaine	Xylocaine (Astra)	2–4 mg/kg IV	CNS excitement
	Procainamide	Pronestyl (Squibb)	4–8 mg/kg/5 min IV	Hypotension
Acute heart failure	Calcium chloride		1 ml 10% sol./10 kg IV	
	Epinephrine	Adrenaline (Parke-Davis)	3–5 µg/kg IV	Hypertension, tachycardia, cardiac arrhythmias
	Dopamine	Intropin (Arnar Stone)	3–10 µg/kg/min IV	
	Dobutamine	Dobutrex (Lilly)	3–10 µg/kg/min IV	
Respiratory failure				
Hypoxia	O₂, nasal catheter; oxygen cage		2–4 L/min	
	Ventilation		Tidal vol. = 14 ml/kg	Decreased venous return, resp. alkalosis
Hypercarbia	Doxapram	Dopram V (Robins)	1.0–2.0 mg/kg	CNS excitement
	Ventilation		Tidal vol. = 14 ml/kg	Decreased venous return, resp. alkalosis
Dyspnea	Tracheostomy Chest tubes Ventilation	Heimlich valve	Tidal vol. = 14 ml/kg	Decreased venous return, resp.

Condition	Treatment	Product (Manufacturer)	Dose	Complications
Sepsis	Surgery			
	Gentamicin	Gentocin (Schering)	4 mg/kg/q 6 h IM	Muscle weakness, renal toxicity
	Kanamycin	Kantrim (Bristol)	10 mg/kg/q 6 h IM	Muscle weakness, renal toxicity
	Ampicillin	Ommipen (Wyeth)	10 mg/kg/q 6 h IV	
Metabolic acidosis	Sodium lactate[a]		Bicarbonate dose = base deficit × 0.3 × wt (kg) or 0.5 mEq/kg/10 min IV to effect	Metabolic alkalosis, hyperosmolarity, CSF acidosis, hyperkalemia, hypocalcemia
	Sodium acetate[a]			
	Sodium bicarbonate			
Hyperkalemia	Sodium bicarbonate		0.5–1.0 mg/kg IV	As above
	NaCl 0.9% solution		10–40 ml/kg/hr IV	Hypervolemia, hypoproteinemia
	Calcium gluconate		0.5 ml/kg of 10% sol. IV	Tachycardia
	Hyperventilation		Tidal vol. = 14 ml/kg	Decreased venous return, resp. alkalosis
Hypoglycemia	Dextrose 50%		1–2 ml/kg IV / 0.5–1.0 g/kg/hr 10% glucose	Hyperosmolarity
Renal ischemia	Fluids	Lactated Ringer's	10–40 ml/kg/hr IV	Hypervolemia, hypoproteinemia, pulm. edema
	Mannitol 20%	Osmitrol (Travenol)	0.5–2.0 mg/kg IV	Hyperosmolality
	Furosemide	Lasix (Hoechst)	1.0–2.0 mg/kg IM, IV	Decreased cardiac output
Hypothermia (<36°C)	Fluids	Lactated Ringer's	10–40 ml/kg/hr warmed to 37°C	Hypervolemia, hypoproteinemia, pulm. edema
	H₂O-filled heating pad		Warmed to 38°C (warm slowly)	
DIC	Correct hypotension	Lactated Ringer's	10–40 mg/kg/hr IV	Hypervolemia, hypoproteinemia, pulm. edema
	Correct hypoxemia	Nasal catheter / Ventilation	2–4 L/min / Tidal vol. = 14 ml/kg	Decreased venous return, resp. alkalosis
	Correct acidosis	Sodium bicarbonate (Lipomed)	0.5–1.0 mg/kg IV	
	Heparin		Dog: 500 units/kg SQ t.i.d. Cat: 250–400 units/kg SQ t.i.d.	Bleeding
Cellular ischemia	Fluids	Lactated Ringer's	10–40 mg/kg/hr IV	Hypervolemia, hypoproteinemia, pulm. edema
	Oxygen	Nasal catheter	2–4 L/min	
	Dexamethasone sodium phosphate	Azium (Schering)	4–6 mg/kg IV	
	Prednisolone sodium succinate	Solu-Delta-Cortef (Upjohn)	>10 mg/kg IV	

[a] Questionable efficacy during severe low-flow states.

of storage components (acid-citrate-dextrose, citrate-phosphate-dextrose), is less desirable. The potential for the development of acidosis, hypothermia, hyperkalemia, hypocalcemia, and prolonged bleeding times must be considered when large volumes of stored blood are used. Prolonged storage of blood reduces platelets, coagulation factors, and 2,3-diphosphoglycerate (2,3-DPG) concentration. A decrease in 2,3-DPG causes an increase in hemoglobin affinity for oxygen, thereby reducing oxygen availability to tissues.

Determination of the volume of fluid required to treat a patient in shock is difficult, particularly when the volume of fluid lost is unknown or fluid loss continues to occur. Clinical evidence of acute hypovolemia does not become evident until 15–20% of the vascular volume has been depleted. Formulas used to calculate fluid needs that estimate the amount of sodium (Na^+) ignore isotonic fluid losses, which may be important in shock patients. Such formulas are therefore inappropriate for the shock patient. A loss of extracellular fluid which results in hemoconcentration, however, allows the extracellular fluid concentration to be calculated from the change in hematocrit (Hct) according to the formula:

$$\text{Extracellular fluid deficit} = 0.3 \times \text{body weight (kg)} \times \frac{\text{Hct measured} - 1}{\text{normal Hct}}$$

Similarly, the amount of blood required to change the Hct of an anemic shock patient to a predetermined value can be calculated from the formula:

Blood requirement

$$= 90 \text{ ml/kg} \times \text{recipient's body weight (kg)} \times \frac{\text{desired Hct} - \text{actual Hct}}{\text{Hct of blood donor}}$$

Patients suffering from acute blood loss, however, generally do not demonstrate changes in Hct, total protein, or electrolyte values. When the amount of blood loss can be estimated, colloidal solutions or stored blood can be used to replace the loss on a one-to-one basis. Three times as much fluid is required to replace blood loss (3:1) when polyionic fluids are used. For example, if a patient is known to have lost 100 ml of blood, 300 ml of polyionic fluids are needed as replacement. Polyionic fluids distribute into a volume (extracellular fluid volume) approximately three times as large as the blood vascular compartment. When the amount of fluid loss cannot be estimated or is unknown, physical findings and the response to fluid therapy guide the amount of fluids administered. Frequent auscultation of the heart and lungs coupled with assessments of the peripheral pulse and measurements of Hct and plasma proteins are excellent indicators of the adequacy of fluid therapy. CVP measurement is a useful guide to the amount and rate of fluid administration. An increase in CVP of 2 cm H_2O over baseline values is an indication that too much fluid is being administered or that the rate of administration is too rapid.

The rate of fluid administration to a shock patient is difficult to determine particularly when the volume of fluid lost and cardiovascular or renal function are unknown. Consequently, CVP, P_{cwp}, and arterial blood pressure measurements are extremely valuable in assessing the rate of fluid administration. Although many emergency manuals recommend fluid administration rates of up to 90 ml/kg/hr for emergency situations, rates in excess of 200 ml/kg/hr are tolerated for short periods providing the cardiovascular and renal functions are normal. Rates of fluid administration as low as 10 ml/kg/hr are capable of producing volume overload and pulmonary edema during cardiogenic shock or renal failure. General guidelines for fluid therapy are discussed further in Chapter 4.

Maintenance of Normal Cardiac Function. Tissue perfusion is dependent on maintenance of an adequate cardiac output and the normal distribution of blood flow (Fig. 2-3). Increases in heart rate, venous return, and cardiac contractility help to maintain or increase cardiac output, whereas increases in peripheral vascular resistance and cardiac arrhythmias decrease cardiac output and tissue perfusion. Optimization of cardiac performance therefore is dependent on ensuring adequate venous return through maintenance of vascular volume, normalizing heart rate and rhythm, maintaining or improving cardiac contractility, and decreasing peripheral vascular resistance. Vascular volume is maintained through appropriate fluid therapy, controlling hemorrhage, and eliminating continued fluid loss. Atropine (0.01 mg/kg IV) or glycopyrrolate (0.005 mg/kg) can be used to treat decreases in cardiac output due to bradycardia. Lidocaine (4 mg/kg IV; 40–80 μg/kg/min IV) and procainamide (4–8 mg/kg IM or IV q.i.d.) are used to treat ventricular arrhythmias, and quinidine (4–8 mg/kg IM q.i.d.) is used to treat atrial fibrillation. Sinus tachycardia can be controlled with appropriate fluid and electrolyte therapy. The administration of potassium chloride (20–40 mEq/L) at rates not exceeding 0.5 mEq/kg/hr is often successful in slowing sinus rate and increasing antiarrhythmic drug efficacy. Digoxin (0.01 mg/kg IV) can also be used to slow sinus tachycardia, decrease ventricular response during atrial fibrillation, and treat atrial arrhythmias. Cardiac contractility is improved by digitalis glycosides or calcium chloride. Dopamine (3–10 μg/kg/min) or dobutamine (3–15 μg/kg/min) are used to increase cardiac rate and contractility when emergency therapy or temporary inotropic support are indicated.

A syndrome characterized by low cardiac output and inadequate response to volume repletion and inotropic agents occasionally develops during the later stages of shock. The CVP is increased, pulse pressure is decreased, mucous membranes are pale, and the extremities are cold. Taken together, these symptoms are indications of an elevated peripheral vascular resistance. Therapy is oriented toward maintaining adequate volume and decreasing vascular constriction. Acetylpromazine (0.05 mg/kg IV, maximum of 4 mg), low dosages of isoproterenol (0.005–0.04 μg/kg/min IV), or low dosages of dopamine (0.05–3 μg/kg/min IV) improve peripheral perfusion by either blocking α-receptors (acetylpromazine) or stimulating β_2 (isoproterenol) or dopaminergic (dopamine) receptors. Pharmacologic dosages of dexamethasone (4–8 mg/kg) or prednisolone sodium succinate (20–50 mg/kg) are useful in returning normal vascular responsiveness to endogenous neurotransmitters.

Maintenance of Vascular Integrity.   Capillary membrane permeability plays a central role in the maintenance of plasma volume and tissue perfusion during shock. Ischemia, hypoxia, acidosis, endotoxins, and increased circulating concentrations of kinins, histamine, and 5-hydroxytryptamine increase capillary membrane permeability, resulting in the loss of plasma proteins from the vascular compartment and interstitial fluid accumulation (edema), which leads to compression and interference with blood flow to surrounding capillary beds. When this process is allowed to progress or involves large amounts of tissue, cell function is dramatically impaired. The causes for increases in capillary membrane permeability have resulted in a wide variety of therapies which may be beneficial, although their efficacy in restoring or improving membrane permeability characteristics has not been proved.

Oxygen therapy is indicated whenever respiratory function is impaired or arterial oxygen tension is reduced. Clinical signs suggestive of a lowered arterial blood oxygen tension include: tachypnea, tachycardia, cyanosis, distress, and occasionally cardiac arrhythmias. Oxygen can be supplied by oxygen cages, nasal catheters, face masks, or anesthetic machines. Patients who are unconscious and hypoventilating should be orotracheally intubated and administered IPPV. Tidal volumes of 14 ml/kg and a respiratory rate of 8–12/min are adequate to maintain normal arterial carbon dioxide tension. Ideally the inspired oxygen concentration is 40–60% of the total gas flow, but not exceeding this range if oxygen therapy is required for long periods of time. These concentrations are easily maintained when using oxygen cages or other open systems. The administration of 100% oxygen from an anesthetic machine for many hours can lead to drying of the mucous membranes, interference with tracheal mucous flow, and decreased surfactant production. The principles of oxygen therapy and artificial ventilation are discussed in more detail in Chapter 3.

The use of glucocorticosteroids for the treatment of shock remains controversial. Their use before and during hemorrhagic, septic, and cardiogenic forms of shock can be beneficial providing appropriate dosages are used. Large (pharmacologic) dosages of dexamethasone (4–8 mg/kg IV) or prednisolone sodium succinate (20–50 mg/kg IV) must be given early in the course of shock for therapy to be beneficial. These dosages can be safely repeated three or four times at 4- to 6-hr intervals. The administration of glucocorticosteroids at these dosages is believed to improve capillary membrane integrity, stabilize lysosomal membranes, produce mild vasodilation, protect against coagulation and complement activation, and help prevent the development of cerebral edema. Antibiotics should be combined with glucocorticosteroid therapy in the treatment of later stages of shock, when septicemia is suspected, and during endotoxic shock. The concurrent administration of glucocorticosteroids with antibiotics helps to prevent the effects of increased endotoxin release associated with the death of gram-negative bacteria. Broad-spectrum antibiotics are recommended based on the even distribution of gram-positive and gram-negative organisms responsible for producing septicemia. Gentamicin (4 mg/kg/q 6 h IM), kanamycin (10 mg/kg/q 6 h IM), and ampicillin (10 mg/kg/q 6 h IV) are the antibiotics of choice at the present time.

Acid-base and electrolyte disturbances and hypoglycemia should be considered during later stages of shock, when shock develops very rapidly, or when shock occurs secondary to a longstanding disease process. Ideally, corrective therapy is based on accurate and frequent determination of blood pH, blood gases, serum electrolytes, and blood glucose. Metabolic acidosis is treated with sodium bicarbonate according to the formula:

Sodium bicarbonate requirement

$$= 0.3 \times \text{body weight (kg)} \times (25 - \text{measured bicarbonate})$$

Trishydroxymethylaminomethane (THAM) is an effective alternate to sodium bicarbonate and is used in severe or longstanding cases of metabolic acidosis. THAM penetrates cell membranes more rapidly than sodium bicarbonate, accepts hydrogen ions from all metabolic acids, and does not increase osmolality appreciably. When blood gases and pH are not available and plasma bicarbonate cannot be determined, sodium bicarbonate 1–2 mEq/kg IV can be administered intravenously at 30-min intervals to treat suspected severe metabolic acidosis. Large amounts of sodium bicarbonate should not be added to polyionic solutions containing calcium (lactated Ringer's) as calcium and bicarbonate combine to form an insoluble calcium carbonate salt. Additional discussion of the therapy of acid-base and electrolyte disturbances can be found in Chapter 4.

Other Therapeutic Considerations. Supplemental glucose, insulin, and potassium solutions may prove to be particularly therapeutic during the latter stages of shock, during endotoxic shock, or when treating the very young animal in shock. Ten percent glucose solutions containing 0.3 units of insulin per gram of glucose and potassium chloride 20–60 mEq/L can be administered at a rate of 0.5–1.0 g glucose/kg/hr to treat hypoglycemia and prevent hypokalemia.

Additional therapeutic adjuncts to the treatment of shock include furosemide (1.0–2.0 mg/kg IM, IV) or mannitol (0.5–2.0 g/kg IV) to promote diuresis and prevent cellular edema, heparin (300–500 units/kg SQ tid) to treat hypercoagulopathies and prevent DIC, and heating units (warm-water circulating blanket) to prevent severe hypothermia.

The drugs, dosages, and techniques currently used to treat shock are constantly being rethought, revised, and expanded. Regardless of the variety of new approaches and specifically oriented therapeutic discoveries aimed at preserving cellular integrity and prolonging cell life, the principal goal of shock therapy remains the restoration of an effective circulating blood volume.

HEART FAILURE

Heart failure refers to the inability of the heart to maintain a cardiac output that is sufficient to satisfy the metabolic needs of tissues during exercise or at rest. Reduced cardiac output can be caused by cardiac malformation or by disease of the active elements (e.g., muscle, impulse forming and conduction

Table 2-4. Common Causes of Heart Failure in Dogs and Cats

Congenital heart disease
Valvular heart disease (congenital/acquired; degenerative/inflammatory)
Aortic stenosis
Pulmonic stenosis
Mitral regurgitation
Tricuspid regurgitation
Aortic regurgitation
Myocardial disease
Congestive (dilated) cardiomyopathy
Hypertrophic cardiomyopathy
Restrictive cardiomyopathy
Excessive moderator bands
Myocarditis/myocardial depression and injury
Infectious, toxic, metabolic (thyrotoxicosis), ischemic, traumatic
Drug-induced
Idiopathic
Pericardial disease
Pericarditis (infective/idiopathic)
Cardiac and heartbase tumors (chemodectoma, hemangiosarcoma, mesothelioma, ectopic thyroid carcinoma)
Cardiac arrhythmias
Heartworm disease

system, blood vessels) or the passive components (e.g., valves and pericardium) of the heart and vascular system (Table 2-4). Heart failure differs from noncardiogenic forms of shock in that venous pressures and cardiac filling are generally increased (Figs. 2-3 and 2-4). Frequently the circulation is able to compensate for inadequate cardiac pumping ability (Fig. 2-5). This is achieved by activation of the sympathetic nervous system, alterations in regional tissue perfusion, renal retention of sodium and water, release of vasoactive chemicals and hormones, and the development of higher-than-normal ventricular filling pressures. Changes in heart size (dilatation) and wall thickness (hypertrophy) represent additional intrinsic methods for the diseased heart to maintain cardiac output.

Pathophysiological Classification of Heart Failure

Heart failure is frequently subdivided into four pathophysiological classes. This classification is clinically useful as the approach to therapy may differ between patients with: (1) myocardial failure; (2) hemodynamic overload; (3) compliance failure; and (4) arrhythmia. Myocardial or contractility failure occurs in dilated cardiomyopathy and is characterized by a reduced capacity to eject blood despite normal or high ventricular volumes. Systolic hemodynamic overloads are initially associated with normal myocardial contractility but an increased demand for ventricular volume or pressure work. Causes of volume overload include mitral and tricuspid valve regurgitation and congenital left-to-right shunts, e.g., patent ductus arteriosus and ventricular septal defect. Pressure overloads are exemplified by congenital stenosis of the pulmonic and aortic valves. These overloading conditions represent ''plumbing'' problems

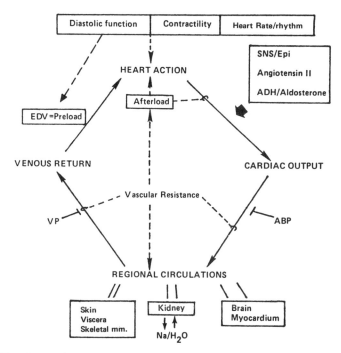

Fig. 2-5. Circulatory dynamics in heart failure. Normal heart action depends on heart rate and rhythm, myocardial contractility, ventricular diastolic (filling) function, and the loading conditions of the heart: preload and afterload. Inadequate cardiac output is compensated by activation of the sympathetic nervous system (SNS) with increased vascular resistance and release of epinephrine (Epi). These changes are enhanced by increased formation of angiotensin II, which modulates sympathetic tone and initiates the release of aldosterone and antidiuretic hormone (ADH). Alterations in vascular resistance lead to changes in regional circulation. Perfusion of the brain and myocardium are maintained at the expense of cutaneous, splanchnic, renal, and skeletal muscle flow. The kidney behaves as in hypovolemia and retains sodium and water—actions that are facilitated by release of aldosterone and ADH. Increased plasma volume and vascular resistance increase venous pressures, which tend to be high behind the failing ventricle. Elevated venous pressures increase ventricular end diastolic volume (EDV), and edema and effusions may occur, leading to clinical signs of congestive heart failure. Ventricular dilation and elevated vascular resistance increase ventricular afterload, resulting in further reductions in ventricular stroke volume.

for the heart and are best treated by surgery whenever possible. Patients with compliance failure have normal muscle contractility but impaired or restricted ventricular filling (Fig. 2-6). Pericardial effusion and hypertrophic cardiomyopathy are examples of diseases characterized by diastolic dysfunction. Cardiac arrhythmias frequently complicate each of the aforementioned types of heart failure; however, it is possible for serious rhythm disturbances alone to result in heart failure. Cardiac arrhythmia produces heart failure by causing a loss of atrial function (e.g., atrial fibrillation), a loss of atrioventricular synchronization

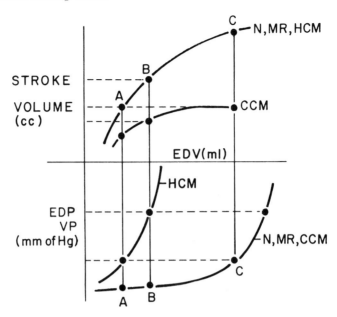

Fig. 2-6. Ventricular systolic (top curves) and diastolic (bottom curves) function. The normal (N) ventricle and hearts with normal myocardial function, as in mitral regurgitation (MR) and hypertrophic cardiomyopathy (HCM), respond appropriately to increased ventricular filling (A to B, B to C). As end-diastolic volume (EDV) increases, ventricular stroke volume is augmented, although much of the blood flows backward in MR. The patient with congestive cardiomyopathy and muscle failure (CCM) develops a relative intolerance to ventricular filling and does not appropriately increase systolic work. Ventricular *diastolic* function may be impaired when a ventricle either dilates or develops excessive hypertrophy. Volume-loading a ventricle (A to C) in animals with MR and CCM produces the following result: The increased volume is well tolerated (B to C) until the ventricle reaches a point at which the end-diastolic ventricular pressure (EDP) and hence the venous pressure (VP) begin to rapidly rise. Excessive hypertrophy (HCM) reduces ventricular compliance and causes small amounts of ventricular filling (A to B) to result in marked increases in EDP and VP.

and dyssynergy (e.g., ventricular tachycardia), bradycardia (e.g., complete atrioventricular block), and tachycardia with inadequate time for ventricular filling.

Clinical Signs of Heart Failure

The clinical signs of heart failure are related to inadequate tissue perfusion, circulatory venous congestion, or both. Depression, syncope, exertional weakness, prerenal azotemia, and pallor of the mucous membranes are attributed to reduced perfusion of the brain, skeletal muscles, kidneys, and skin (Fig. 2-5). Symptoms of congestive heart failure—dyspnea, tachypnea, cough, ascites, jugular venous distention, and edema—occur secondary to elevation of venous pressure behind a failing ventricle (Fig. 2-7). Increased vascular pressure can

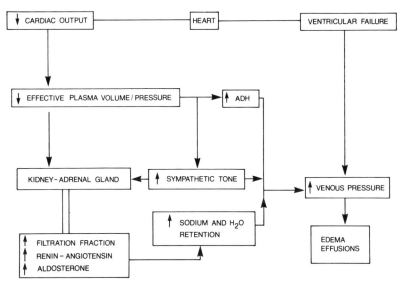

Fig. 2-7. The pathogenesis of edema and effusions in heart failure can be explained by the interaction of ventricular failure and activation of potent mechanisms of sodium retention by the kidney. Sodium and water retention are further enhanced by aldosterone and ADH, which are released in heart failure. Expansion of the blood volume and increases in sympathetic activity act to promote elevated venous pressures during ventricular failure. (Reproduced by permission from Bonagura JD: Fluid and electrolyte management of the cardiac patient. p. 501. In Schaer M (ed): Symposium on Fluid and Electrolyte Balance. Veterinary Clinics of North America. W. B. Saunders, Philadelphia, 1982, Vol. 12.)

be verified by placing a flow-directed balloon catheter and measuring the CVP and P_{cwp} (Fig. 2-4).

Diagnosis of Heart Failure

Identification of heart failure requires a careful medical history, physical examination, evaluation of radiographs, ECGs, routine laboratory tests, and occasionally specific studies, e.g., angiograms and echocardiograms. Heartworm tests are indicated in many geographic locations. Reliable signs of heart disease include loud cardiac murmurs, gallop rhythms, arrhythmias, and ECG and radiographic evidence of cardiomegaly. Jugular venous distention, hepatosplenomegaly, ascites, and pleural effusion are suggestive of right heart failure. Auscultatory and radiographic evidence of pulmonary edema, associated with radiographic and clinical signs of left heart disease, are typical findings of left heart failure. The identification of cardiac murmurs or cardiac arrhythmias, e.g., atrial fibrillation, is strong evidence of serious underlying heart disease.

The clinician must be cognizant that heart disease may coexist with noncardiac disorders which produce clinical signs similar to those of heart failure. Thus pleural and abdominal effusions should be evaluated cytologically and neoplasia and hypoproteinemia ruled out as causes of serous cavity transudation. The respiratory system must be carefully assessed. Of equal importance during clinical evaluation is the identification of abnormalities that lead the clinician away from a diagnosis of heart failure and suggest noncardiac problems, e.g., bronchitis, pneumonia, and pulmonary neoplasia.

Treatment of Heart Failure

Treatment of severe heart failure is divided into symptomatic and specific therapy. Symptomatic therapy includes reducing activity and anxiety, improving blood and tissue oxygenation, reducing edema and effusions, and increasing cardiac output. Specific treatment refers to measures that correct the underlying disorder and includes surgical repair of a congenital heart defect, surgical removal of a diseased pericardium, chemotherapy of dirofilariasis, and drug therapy for malignant cardiac arrhythmia. Patients in congestive heart failure (CHF) are placed at strict cage rest and treated in an oxygen-enriched environment of 40–60% oxygen for 24–48 hr if necessary. Adequate cage ventilation and avoidance of high humidity are important when managing the dyspneic patient. Anxiety in dogs can be reduced by subcutaneous administration of morphine sulfate (0.1–0.2 mg/kg). Morphine also decentralizes blood volume, thereby reducing the tendency toward the development of pulmonary edema. Cats can be mildly sedated with low dosages of phenothiazine tranquilizers (acetylpromazine 0.05–0.1 mg/kg) provided the rectal temperature is greater than 98°F. Promazine tranquilizers are peripheral vasodilators (α-antagonists); therefore hypotension and hypothermia may occur with overdosages. Antiarrhythmic drugs are administered as needed (see below).

Improving Gas Exchange. Specific measures are taken to improve pulmonary gas exchange in addition to sedation and increasing the inspired oxygen concentration. Animals with large pleural effusions benefit from immediate thoracocentesis, which permits reexpansion of atelectatic lungs. A 19- to 21-gauge butterfly catheter facilitates thoracentesis and allows the procedure to be accomplished with the patient in a standing or sternally recumbent position. Needle drainage is not usually necessary for ascitic effusions unless they are refractory to drugs or so great in volume as to result in diaphragmatic displacement and dyspnea. Aminophylline is a bronchodilator that may reduce bronchospasm in animals with acute severe pulmonary edema; however, this drug should be dosed carefully (4–6 mg/kg IM or IV) in order to avoid sensitizing the heart to arrhythmias.

Reducing Venous Pressures. Both pulmonary edema and pleural effusion can be decreased by drugs that reduce capillary hydrostatic pressure. Diuretics and venodilators are commonly employed treatments that are successful in reducing venous pressures. Furosemide is almost always the diuretic of choice in the dog and cat and is administered parenterally during the first 24–48 hr of treatment. Because furosemide decreases plasma volume and causes the loss of serum electrolytes, potential adverse effects include dehydration, hypokalemia, alkalosis, prerenal azotemia, and reduced cardiac filling. These adverse

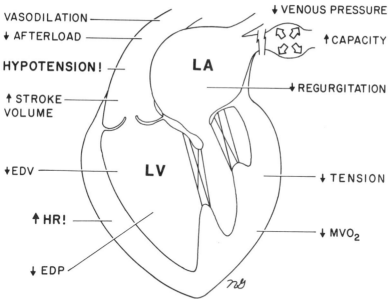

VASODILATION
↓ AFTERLOAD
HYPOTENSION!
↑ STROKE VOLUME
↓ EDV
↑ HR!
↓ EDP

LA
LV

↓ VENOUS PRESSURE
↑ CAPACITY
↓ REGURGITATION
↓ TENSION
↓ MVO₂

Fig. 2-8. Composite effects of vasodilator therapy on the left heart. Systemic veno-dilators, e.g., nitroglycerine and sodium nitroprusside, increase systemic venous ca-pacity (upper right), permitting translocation of pulmonary blood to the systemic veins and lowering both pulmonary and systemic venous pressures. This decreases the ten-dency to form edema. Systemic arteriolar vasodilators, e.g., hydralazine, cause va-sodilation and a decreased left ventricular afterload, and permit an increased left ven-tricular stroke volume. If the ventricle is initially dilated, the end-systolic and end-diastolic (EDV) volumes decrease along with the end-diastolic ventricular pressure (EDP). Systolic wall tension is reduced with an accompanying decline in myocardial oxygen consumption (MVO_2). Important adverse effects include excessive vasodilation with hypotension and reflex sinus tachycardia (HR). (Reproduced by permission from Bonagura JD: Cardiopulmonary disorders in the geriatric dog. p. 705. In Wingfield WE (ed): Symposium on Emergency Medicine. Veterinary Clinics of North America. W. B. Saunders, Philadelphia, 1981, Vol. 11.)

effects may be more important with chronic diuretic administration, particu-larly when the patient is not eating or receiving adequate fluid and electrolytes.

The direct-acting venodilator nitroglycerine (2% ointment) can effectively lower systemic venous pressure when applied to the skin. After its absorption into the circulation, nitroglycerine increases systemic capacitance and allows for a translocation of blood out of the pulmonary circulation into the systemic veins (Fig. 2-8). The net effect is a lowering of both pulmonary capillary and central venous pressures. Decreases in pulmonary capillary pressure reduces the formation of edema in capillary beds (Fig. 2-3) and complements the effect of diuretic therapy. Nitroglycerine can be administered safely when there is objective evidence of venous congestion, as demonstrated by thoracic radiog-raphy, observation of jugular venous distention, or direct measurement of CVP or P_{cwp}. Other drugs with venodilator effects include prazosin, sodium nitro-

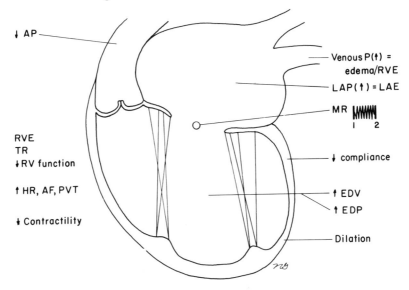

Fig. 2-9. Proposed pathophysiology of dilated (congestive) cardiomyopathy. The essential abnormality of the dilated cardiomyopathies is a reduction in ventricular contractility. This leads to decreased systolic function, low cardiac output, and possible reductions in arterial blood pressure. Cardiac abnormalities include marked left ventricular and left atrial dilation, elevated ventricular end-diastolic volume (EDV) and end-diastolic pressure (EDP), and mitral regurgitation (MR) due to annulus enlargement causing holosystolic murmurs or distortion of ventricular or papillary muscle geometry. The ventricle may be stiff due to dilation and fibrosis and may exhibit decreased diastolic compliance. Chronic elevations in left atrial pressure (LAP) and venous pressure predispose to pulmonary edema. Right ventricular function may also be affected with associated right ventricular enlargement (RVE), tricuspid regurgitation (TR), and biventricular failure. Dilated cardiomyopathies are frequently complicated by serious arrhythmias, e.g., atrial fibrillation (AF) and sustained or paroxysmal ventricular tachycardia (PVT).

prusside, and captopril. These agents are discussed under "Vasodilator Therapy."

Additional therapeutic measures designed to reduce venous pressure include improving ventricular function with inotropic drugs and systemic vasodilators. Phlebotomy, although potentially lifesaving, is rarely performed to acutely reduce venous pressure.

Positive Inotropic Agents. Digitalis, dobutamine, dopamine, and milrinone are drugs that increase myocardial contractility. As such, they are most useful for the treatment of heart failure caused by a decreased myocardial inotropic state. Dilated, or congestive, cardiomyopathies of the dog and cat are important examples of this type of heart failure (Fig. 2-9) and may respond well to inotropic drugs. Positive inotropic drugs are not indicated for syndromes of diastolic dysfunction, e.g., hypertrophic cardiomyopathy (Fig. 2-10) or per-

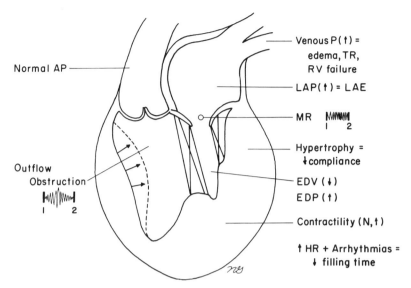

Normal AP

Venous P (↑) =
edema, TR,
RV failure

LAP(↑) = LAE

MR

Hypertrophy =
↓compliance

Outflow
Obstruction

EDV (↓)
EDP (↑)

Contractility (N, ↑)

↑ HR + Arrhythmias =
↓ filling time

Fig. 2-10. Proposed pathophysiology of hypertrophic cardiomyopathy. Marked left ventricular hypertrophy is associated with normal left ventricular systolic function but marked reductions in ventricular diastolic function and reduced ventricular compliance. Contractility is normal to increased, but the stiff ventricle has a small end-diastolic volume and must be filled at higher than normal left atrial and ventricular end-diastolic pressures. Left atrial enlargement is typical. If venous pressure is chronically elevated, the patient is predisposed to pulmonary edema. Pulmonary edema is hastened by concurrent mitral regurgitation caused by deformation of ventricular geometry and by periods of tachycardia or arrhythmia which reduce ventricular filling time and elevate atrial pressures. Secondary right heart failure occurs in chronic cases and is probably due to the increased right ventricular work needed to eject blood through the lung and into the stiff left ventricle. Atrial gallops and murmurs of mitral regurgitation or dynamic left ventricular outflow can be heard in many cases. Abbreviations as per Figure 2-6.

icardial tamponade (Fig. 2-11), as these conditions are not characterized by a reduced contractile state. The use of inotropic agents for the treatment of volume- or pressure-overload causes of heart failure is controversial inasmuch as myocardial contractility may be normal, or nearly so, in most forms of valvular and congenital heart disease. Experimental studies and clinical experiences in man and animals suggest that positive inotropic drugs can exert a beneficial effect in the volume-overloaded ventricle, particularly when there are superimposed atrial tachyarrhythmias. Thus most patients with heart failure caused by atrioventricular valvular insufficiency, dirofilariasis, and patent ductus arteriosus are first stabilized with rest and then administered diuretics (and venodilators if needed). When heart failure does not respond to these measures or if there are significant atrial arrhythmias, a positive inotrope, e.g., digitalis, is added to the therapeutic regimen.

Digitalis glycosides are the most commonly used positive inotropic agents. Because of their low therapeutic index, they must be used cautiously even in

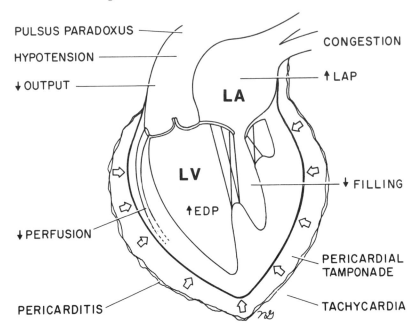

Fig. 2-11. Pathogenesis of pericardial tamponade. Pericardial effusion may develop as the result of pericarditis or intrapericardial tumors. When intrapericardial pressures elevate and prevent ventricular filling, pericardial tamponade is present. Reduced ventricular filling results in decreased cardiac output, possible hypotension, and elevated ventricular end-diastolic pressures (EDP). Impeded ventricular filling coupled with compensatory retention of sodium and water elevates atrial pressures and causes venous congestion. Both ventricles are affected, although the right ventricle tends to be more influenced by pericardial tamponade. Variable filling of the heart can lead to a fluctuating arterial pulse pressure (pulsus paradoxus), and high intrapericardial pressures can actually reduce coronary perfusion.

emergency situations. The principle indication for loading doses of digitalis is the presence of severe CHF or hypotension associated with atrial tachycardia or atrial fibrillation or flutter. Intravenous or oral loading dosages of digoxin (Table 2-5) can be used in an attempt to slow ventricular response and improve ventricular filling. Loading doses should be monitored electrocardiographically. In less critical patients, digitalis glycosides are administered orally using maintenance dosage guidelines.

Cats and dogs with dilated cardiomyopathy may be presented in cardiogenic shock with severe congestion and concurrent hypotension. Such patients are best supported with potent inotropic drugs that are administered by intravenous infusion. Dopamine HCl is a precursor to norepinephrine and can stimulate α, β, and dopaminergic receptors. Dopamine is a potent positive inotrope and a pressor agent that can elevate arterial blood pressure (see "CPR"). Dobutamine is a synthetic catecholamine with potent β-adrenoceptor and dose-dependent α-adrenergic effects. Dobutamine produces effects similar

Table 2-5. Drugs Used to Treat Heart Failure and Cardiac Arrhythmias in Dogs and Cats

Generic Name	Commonly Used Preparations	Approximate Dosage (Canine Unless Otherwise Noted)
Digitoxin	Crystodigin, Foxalin	*Oral maintenance*: 0.04–0.1 mg/kg divided b.i.d. to t.i.d. *Rapid IV digitalization*: 0.01–0.03 mg/kg; administer 1/2 of calculated dose IV, wait 30–60 min and administer 1/4 of dose, wait 30–60 min and administer remaining dose if necessary
Digoxin	Lanoxin, Cardoxin	*Oral maintenance*: 0.01–0.02 mg/kg divided b.i.d. *Rapid IV digitalization*: 0.01–0.02 mg/kg IV as per digitoxin *Rapid oral digitalization*: 0.02–0.06 mg/kg divided b.i.d. for 1 day **For the cat** *Rapid IV digitalization*: 0.01 mg/kg (administer 1/4 of the calculated dose q 1 h *Oral maintenance*: 0.007–0.015 mg/kg/day (or every other day if BUN >40 mg/dl) *Commonly used dose*: 1/4 of a 0.125 mg Lanoxin tablet o.d. to b.i.d. (every other day if BUN >40 mg/dl)
Dobutamine	Dobutrex	3–20 µg/kg/min IV
Dopamine	Intropin	3–10 µg/kg/min IV
Furosemide	Lasix	2–4 mg/kg (IV, IM, SQ, PO); repeat b.i.d. or t.i.d. if needed **For the cat** 1–2 mg/kg *Maintenance dose*: 0.5–2 mg/kg/day divided b.i.d.
Nitroglycerine (2% ointment)	Nitrol, Nitrobid	1/4–3/4 inch, cutaneously, q 6–8 h **For the cat** 1/4 inch q 6–8 h
Hydralazine	Apresoline	
Captopril	Capoten	0.5–2 mg/kg PO t.i.d. **For the cat** 6.25 mg b.i.d.-t.i.d.
Theophylline	Aminophylline	4–6 mg/kg IV **For the cat** Same dose
Atropine sulfate	Atropine, USP	0.01–0.02 mg/kg IV, IM; 0.02–0.04 mg/kg SQ **For the cat** Same dose
Glycopyrrolate	Robinul	0.005–0.01 mg/kg IV, IM; 0.01–0.02 mg/kg SQ **For the cat** Same dose
Isoproterenol	Isuprel	0.5–1 mg in 250 ml D_5W: drip slowly to effect **For the cat** Same dose
Lidocaine 2%	Xylocaine	2–4 mg/kg IV slowly, repeat to maximum of 8 mg/kg *Constant rate infusion for the dog*: 25–75 µg/kg/min **For the cat** 0.25–0.5 mg/kg IV over 5–10 min (with great caution due to neurotoxicity in this species)

CRI = constant rate of infusion.

Table 2-5. (*continued*)

Generic Name	Commonly Used Preparations	Approximate Dosage (Canine Unless Otherwise Noted)
Procainamide	Pronestyl	6–8 mg/kg IV over 5 min; CRI: 25–40 µg/kg/min; 6–20 mg/kg IM q 4–6 h (see text) Tablets: 8–20 mg/kg q 6 h Procan SR: 8–20 mg/kg q 8 h
Quinidine gluconate sulfate	Quinidine, USP	6–20 mg/kg IM, q 6 h (see text); 6–16 mg/kg PO q 6 h
Propranolol HCl	Inderal	0.04–0.06 mg/kg IV slowly; 0.1–1.0 mg/kg PO t.i.d. **For the cat** 0.04–0.06 mg/kg IV over 5–10 min *Oral maintenance*: 2.5 mg b.i.d. to t.i.d. or 5 mg b.i.d.

to those of dopamine but is less likely to raise peripheral resistance or result in tachycardia. Both dopamine and dobutamine, given in excess, cause sinus tachycardia and atrial, junctional, and ventricular premature complexes.

The principle indication for either dopamine or dobutamine is life-threatening or refractory ventricular failure. Both drugs are diluted in 5% dextrose solution or 2.5% dextrose in 0.45% NaCl solution and administered with an infusion pump, beginning at the lower range of the infusion rate (Table 2-5). The clinician must monitor fluid volume when using these drugs. Clinical monitoring involves frequent checking of heart rate and rhythm, blood pressure, character of the arterial pulse and precordial impulse, urine output, and the patient's level of consciousness. These drugs are typically given for 24–48 hr. Propranolol and other β-adrenoceptor blocking drugs should not be given with catecholamines as each negates the other's effects. If dobutamine is given to a dog with atrial fibrillation, intravenous digitalization may be necessary to slow the ventricular rate, which may be increased by the catecholamine. Infusions of dobutamine and dopamine represent relatively aggressive methods for stabilizing patients with severe CHF.

The recent development of orally active catecholamines, e.g., pirbuterol, and the noncatecholamine inotropic agents, e.g., amrinone and milrinone, may provide the clinician with additional modes of therapy for myocardial failure. Milrinone, a potent inotropic agent with arterial vasodilator properties, has been successfully used in dogs with refractory CHF due to cardiomyopathy and valvular heart disease (0.5–1.0 mg/kg PO b.i.d. to t.i.d.). Although milrinone may represent a new mode of therapy for refractory heart failure, it is unlikely to be of great value in the initial treatment of acute fulminant heart failure.

Vasodilator Therapy.   The stroke volume of the ventricle is dependent on cardiac contractility and the loading conditions of the heart. Venous return helps to determine the ventricular preload, whereas arterial resistance contributes to the ventricular afterload (Fig. 2-3). Because increasing degrees of peripheral vasoconstriction actually reduce left ventricular output, considerable attention has been directed to lowering ventricular impedance via systemic arteriolar vasodilation. Hydralazine (a direct smooth muscle dilator), prazosin (an α-adrenergic blocking drug), captopril (an angiotensin II converting enzyme inhibitor), and sodium nitroprusside (a smooth muscle dilator) have all been used in the management of severe heart failure in the dog.

Excessive vasodilation, leading to symptomatic hypotension and reflex tachycardia, is a great concern when deciding to administer an arteriolar vasodilator. Proper therapy is facilitated by appropriate patient selection, conservative use of vasodilating drugs, and objective hemodynamic monitoring of venous and arterial blood pressures. The patient with marked elevation of venous pressure, significant ventricular dilatation, mitral regurgitation, and normal baseline arterial blood pressure is mose likely to benefit from administration of an arteriolar vasodilator (Fig. 2-8). Vasodilators should not be given to hypotensive patients and must be administered very carefully whenever blood pressure cannot be accurately monitored.

Sodium nitroprusside and prazosin are deemed "balanced" vasodilators based on their ability to cause both arteriolar and systemic venodilator effects. Nitroprusside can be given only by infusion and is so potent that its use is precluded unless invasive monitoring of P_{cwp} (Fig. 2-4) and arterial blood pressures is employed. During emergency situations, sodium nitroprusside produces a rapid decrease in pulmonary venous pressure and an increase in cardiac output.

Patients with chronic decompensated CHF are frequently treated with oral vasodilators, e.g., hydralazine, prazosin, or captopril, in an attempt to increase cardiac output. Because captopril inhibits formation of angiotensin II, it may prevent sodium retention and edema. This type of oral vasodilator therapy is best initiated in the hospital. The vasodilator must be given in conjunction with a diuretic. Diuretics retard renal retention of sodium secondary to vasodilator-induced hypotension and reduce perivascular edema, which could prevent an adequate vasodilator response. The following parameters are assessed before and after (1, 2, and 4 hrs) administration of a vasodilator: level of activity and consciousness, muscle strength, arterial pulse pressure, capillary refill time, heart rate, arterial blood pressure, and urine output.

Transition from Acute to Chronic Therapy. Most pharmacologic agents used in the treatment of acute heart failure are effective in the management of chronic heart failure. Once the patient's emergency situation has been stabilized, oral maintenance therapy with furosemide, dietary sodium restriction and rest, positive inotropic agents (if indicated), and vasodilator drugs can be selected on an individual basis. Additional therapy generally depends on the cause of heart failure, the overall prognosis, and the patient's response to previous treatments. Successful management of the patient with severe CHF frequently depends on prompt recognition of heart failure, efficient delivery of symptomatic therapy, and the ability to monitor and change therapy when necessary.

PERICARDIAL TAMPONADE

Pericardial tamponade is the impairment of ventricular filling caused by the development of pericardial effusion or hemorrhage. Intrapericardial pressures are elevated in pericardial tamponade and must be reduced by pericardiocentesis if the animal is to be successfully treated. Intrapericardial pressures may quickly decline when only small amounts of intrapericardial fluid are removed; this aspect is best explained by the observation that intrapericardial pressure rises abruptly when the elastic limits of the parietal pericardium are exceeded. Thus the clinician need not fully drain the pericardium in order to provide lifesaving treatment. Common causes of pericardial tamponade are listed in Table 2-4.

Clinical Signs and Diagnosis

Clinical recognition of pericardial tamponade is usually straightforward because of its association with muffled heart sounds, jugular venous distention, hepatomegaly, ascites, and pleural effusion. Right ventricular failure is common in pericardial tamponade, although pulmonary edema may coexist. Systemic arterial hypotension is the result of impeded filling of both ventricles and a reduced stroke volume (Fig. 2-11). Radiography (globoid heart), electrocardiography (decreased amplitude complexes, ST-T segment elevation, electrical alternans), and echocardiography are useful in the diagnosis of pericardial tamponade.

Treatment

The specific emergency therapy of cardiac tamponade is needle or catheter drainage of the pericardial effusion. Pericardiocentesis can be done from either hemithorax. Left lateral recumbency facilitates puncture at the lower right 4th to 5th intercostal space, just above the sternum, with the needle directed craniomedially. Puncture of the ventricle (but not the atrium) can usually be determined by watching an ECG monitor or by detecting increased resistance or movement of the needle. Most effusions are quite bloody and therefore should not be assumed to indicate cardiac puncture. A variety of equipment can be used for pericardiocentesis. Butterfly catheters (19 to 23 gauge) are safe and effective for most animals—even large dogs. Angiography catheters with added side holes (Angiocath) permit rapid drainage and further radiographic studies, e.g., pneumopericardiography.

Clinical signs rapidly improve after pericardiocentesis in animals with massive edema. The concurrent use of furosemide and topical nitroglycerine (as per heart failure) can be helpful when edema is present. Dehydration must be avoided in order to prevent serious hypotension due to inadequate cardiac filling and volume depletion. Although vasodilators have been shown to improve cardiac output during pericardial tamponade, such therapy is inferior to pericardiocentesis. After stabilization, the cause of pericardial effusion must be sought and more specific therapy applied.[13]

CARDIAC ARRHYTHMIAS

Cardiac arrhythmias are disorders of cardiac rate, rhythm, and conduction, and can be life-threatening or lead to physical impairment. The ability of the heart to pump blood is initially dependent on normal electrical activity in cardiac muscle. Patients with cardiac arrhythmias may exhibit profound alterations in circulatory function leading to depression, weakness, hypotension, syncope, congestive heart failure, renal failure, progressive deterioration of cardiac rhythm, and sudden death. The clinician must be able to recognize cardiac arrhythmias and ascertain the hemodynamic significance of the disorder in order to direct prompt and appropriate antiarrhythmic therapy. The reader is directed to other sources for discussions of ECG diagnosis and etiologic considerations.[1]

Sinus Bradycardia

Sinus bradycardia (Fig. 2-12A) is associated with numerous clinical disorders, including sick sinus syndrome, increased vagal activity, CNS disease, hypoadrenocorticism, hypoglycemia, hypothermia, and drug administration. In general, sinus bradycardia is a self-limiting arrhythmia, resolving with correction of the underlying disorder. Therapy is usually not necessary unless the heart rate decreases to less than 50 beats/min or the animal is symptomatic for bradycardia. Treatment for sinus bradycardia includes correction of the underlying problem, administration of supportive intravenous fluids to maintain blood pressure, correction of acid-base and electrolyte disturbances (sodium bicarbonate), and administration of vagolytic or sympathomimetic drugs. Atropine or glycopyrrolate (Table 2-5) are appropriate as initial therapy. Parasympatholytic drugs should be given intramuscularly or intravenously when a rapid response is required. The sinus node may be driven by the administration of catecholamines, e.g., epinephrine or dopamine (see "CPR"), or the heart paced via a transvenous pacing wire during cardiac or circulatory collapse.

Sinus Arrest and Atrial Standstill

Sinus arrest and atrial standstill are associated with a variety of diseases. Organic heart disease results in periods of sinoatrial arrest in schnauzers and dachshunds with sick sinus syndrome. Atrial standstill can be temporary during hyperkalemia (Fig. 2-12B) or persistent in severe dilated cardiomyopathy, atrial myocarditis, and the muscular dystrophy of springer spaniels.

Short periods of sinus arrest often result in syncope; however, these are seldom lethal events and generally are not emergency situations. Cage rest, intramuscular atropine or glycopyrrolate, and client reassurance are usually

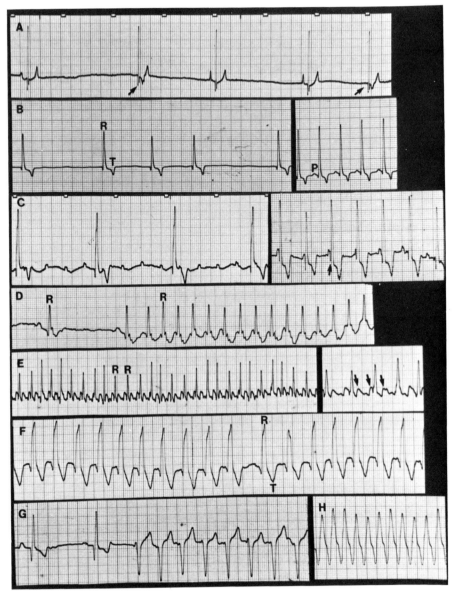

Fig. 2-12. Cardiac arrhythmias in the dog. **(A)** A dachshund with sick sinus syndrome, showing sinus bradycardia and sinus arrest. Two junctional escape complexes with retrograde atrial activation are shown (arrows). Paper speed 25 mm/sec; 1 cm = 1 mV. **(B)** A 1-year-old English pointer with Addison's disease. The left panel shows probable sinoventricular rhythm with atrial standstill. No P-waves are evident. After therapy with sodium bicarbonate, glucocorticoids, and intravenous saline (right panel) sinus tachycardia is noted. Paper speed 25 mm/sec; 1 cm = 1 mV. **(C)** Complete AV block (left panel) in a weimaraner. A ventricular escape rhythm is evident. The right panel was recorded after insertion of a transvenous pacing catheter into the right ventricle.

adequate and allow time for more detailed ECG studies and, if necessary, insertion of a pacemaker.

Atrial standstill caused by hyperkalemia is approached by attempting to determine the cause of the problem (e.g., urinary obstruction, ruptured bladder, Addison's disease) and by beginning therapy aimed at lowering serum potassium. Correction of the underlying problem is essential, and intravenous 0.9% saline and bolus injections of sodium bicarbonate are effective in improving the ECG. Sodium bicarbonate, dosed at 0.5–1 mEq/kg IV over 5 min (repeated at 10-min intervals), is the first drug administered. If alkalinization (up to 3 mEq/kg during a 30-min period) does not improve the ECG, calcium chloride (1 ml of a 10% solution per 10 kg body weight, IV, over 10 min) is administered. Insulin-dextrose infusions are rarely necessary to treat hyperkalemia. The management of hyperkalemia is described further in Chapter 4.

Atrioventricular Block

Complete atrioventricular (AV) block generally indicates severe drug toxicity or organic disease of the conduction system. Complete AV block is often preceded by high-grade second-degree AV block (> 3:1 P:QRS). The ECG often shows alternating periods of second-degree and complete AV block (Fig. 2-12C) Syncope and congestive heart failure are common sequelae of these arrhythmias.

High-grade second-degree and complete AV block are usually refractory to therapy with glucocorticoids, atropine, or isoproterenol (although this drug may increase the ventricular escape rate). These conduction defects are best managed with a cardiac pacemaker. High-grade second-degree and complete AV block are occasionally responsive to high doses of oral isoproterenol, al-

←——————————————————

Small pacing artifacts (arrow) are noted just in front of the QRS complexes. The ventricular rate is now higher owing to the external pacing device. P waves are nonconducted throughout the ECG. (**D**) Example of narrow-QRS tachycardia recorded from a 10-year-old poodle with cardiomegaly. The first two QRS complexes are sinus in origin; however, these complexes are followed by a supraventricular tachycardia of greater than 380 beats/min. (Transtelephonic ECG recorded at 50 mm/sec.) (**E**) Sustained atrial tachycardia (or flutter) in a 5-month-old Great Dane with tricuspid valve dysplasia. The rate of atrial activation is greater than 450/min, and the ventricular response is irregular owing to physiological block of some P waves in the AV node. In the right panel, the paper speed has been increased from 25 to 50 mm/sec and the P waves are now more obvious (arrows). Lead aVF, 1 cm = 1 mV. (**F**) ECG from a Doberman pinscher with cardiomyopathy. The rhythm is atrial fibrillation with a rapid ventricular response. Fibrillation waves are not apparent. Widening of the QRS complexes is due to myocardial disease and intraventricular conduction delay. Lead 2 ECG recorded at 50 mm/sec; 1 cm = 1 mV. (**G**) Paroxysmal ventricular tachycardia. (**H**) Record from a dog with nonparoxysmal ventricular tachycardia. This dog developed ventricular flutter and fibrillation shortly after this record was obtained (paper speed 50 mm/sec for both records).

though this type of treatment is usually ineffective and unnecessarily prolongs the period between diagnosis and implantation of a pacemaker.

Transvenous pacing (Fig. 2-12C) is the method of choice for temporary control of heart failure caused by complete AV block. If cardiac transvenous pacing is not feasible, the patient should be placed at strict cage rest and given furosemide (1–2 mg/kg IM) to prevent congestive heart failure and a trial dosage of atropine (0.03 mg/kg IM) to observe the effect on the cardiac rate. Therapy is generally unnecessary when the patient's heart rate is greater than 50 beats/min. Isoproterenol (1 mg in 250–500 ml of 5% dextrose) is administered by infusion to treat profound bradycardia. The purpose of isoproterenol therapy is to increase the ventricular escape rate to 50–60/min while avoiding the development of new ventricular arrhythmias secondary to catecholamine infusion. The catecholamine infusion rate is thus adjusted to provide the optimal response. Dopamine has also been used to increase the rate of ventricular escape rhythm. Permanent pacemaker implantation provides the best long-term therapy for complete AV block.

Supraventricular Tachycardia, Atrial Fibrillation, Atrial Flutter

Supraventricular tachycardia is a general term used to describe a rapid heart rate caused by abnormal impulse generation in the atrial and AV junctional tissues (Fig. 2-12D). Sinus tachycardia, atrial fibrillation, and atrial flutter are usually not included in this group of arrhythmias, although they also constitute types of supraventricular tachyarrhythmias. Sustained, nonparoxysmal supraventricular tachycardias are particularly serious and can cause severe hypotension or congestive heart failure (Fig. 2-12E). A detailed description of the electrophysiology and electrocardiography of supraventricular tachyarrhythmias is beyond the scope of this chapter. General principles of emergency therapy are enumerated below.

The first step in treating a patient with narrow-QRS tachycardia is to determine if atrial fibrillation or atrial tachycardia is present. Atrial fibrillation is usually characterized by a rapid, irregular ventricular rate and the absence of organized atrial activity (Fig. 2-12F). Atrial tachycardia is associated with a rapid atrial rate (often 280–360/min) which may have a regular or irregular ventricular response. Atrial flutter is electrocardiographically similar to atrial tachycardia, although there is a greater tendency for the R-R intervals to be more regular. Regular, narrow-QRS tachycardias without obvious P waves are generally caused by sinus tachycardia and fusion of the P wave with the previous T wave, by atrial flutter, or by junctional (or reentrant) tachycardias with buried P waves (Fig. 2-12E).

A vagal maneuver (10–30 sec of ocular or carotid sinus pressure) is helpful in distinguishing the cause of the tachycardia. Rarely, this converts the arrhythmia to normal sinus rhythm. More often there is no effect or periods of irregular ventricular activation between which P waves or flutter waves are observed. Patients who abruptly convert to sinus rhythm with vagal maneuvers but who subsequently regress to supraventricular tachycardia are probably candidates for therapy with verapamil (0.05–0.2 mg/kg IV over 5 min). Patients who do not respond to vagal maneuvers can be treated as described below for atrial tachycardia and atrial fibrillation.

The majority of animals with atrial tachycardia, flutter, or fibrillation have serious underlying cardiac disease. Many of these animals are in congestive heart failure and require concurrent medication for edema. When one of these atrial dysrhythmias is identified, the usual approach involves controlling the ventricular rate, with less effort directed toward actual conversion of the arrhythmia to a normal sinus rhythm. Digoxin and propranolol are the agents most often used to slow AV conduction and ventricular rate. Propranolol is a potent negative inotropic agent and, as such, is reserved for refractory tachyarrhythmias or arrhythmias caused by increased sympathetic tone. Digoxin is the drug of choice for atrial tachyarrhythmias and is given orally or intravenously (Table 5-5). It may take 6–24 hr to observe a slowing of the ventricular rate after oral digoxin administration; however, intravenous digoxin given in divided doses produces a faster response. Digoxin is continued as a maintenance dose after the initial administration.

Propranolol should be diluted with saline to a 0.1 mg/ml concentration and given at a rate of 0.1 mg/min until the calculated dose is administered. The dosages listed in Table 5-5 are general guidelines and were designed to assist the clinician in the early management of supraventricular tachycardias. Alternative approaches using quinidine, verapamil, and vagomimetic drugs are possible and are described in greater detail elsewhere.[2]

Ventricular Tachycardia

Ventricular tachycardia can be sustained or paroxysmal (nonsustained) (Fig. 2-12G). Sustained ventricular tachycardia requires immediate medical attention because it frequently produces hypotension, myocardial ischemia, and electrical instability and may predispose to ventricular fibrillation (Fig. 2-12H). This arrhythmia is particularly worrisome when reduced myocardial contractility or hypovolemia are present. Clinical assessment of ventricular tachycardia is covered elsewhere, but guidelines for initiating therapy can be summarized as follows: Antiarrhythmic therapy is indicated when there is hypotension, shock, multiform ventricular premature complexes, ventricular rates greater than 140/min, or previous ventricular fibrillation.

Initial treatment of ventricular tachycardia generally involves oxygen, intravenous fluids, replacement of potassium deficits, and the control of acidosis. Hypokalemia and acidosis can reduce the response to antiarrhythmic drugs. Digitalis glycosides should not be given to patients with ventricular tachycardia. ECG monitoring is imperative for assessing therapy.

Lidocaine hydrochloride is almost always the agent of choice for immediate control of sustained ventricular tachycardia. Lidocaine has minimal adverse hemodynamic effects, and the neurotoxic signs associated with higher doses are readily controlled by diazepam. Lidocaine doses of 2–3 mg/kg IV for dogs (for cats: 0.25–1.0 mg/kg IV over 5 min) are generally effective within 2–3 min of administration. Lidocaine in doses up to 8 mg/kg IV can be given to dogs during a 20-min period. Because of the rapid redistribution and clearance of lidocaine in the dog, the antiarrhythmic effect is transient unless repeated boluses or a constant-rate infusion is administered. A constant infusion of lidocaine is used to maintain normal sinus rhythm when initial lidocaine boluses are effective. Four or five hours may be required before lidocaine reaches a steady-state plasma concentration. Supplemental intravenous boluses (0.5–1.0 mg/kg) may be needed during this period to maintain the sinus rhythm. Lidocaine infusions can be continued for 2–3 days or gradually replaced with intramuscular or oral quinidine or procainamide when the dog is in stable condition. The lidocaine infusion rate is decreased by 50% and continued for 6 hr, then halved and continued for 6 hr, and finally totally discontinued if normal sinus rhythm is maintained.

Alternative antiarrhythmic drugs include procainamide, propranolol, and quinidine. Propranolol is the second-choice drug in the cat and is the third-choice drug in the dog when intravenous lidocaine (and procainamide) therapy is unsuccessful. Some clinicians prefer propanolol over lidocaine in the cat and use this agent as the drug of first choice. The ECG must be frequently reevaluated in animals with refractory ventricular tachycardia in order to rule out supraventricular tachycardia with aberrant conduction. Serum electrolyte and acid-base values are reexamined periodically for uncorrected abnormalities. Procainamide, quinidine, and propranolol are potentially hypotensive agents and must be used with caution in shocky patients. After initial parenteral stabilization and determination of the cause of the rhythm disturbance, long-term therapy can be directed as necessary.[1,2]

CARDIOPULMONARY RESUSCITATION

Cardiopulmonary resuscitation (CPR) is the implementation of procedures, both mechanical and pharmacologic, which restore life. The lifesaving procedures involved are generally performed on patients in whom a relatively acute catastrophic event has resulted in sudden cessation of ventilation or blood flow. The primary goals of CPR are to restore adequate ventilation and normal circulation and to prevent the consequences of the emergency situation from causing potentially lethal effects.[6,11] These goals can be accomplished only if the personnel performing CPR are totally familiar with CPR techniques, the patient's clinical history, and the use of emergency drugs and equipment. Anticipation of potential problems, preparedness, and the experience of the personnel involved are other factors which determine the success of CPR.

Etiology

The causes for respiratory distress and arrest are the subject of Chapter 3 and are not discussed here. Any situation which leads to the acute inability to exchange adequate quantities of oxygen and carbon dioxide is considered

Table 2-6. Factors Predisposing to Cardiac Arrest

1. Respiratory failure—hypoxia
    a. Hypoventilation
    b. Low inspired O_2
    c. Ventilation-perfusion inequalities
    d. Shunt
    e. Diffusion impairment
2. Acid-base imbalance
    a. Respiratory acidosis
    b. Metabolic acidosis—myocardial depression
    c. Respiratory alkalosis
    d. Metabolic alkalosis—myocardial irritability
3. Electrolyte imbalance
    a. Hypokalemia—tachycardia
    b. Hyperkalemia—bradycardia
    c. Decreased $[Na^+]:[K^+]$ (Addison's disease)
4. Autonomic imbalance
    a. Increased sympathetic tone (tachyarrhythmias)
    b. Increased parasympathetic tone (bradyarrhythmias)
5. Hypothermia
6. Sepsis
7. Trauma
8. Shock
9. Congenital or acquired heart disease
10. Cardiac arrhythmias
    a. Bradyarrhythmias
    b. Ventricular tachycardia
11. Iatrogenic
    a. Drug overdose (anesthetics)
    b. Inappropriate drug administration (epinephrine during halothane anesthesia)
    c. Drug sensitivities or toxicity

a respiratory emergency and should be corrected rapidly and effectively. Similarly, any acute situation which interferes with the ability of the heart to deliver adequate quantities of blood to peripheral tissues is potentially capable of causing shock or death and must be treated. Although the factors responsible for acute dramatic reductions in blood flow are varied, the specific mechanisms involved are relatively limited (Table 2-6). Those mechanisms responsible for sudden cardiac death include ventricular tachycardia, ventricular fibrillation, severe bradyarrhythmias, asystole, and electromechanical dissociation. It is very important that the veterinary clinician be able to distinguish between the mechanisms responsible for sudden cardiac arrest if rational therapy is to be instituted.

Clinical Signs and Diagnosis

Table 2-7 lists the signs which are indicative of cardiopulmonary distress or arrest. The sudden development of an acute cardiorespiratory emergency is usually heralded by respiratory distress, excitement, or depression, and occasionally vocalization. This is followed by collapse, unconsciousness, and apnea. Some animals urinate or defecate during this period. The pupils begin to dilate almost immediately after the animal has become unconscious but con-

Table 2-7. Signs of Cardiopulmonary Distress or Arrest

1. Altered consciousness or coma
2. Changes in ventilatory rate or rhythm
    a. Tachypnea
    b. Dyspnea
    c. Gasps
    d. Apnea
3. Loss of a palpable pulse or irregular pulse
4. Absent or muffled heart sounds
5. Altered peripheral perfusion
        a. Change in color (red, white, cyanotic)
        b. Prolonged capillary refill time
        c. Absence of bleeding
6. Pupillary dilation

strict if the circulation is restored. The pupillary response should not be used to indicate the adequacy of cerebral blood flow, however, particularly if anticholinergic drugs (atropine, glycopyrrolate) have been administered. Palpation of a peripheral artery is unproductive or indicates a slow or a rapid weak pulse. Palpation of the thoracic cavity over the heart is usually unproductive but may reveal an almost imperceptibly slow or extremely rapid cardiac impulse. The heart sounds may be infrequent, rapid and irregular, muffled, or absent. The capillary refill time usually remains normal (less than 1.5 sec) initially after cardiac arrest but then gradually prolongs. Mucous membranes are usually pale pink or white after cardiac arrest because of intense peripheral vascular constriction, but they can be injected (bright red) when significant hypercarbia or sepsis is present. Cyanosis is present or develops when hypoxia is responsible for the cardiac arrest or when arterial oxygenation cannot be maintained.

The ability to distinguish between the various acute mechanisms responsible for sudden cardiac failure is frequently difficult but can be facilitated by physical findings, the ECG (Fig. 2-13), and direct observation (Table 2-8). A hypodermic needle can be pushed through the chest wall and into the myocardium to help distinguish between periodic ventricular contractions, ventricular fibrillation, and ventricular arrest when an ECG is not available. Ventricular fibrillation causes the hub of the needle to vibrate weakly and continuously as opposed to the periodic jerking which occurs with periodic cardiac contraction. Regardless of practicality, however, this technique does not indicate the pattern or the force of ventricular contraction. Furthermore, there is the possibility of lacerating the lung and producing pneumothorax or puncturing a coronary artery and producing hemopericardium. An alternative to the hypodermic needle technique is direct visualization of the heart after performing a thoracotomy. This technique is unquestionably more heroic, but it can be lifesaving, particularly when there has been a lack of response to initial mechanical and pharmacologic resuscitative attempts. Direct visualization of cardiac color, pattern of contraction, force of contraction, and the regularity of cardiac contraction is the best information available for determining appropriate therapy.

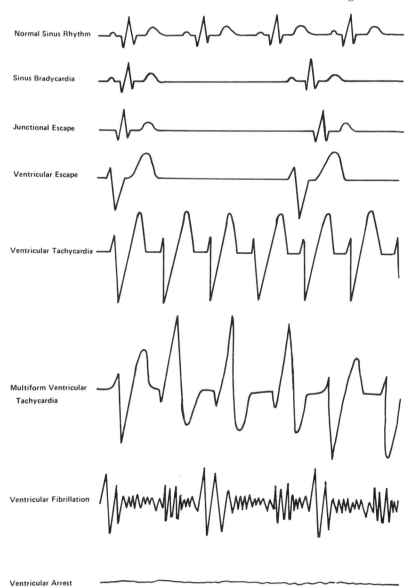

Fig. 2-13. Various types of cardiac rhythm disturbances associated with poor cardiac output. Sinus bradycardia, junctional escape, and ventricular escape rates less than 50 beats/min are associated with a low cardiac output.

Treatment

The initial approach to the patient suffering from cardiopulmonary arrest is the same regardless of cause and includes the restoration of ventilation after orotracheal intubation or tracheostomy and the restoration of circulation by external chest compression. Attempts should be made to determine the exact

Table 2-8. Distinguishing Characteristics of Several Types of Cardiac Failure or Arrest

Cause	Peripheral Pulse	Auscultation of Heart Sounds	ECG	Visual Observation
Ventricular tachycardia	Rapid, irregular, pulse deficit	Muffled, may be variable intensity	Wide QRS-T complexes; absence of P-QRS relationship	Disorganized, rapidly beating heart
Ventricular fibrillation	None	None	Absence of QRS-T complexes; fibrillation waves	Fine to coarse rippling of the ventricular myocardium
Bradycardia	Slow, may be irregular	Slow	Infrequent or irregular P-QRS-T complexes; junctional or ventricular escape complexes	Infrequent coordinated ventricular contractions
Ventricular asystole	None	None	Absence of QRS-T complexes; straight-line ECG	No cardiac improvement
Electromechanical dissociation	None	None	Normal P-QRS-T complexes	Feeble or absent cardiac contractions

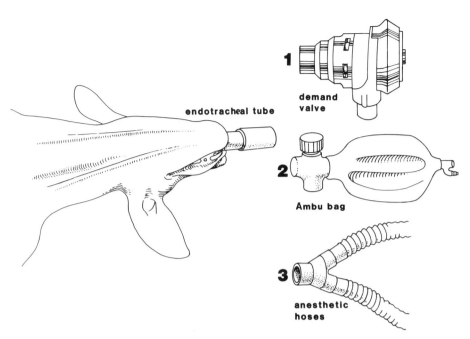

Fig. 2-14. Various methods used to respirate an animal. An oxygen demand valve (1) delivers oxygen at a flow rate up to 50 L/min. A self-inflating Ambu bag (2) can be used to deliver oxygen or room air. The Y-piece (3) from an anesthetic machine can be connected to a properly placed endotracheal tube.

cause of cardiopulmonary arrest. If the presence of ventricular fibrillation can be ascertained, the patient should be immediately defibrillated. Other therapeutic goals include the restoration of normal sinus rhythm, arterial blood pressure, and cardiac output. Any patient suffering from cardiopulmonary arrest is treated for cardiogenic shock (see "Shock"). The following discussion describes a specific approach to the various types of cardiac arrest. For obvious reasons these steps have been termed the A (airway), B (breathing), C's (circulation) of cardiopulmonary resuscitation.

Airway. The first essential step in performing resuscitation is the establishment of an airway and oxygenation, which are discussed in more detail in Chapter 3. The most effective way to achieve this goal is by endotracheal intubation and the use of 100% oxygen. Occasionally animals become cyanotic and unconscious because foreign material, e.g., food or soft tissue structures (soft palate, tongue), obstruct the upper airway. The latter problem is particularly common in brachycephalic breeds recovering from anesthesia. Food, liquid, or excessive mucus are removed manually or by suction. Ventilation and oxygenation can be accomplished by a self-inflatable bag (Ambu bag), demand valve, or anesthetic machine (Fig. 2-14). When airway obstruction cannot be removed, a tracheostomy is performed, as described in Chapter 3. Transtracheal catheter ventilation, an alternative to tracheostomy, is less traumatic and does not predispose to infection. Ventilation is achieved by placing a 14-gauge plastic intravenous catheter in the trachea by percutaneous puncture as depicted in Figure 3-1.

Mouth-to-nose resuscitation is performed when endotracheal tubes and ventilatory assist devices are not available. This is accomplished by cupping both hands around the animal's muzzle, placing the operator's mouth against the thumbs (attempting to produce an airtight seal), and blowing air into the animal's mouth. Unintentional inflation of the stomach with air may occur but can be avoided by pushing the larynx dorsally in order to occlude the esophagus.

Breathing.   The pulmonary resuscitation portion of CPR is detailed in Chapter 3. Carbon dioxide elimination and arterial oxygenation is best accomplished by connecting an endotracheal tube to a self-inflating bag (Ambu bag), various anesthetic apparatuses (T-system, Y-piece), or an anesthetic machine (Fig. 2-14). The respiratory rate should be between 8 and 14 breaths/min and simultaneous with chest compression. Two popular breathing/cardiac compression ratios are 1:5 or 2:10–15. The amount of gas volume delivered should approximate 14–20 ml/kg at an inspiratory pressure of 30 cm H_2O. In practice, this volume is generally delivered with minimum expansion of the chest and lifting of the abdomen. There is a great tendency to overinflate the lungs in cats, neonates, and patients with restrictive forms of lung disease (pulmonary fibrosis, diaphragmatic hernia). Lung overexpansion can lead to pulmonary barotrauma, pulmonary hemorrhage, and pneumothorax. Smaller tidal volumes at greater respiratory rates should be used in these situations. Inspiratory time should be kept to less than 1.5 sec. Prolonged inspiratory time or the maintainance of positive end-expiratory pressure (PEEP) increases intrathoracic pressure, thereby decreasing venous return, cardiac output, and arterial blood pressure. Small amounts of PEEP (3–5 cm H_2O), however, may improve oxygenation and are not harmful if the thoracic cavity is open to the atmosphere (open pneumothorax) or during internal cardiac massage. Mechanical artificial respiratory assist devices, particularly pressure-cycled ventilators, perform poorly during CPR. The intrathoracic pressure fluctuations produced by closed-chest cardiac massage causes mechanical respirators to prematurely initiate or terminate their inspiratory cycle, resulting in inadequate tidal volumes. Coordination of respiratory cycles with chest compression when using respirators is also difficult.

Once the circulation is restored and the patient begins to show signs of spontaneous ventilation, ventilatory support is not stopped. IPPV is usually necessary until the patient regains consciousness. Listening to the end of the endotracheal tube, watching for normal ventilatory movements of the chest wall, and continued monitoring of mucous membrane color and capillary refill time help to assess the adequacy of ventilation.

Circulation.   The restoration of normal cardiac electrical and mechanical activity is dependent on the early generation and maintenance of peripheral blood flow. The latter can be initiated and maintained by either chest compression or intrathoracic cardiac compression. Blood flow is maintained during

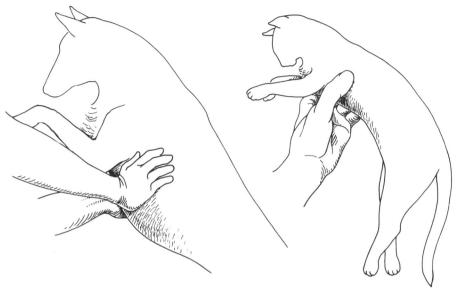

Fig. 2-15. Illustration of hand positions used for chest compression in the dog and cat.

chest compression by the phasic increase in intrathoracic pressure, rarely from direct cardiac compression. The ideal compression rate in dogs or cats should be 70–100 compressions/min with a compression duration of approximately 0.4 sec. Effective chest compression in small animals is accomplished with the animal in lateral recumbency by compressing the chest wall from side to side (Fig. 2-15). The heel of one hand can be used to compress one side of the chest wall while the palm of the other hand or a sand-filled pillow is placed under the opposing chest wall. The thumb and forefinger can be used to accomplish the same maneuver in cats and very small dogs. The rescuer's attention should be focused on how fast the heel of the hand compresses the thorax, not the force necessary to compress the chest, although enough force must be generated to produce an obvious indentation of the chest wall.

The ideal ratio between the number of chest compressions and ventilations has been debated for many years. One approach is to interpose one ventilation between every fifth or sixth chest compression. A second popular technique delivers two or three ventilations every 10–15 chest compressions. Recent evidence, however, suggests that blood flow to the brain, heart, and kidneys is more effectively maintained by administering chest compressions simultaneously with ventilations at relatively high airway pressures (30–40 cm H_2O) and with abdominal binding.[8,10] The lung is not traumatized using this technique, providing that airway pressures do not become excessive (greater than 60 cm H_2O) and that significant lung pathology is not present prior to resuscitation attempts. Intermittent slow abdominal compression (counterpressure) seems to be an effective means of improving peripheral perfusion during resuscitative efforts. Abdominal counterpressure during CPR is accomplished by having a second person use the palms of both hands to slowly compress the abdominal cavity at approximately 15-sec intervals. The abdomen may be temporarily bound during CPR with an elastic bandage or towel if extra help is not available.

Signs of restoration of effective peripheral blood flow include improvement in mucous membrane color, a decrease in capillary refill time, a reduction in pupil size, and the restoration of a peripheral arterial pulse. The latter should be evaluated during a short pause in chest compressions. Attempts to palpate and evaluate the peripheral pulse during chest compression usually results in erroneous findings based on the production of shock waves which are carried into the femoral veins simultaneous with chest compression.

Attempts to maintain peripheral blood flow by chest compression should not be maintained indefinitely. If signs of successful resuscitation do not become evident or continue to improve, leading to the generation of an effective spontaneous cardiac contraction, or if a normal circulation cannot be restored within approximately 20–30 min, the chest should be opened and internal cardiac massage initiated. Severe chest trauma, fractured ribs, pneumothorax, hemothorax, pericardial effusion, diaphragmatic hernia, and other primary thoracic diseases (neoplasms, foreign bodies) are additional reasons for bypassing chest compression and immediately opening the chest. The chest is opened by creating a left lateral incision from the top of the scapula to approximately 4 cm from the sternum on the anterior surface of the fifth rib. The hair should be clipped and antiseptic solution applied to this site prior to the skin incision. Care must be taken not to damage the lung when entering the thoracic cavity. Once the chest is entered, the fourth and fifth ribs are spread apart, the lungs are reflected dorsally and caudally, and the pericardium is grasped and opened near the apex of the heart. The pericardium is torn dorsally, in order to expose the ventricles, taking care not to damage the phrenic nerve. The heart is then grasped with either hand between the thumb and forefingers and internal cardiac massage initiated at a rate of approximately 60–80 compressions/min. The majority of effort should be focused on compressing the left ventricle and the rate with which the ventricles are compressed, not the force necessary to compress the heart. Excessive force during internal cardiac compression can result in the development of severe cardiac trauma, cardiac arrhythmias, and ventricular fibrillation. The aorta can be compressed dorsally against the spine with the thumb of the opposite hand in order to improve blood flow to the heart and brain. Internal cardiac compression is twice as effective as external chest compression in maintaining cardiac output but requires surgical intervention and predisposes to infection.

The color, tone, and rhythm of the heart can be evaluted during internal cardiac massage. Color can be improved by appropriate ventilation and cardiac compression. Cardiac tone and rhythm can be improved by normalizing acid-base and electrolyte abnormalities and administering cardiotonic or antiarrhythmic drugs. Table 2-9 lists the equipment that should be immediately available in order to perform CPR, and Table 2-10 gives the drugs which are poten-

Table 2-9. Equipment Necessary for CPR

Cuffed endotracheal tubes
  Small
  Medium
  Large
Lighted laryngoscope with small, medium, and large tongue blades
Tongue depressors
Ambu bag or demand valve and oxygen
Chest tube—Heimlich valve
Syringes, 5 each
  3 cc
  5 cc
  12 cc
  30 cc
Three-way valve
Roll 1-inch adhesive tape
Pack of sterile 4 × 4 gauze pads
Roll elastic bandage
Blood administration set
Needles, five each
  20 gauge
  18 gauge
  16 gauge
"Butterfly" administration needles, 2 each
  21 gauge
  19 gauge
IV fluid administration set
Sterile emergency surgery pack
  Scalpel handle
  Blades: two No. 10, two No. 15
  Two small hemostats
  Thumb forceps
  One pair Metzenbaum scissors
  One pair curved forceps
  Several packages of sutures of your preference with swedged on needles
  Needle holders
  One set medium-sized rib retractors
Intravenous catheters: one 16 gauge, one 18 gauge

tially useful during CPR as well as their indications, adverse side effects, and doses. Figure 2-16 is an algorithm describing a logical approach to CPR.

Restoration of Normal Sinus Rhythm

At least one of five rhythms is observed after the development of a cardiac emergency (Table 2-8):

Rapid Ventricular Tachycardia with Severe Hypotension or Ventricular Fibrillation. Rapid ventricular tachycardia resulting in an imperceptible peripheral pulse is difficult to diagnose without the aid of an ECG. Lidocaine is administered intravenously to reestablish normal sinus rhythm, and intravenous fluids are given to increase the effective circulating blood volume. Intravenous procainamide is an alternative antiarrhythmic therapy when lidocaine is not effective in restoring normal sinus rhythm. Calcium chloride or epinephrine is administered to increase the force of cardiac contraction. In-

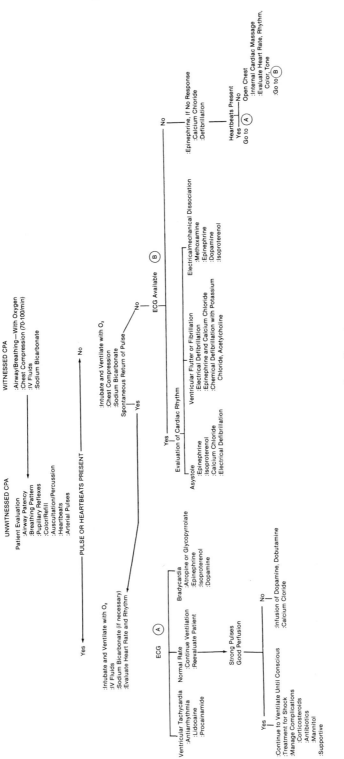

Fig. 2-16. Management of cardiopulmonary arrest.

Table 2-10. Essential Drugs Used in the Management of Cardiopulmonary Arrest

Generic Name	Trade Name	Beneficial Effects (Recommended Use)	Adverse or Side Effects	Dose and Route of Administration
Vasoactive and cardiostimulatory agents				
Epinephrine HCl	Adrenaline	Positive inotrope. Initiates heartbeats. Increases heart rate and cardiac output. Initially increases, then decreases mean arterial blood pressure and coronary blood flow.	Intense vasoconstriction of renal and splanchnic vasculature. Causes decreased perfusion of these tissues. Increases myocardial oxygen consumption and cardiac work. Arrhythmogenic.	0.5–5 μg/kg IC 15–20 μg/kg IV
Isoproterenol HCl	Isuprel	Positive inotrope. Initiates heartbeats, increases heart rate and cardiac output. Vasodilation.	Lowers mean arterial pressure, requiring concurrent blood volume expansion. May decrease coronary perfusion. Increases myocardial workload and oxygen consumption. Arrhythmogenic.	0.5–5 μg/kg IC 5–10 μg/kg IV 0.01–0.04 μg/kg/min
Dopamine HCl	Intropin	Positive inotrope. Increases heart rate, cardiac output, and mean arterial blood pressure. Improves blood flow to coronary, renal, and mesenteric circulations.	May produce severe tachycardia if given rapidly. Arrhythmogenic. Vasoconstriction at higher doses.	Add 5.0 mg to 250 cc 5% dextrose. Drip slowly at rate of 2–10 μg/kg/min
Dobutamine HCl	Dobutrex	Positive inotrope. Lesser chronotropic and vasopressor effect than dopamine.	Tachyarrhythmias, vasoconstriction, and arrhythmias at higher dosages.	2–15 μg/kg/min
Methoxamine HCl	Vasoxyl	Vasopresser. Increases systolic, diastolic, and mean blood pressure.	Hypertension, reflex bradycardia.	0.2–0.5 mg/kg IV
Drugs to specifically increase contractility				
Calcium chloride		Positive inotrope.	May cause arrhythmias or asystole.	0.05–0.1 cc/kg of the 10% solution IV, IC
Digoxin	Lanoxin	Positive inotrope. Increases vagal tone. *Only* used in patients with CPA caused by congestive heart failure.	Arrhythmogenic. Increases oxygen consumption. Causes vasocontriction when given IV.	0.02–0.04 mg/kg IV. Given in 4 divided doses, dosed every 1–2 hr to effect. Monitor ECG.

Table 2-10. *(continued)*

Generic Name	Trade Name	Beneficial Effects (Recommended Use)	Adverse or Side Effects	Dose and Route of Administration
Drugs to combat acidosis				
Sodium bicarbonate		Corrects metabolic acidosis. Allows more effective defibrillation.	Excessive administration may produce alkalosis, hyperosmolarity, paradoxical CSF acidosis.	0.5 mEq/kg/10–15 min IV or 1–2 mEq/kg IV to effect
Trihydroxymethyl-aminomethane	THAM	Corrects severe metabolic acidosis.	Metabolic alkalosis. Irritating when given extravascularly. Diuresis.	1–4 mEq/kg IV
Drugs to treat acute cardiac arrhythmias				
Atropine sulfate		Parasympatholytic effects. May correct supraventricular bradycardia or a slow ventricular rhythm by stimulating supraventricular pacemakers.	May cause excessive tachycardia. Increases myocardial oxygen consumption. Lowers ventricular fibrillatory threshold. May predispose to sympathetic induced arrhythmias.	0.1–0.2 mg/kg IV
Glycopyrrolate	Rubinul-V	Parasympatholytic (anticholinergic). May correct supraventricular bradycardia.	May cause excessive tachycardia.	0.005–0.01 mg/kg IV
Propranolol HCl	Inderal	β-Adrenergic blocker. Antiarrhythmic. May correct supraventricular and ventricular tachycardias.	Decreases contractility, bradycardia. May increase airway resistance.	0.1–0.3 mg/kg
Lidocaine	Xylocaine	Ventricular antiarrhythmic.	CNS toxicity, nausea, vomiting.	2–6 mg/kg IV. Dogs 0.25–1 mg/kg IV. Cats 40–80 µg/kg/min IV.
Procainamide	Pronestyl	Ventricular antiarrhythmic.	Hypotension, depression.	4–8 mg/kg IV; 40–60 µg/kg/min
Bretylium tosylate	Bretylol	Chemical ventricular antifibrillatory drug.	Of questionable value for treating ventricular fibrillation in dogs and cats.	??
Acetylcholine KCl cocktail		Chemical ventricular antifibrillatory drug.	Parasympathomimetic side effects.	ACh 6 mg/kg + KCl 1 mEq/kg IC
Drugs to stimulate ventilation				
Doxapram HCl	Dopram	Direct stimulant action on respiratory centers in the medulla. Antagonizes CNS depression caused by xylazine	Respiratory alkalosis—hyperkalemia, convulsions.	1–2 mg/kg IV

Drug	Trade name	Action	Precautions	Dosage
Methetharimide	Mikedimide	CNS stimulant effective in treating barbiturate-induced respiratory depression.	Overdose causes convulsions.	0.4–0.8 mg/kg IV (can repeat)
Drugs to combat cerebral edema				
Oxygen		Prevents hypoxia and CNS vascular dilation.	Decreases surfactant production. May suppress ventilatory drive.	2–4 L/min
Mannitol	Osmitrol 20%	Osmotic diuretic. Prevents cerebral edema.	Volume overload. Hyperosmolality.	1–2 g/kg IV
Dexamethasone	Azium	Stabilizes lysosomal membranes, induces vasodilation.		30 mg/kg IV
Steroids				
Prednisolone sodium succinate	Solu-Delta-Cortef	Stabilizes lysosomal membranes, induces vasodilation. Regulates fluid and electrolyte homeostasis.		30 mg/kg IV
Dexamethasone	Azium	Increases cardiac output.		8 mg/kg IV
Fluids				
Isotonic intravenous Fluids: Lactated Ringer's 0.9% saline, 5% dextrose in water, acetated Ringer's		Expand blood volume. Treat hypotension. Improve tissue perfusion.	Fluid administration rate generally should not exceed 90/ml/kg/min. Administer at high rates initially to improve venous return.	40–90 ml/kg/hr to effect
Specific drug antagonists				
Nalorphine	Nalline	Narcotic antagonist.	Narcotic-like effects at increased dosages.	0.4 mg/kg
Levallorphan	Lorfan	Narcotic antagonist.	Narcotic-like effects at increased dosages.	1 mg followed by 0.5 mg if necessary
Naloxone	Narcan	Narcotic antagonist.	None.	50 μg/kg
Neostigmine	Prostigmin Stiglyn	Cholinesterase inhibitor—used to reverse nondepolarizing neuromuscular blocking agents.	Cholinergic effects—atropine or glycopyrrolate must be given prior to drug administration.	0.01–0.04 mg/kg
Pyridostigmine	Regonol	Cholinesterase inhibitor—used to reverse nondepolarizing neuromuscular blocking agents.	Cholinergic effects—atropine or glycopyrrolate must be given prior to drug administration.	0.1 mg/kg

Table 2-11. Defibrillation Techniques

Ventricular tachycardia with severe hypotension or ventricular fibrillation
Direct-current defibrillators: 0.5–2.0 watt-seconds (ws)/kg internal; 5–10 ws/kg external
  Small patient (< 7 kg)
    5–15 ws internal
    50–100 ws external
  Large patient (> 10 kg)
    20–80 ws internal
    100–400 ws external
Alternating-current defibrillators
  Small patient
    30–50 V internal
    50–100 V external
  Large patient
    50–100 V internal
    150–250 V external
Chemical defibrillation[3]
  1 mg potassium chloride and 6 mg acetylcholine/kg followed by 10% calcium chloride
  1 ml/10 kg
Unresponsive ventricular fibrillation
  Evaluate ventilation
  Evaluate chest or cardiac compression
  Repeat epinephrine and calcium chloride administration (see Table 2-5)
  Repeat sodium bicarbonate administration
  administer lidocaine
  Repeat electrical defibrillation (direct-current; see above)

travenous sodium bicarbonate 0.5 mEq/kg is given at 10 to 15-min intervals; otherwise administration is based on frequent arterial pH and blood gas determination.

Electrical defibrillation is the therapy of choice for ventricular tachycardia which is unresponsive to pharmacologic intervention and is the first therapeutic technique used when ventricular fibrillation is diagnosed. Table 2-11 lists the various methods of electrical defibrillation available. Lidocaine is not capable of converting ventricular fibrillation to normal sinus rhythm but can be used to prevent the deterioration of cardiac rhythm after defibrillation. The persistence or recurrence of ventricular fibrillation after repeated attempts to defibrillate the heart is an indication of myocardial hypoxia, acidosis, myocardial depression, or severe systemic disease. The adequacy of ventilation, chest or cardiac compression, and drug therapy is then reevaluated. Intravenous or intracardiac epinephrine and calcium chloride are administered prior to repeated attempts to defibrillate the heart. Occasionally, intracardiac injections of drugs are deliberately made into the left ventricle in order to hasten their delivery to the coronary arteries and ventricular myocardium. Cardiac injections through the chest wall are infrequently required but when given can cause pneumothorax, hemopericardium, or intramyocardial injection, leading to cardiac arrhythmias.

Ventricular Bradycardia. Bradyarrhythmias are common immediately before cardiac arrest or after successful cardiopulmonary resuscitation. Sinus bradycardia and junctional escape rhythms are frequently observed before ventricular asystole or fibrillation, whereas junctional and ventricular (idioventricular) escape rhythms develop after defibrillation (Fig. 2-13). These rhythm disturbances are impossible to distinguish from one another without an ECG. Their hemodynamic consequences are identical and are characterized by inadequate cardiac output and arterial blood pressure. Patients who present with junctional or idioventricular escape rhythms should be suspected of having disease of the AV node or hyperkalemia. Therapy in these instances may require a pacemaker or specific techniques to lower serum potassium. Saline, sodium bicarbonate, calcium chloride, and hyperventilation are indicated when acute hyperkalemia is responsible for bradyarrhythmia. When the cause of bradycardia is unknown, the first step is to evaluate the adequacy of ventilation, begin chest compression, and correct acidosis. The administration of inhalation or intravenous anesthetics is discontinued. If chest compression is not successful in restoring sinus tachycardia, atropine or glycopyrrolate is administered IV. Epinephrine is given IV when the heart rate is rapidly slowing and peripheral pulses are not palpable. Stable bradyarrhythmias (20–50 beats/min for the dog, 30–60 beats/min for the cat) can be treated by infusion of isoproterenol, adjusting the infusion rate to maintain a ventricular rate between 60–100 beats/min in dogs and 80–120 beats/min in cats. Increases in ventricular rate should restore peripheral blood flow and pressure. Calcium chloride or dobutamine can be given to improve the force of cardiac contraction.

Ventricular Asystole. Ventricular asystole generally occurs secondary to drug overdose (anesthesia, adverse reaction), severe hypoxia, and acidosis, or after electrical defibrillation. An airway, breathing, and chest compression must be instituted immediately. All cardiovascular anesthetic drugs are discontinued and epinephrine and sodium bicarbonate administered intravenously. Calcium chloride or dobutamine can be given if a palpable pulse is restored. Epinephrine is readministered at 5-min intervals if asystole persists. External electrical defibrillation is attempted when administration of epinephrine is not successful in initiating a heartbeat if ventricular fibrillation cannot be distinguished from ventricular asystole (no ECG). Ventricular asystole usually results from severe myocardial depression and is associated with a poor prognosis.

Electromechanical Dissociation. Electromechanical dissociation is difficult if not impossible to distinguish from ventricular fibrillation or asystole without an ECG. It is characterized by ECG evidence of organized electrical activity (P-QRS-T) but without effective myocardial contraction (Table 2-8). This disorder is observed in association with anesthetic drug overdose, acute hypoxia, severe acidosis, and cardiogenic shock. Severe hypovolemia, tension pneumothorax, and pericardial effusions can mimic electromechanical dissociation and must be ruled out prior to therapy. Therapy with ventilation, chest compression, correction of acidosis, and epinephrine and calcium chloride is begun immediately. The administration of shock doses of fluids is vital in the treatment of this disorder. Recent evidence suggests that the most efficacious treatment for electromechanical dissociation in dogs is the administration of methoxamine, a peripheral vasoconstrictor (adrenoceptor agonist). The administration of methoxamine and fluids was shown to be as effective as epinephrine in restoring cardiac rhythm during asystole and twice as effective as epinephrine in resuscitation from ventricular fibrillation.[12] These studies require clinical verification but suggest alternatives to currently accepted therapeutic techniques.

The decision to discontinue resuscitative efforts is based on the patient's medical history, the duration of cardiopulmonary arrest prior to initiating CPR, the cause of cardiopulmonary arrest, and long-term economic considerations. Resuscitative attempts in dogs or cats with severe metabolic disturbances or cardiac disease are often unsuccessful. Dogs and cats who cannot be effectively resuscitated within 10–15 min of initiation of CPR usually suffer neurologic deficits and require days of close supervision and therapy. In general, dogs or cats who do not respond to CPR within 30 min cannot be resuscitated or will die from shock within 24–48 hr.

Proper postresuscitation monitoring and therapy is as critical as the resuscitation period itself if the patient is to survive. The period of hypoxia and ischemia, regardless of how brief, results in metabolic acidosis an increase in capillary and blood-brain barrier permeability, and intense peripheral vascular constriction. These effects can lead to temporary or permanent blindness, neurologic deficits, cerebral or pulmonary edema, gastrointestinal mucosal sloughing, renal failure, hypothermia, and shock. Careful monitoring of CNS signs, heart rate and rhythm, the peripheral pulse, acid-base and electrolyte status, urine volume, and ventilation must be continued for many hours post resuscitation in order to ensure success. Infusions of dopamine and dobutamine are useful in maintaining cardiac contractile force and peripheral blood flow during the postresuscitation period. The judicious use of polyionic salt solutions containing lactate with frequent auscultation of the chest and measurement of CVP and urinary output are important. Mannitol and furosemide can be used to prevent cerebral edema. Antibiotics can be used to treat infection and steroids administered to combat shock (see "Shock"). Preparedness and total familiarity with resuscitative techniques are the key factors to successful CPR.

REFERENCES

1. Bonagura JD: Therapy of cardiac arrhythmias. p. 360. In Kirk RW (ed): Current Veterinary Therapy VIII — Small Animal Practice, W. B. Saunders, Philadelphia, 1983
2. Bonagura JD, Muir WW: Therapy of cardiac arrhythmias. In Tilley LP (ed): Essentials of Canine and Feline Electrocardiography. Lea & Febiger, Philadelphia, 1984
3. Breznock DM, Kagan KG, Attix ES: Effects of ionic salts or acetylcholine, or both, on electrically induced ventricular fibrillation in dogs. Am J Vet Res 39:977, 1978
4. Chaundry IH: Cellular mechanisms in shock and ischemia and their correction. Am J Physiol 245:R117, 1983
5. Hackel DB, Ratliff NB, Mikat E: The heart in shock. Circ Res 35:805, 1974
6. Haskins SC: Cardiopulmonary resuscitation. Compend Contin Educ 4:170, 1982

7. Haskins SC: Shock (the pathophysiology and management of the circulatory collapse states). p. 2. In Kirk RW (ed): Current Veterinary Therapy VIII — Small Animal Practice. W. B. Suanders, Philadelphia, 1983
8. Koehler RC, Chandra N, Guerci AD, et al: Augmentation of cerebral perfusion by simultaneous chest compression and lung inflation with abdominal binding after cardiac arrest in dogs. Circulation 67:266, 1983
9. Kolata RJ, Burrows CF, Soma LR: Shock: pathophysiology and management. p. 32. In Kirk RW (ed): Current Veterinary Therapy VII — Small Animal Practice. W. B. Saunders, Philadelphia, 1983
10. Luce JM, Rose BK, O'Quin RJ, et al: Regional blood flow during cardiopulmonary resuscitation in dogs using simultaneous and nonsimultaneous compression and ventilation. Circulation 67:258, 1983
11. Morgan RV: Cardiac emergencies Part II. Compend Contin Educ 3:838, 1981
12. Redding JS, Haynes RR, Thomas JD: Drug therapy in resuscitation from electromechanical dissociation. Crit Care Med 11:681, 1983
13. Thomas WP: Pericardial disease. In Ettinger SJ (ed): Textbook of Veterinary Internal Medicine. 2nd Ed. Saunders, Philadelphia, 1983
14. Weil MH, Henning RJ: New concepts in the diagnosis and fluid treatment of circulatory shock. Anesth Analg 58:124, 1979

3 | Respiratory Emergencies

Robert G. Sherding

There are several respiratory emergency situations in veterinary medicine. The most important are acute respiratory failure, respiratory arrest, acute upper airway obstruction, lower airway obstruction (including asthma), problems related to thoracic trauma, pulmonary edema, and acute bacterial bronchopneumonia.

ACUTE RESPIRATORY FAILURE

Mechanisms of Abnormal Gas Exchange and Hypoxemia

Failure of respiratory function is one of the most common life-threatening emergencies encountered in the dog and cat. The respiratory system is a two-way gas exchanger with two life-sustaining functions: (1) the transfer of oxygen from inspired air to arterial blood for delivery to body tissues; and (2) the excretion of carbon dioxide (CO_2), a by-product of body metabolism. Therefore the ultimate purpose of the respiratory system is to meet the needs of peripheral body tissues for oxygenation and CO_2 elimination. Effective gas exchange depends on normal function of each of the following processes[41]:

1. Ventilation—the mass movement of air into and out of the lungs
2. Distribution—the even distribution of incoming air to each of millions of alveoli
3. Perfusion—the even matching of pulmonary capillary perfusion with ventilated alveoli
4. Diffusion—the actual exchange of gas across the alveolar-capillary membranes

95

The malfunction of these respiratory processes results in failure of the lung to adequately oxygenate arterial blood and/or prevent CO_2 retention. Thus the hallmark of respiratory failure and all types of respiratory emergency is arterial hypoxemia. The four basic pathophysiological mechanisms of abnormal gas exchange and hypoxemia are hypoventilation, ventilation-perfusion inequality, right-to-left shunt, and diffusion impairment.[10,45] It is important to understand these four types of hypoxemia because each may indicate a different underlying cause and require a different therapeutic approach. These mechanisms and the corresponding arterial blood gas responses are described in Table 3-1. In many cases of respiratory failure, combinations of these four mechanisms probably contribute to the severe hypoxemia; however, by far the most important factor is ventilation-perfusion inequality.[41,45]

The first mechanism of hypoxemia, hypoventilation, is characterized by reduced flow of inspired gas to the alveoli per unit of time such that ventilation is insufficient to prevent CO_2 retention.[10,45] The cardinal features of hypoventilation include hypoxemia that is readily abolished with increased inspired oxygen and a consistent elevation of arterial CO_2 level (CO_2 retention). In most cases of pure hypoventilation the lungs themselves are normal. The causes are mostly extrapulmonary, e.g., abnormal central nervous system (CNS) or neuromuscular control of respiration (drug-induced CNS depression, brainstem disease or injury, and paralysis, fatigue, or spasm of respiratory muscles), abnormal bellows function of the thoracic cage (flail chest), pleural space encroachment (pleural effusion, pneumothorax, diaphragmatic hernia), and upper airway obstruction.

The second and most important mechanism of hypoxemia is ventilation-perfusion inequality.[10,41,45] Under normal resting conditions ventilation and perfusion are fairly evenly matched, approximating a 1:1 ratio. A moderately low ratio (mismatch) results when ventilation is distributed unevenly within various regions of the lung relative to perfusion (maldistribution), mostly because of localized, nonuniform changes in lung compliance and airway resistance.[41] When nonuniform airway obstruction increases regional airway resistance, e.g., in asthma or bronchitis, maldistributed ventilation results from preferential distribution of inspired air to those airways with more normal resistance. When there is a nonuniform decrease in regional lung compliance, e.g., in many forms of diffuse interstitial disease, maldistributed ventilation results from preferential distribution of inspired air to those lung units with more normal compliance. When there is a nonuniform increase in regional lung compliance, e.g., with disrupted elastic support from emphysema, maldistributed ventilation results from air exchange in more normal regions whereas inelastic areas remain distended with a fixed volume of air.[41]

On the other end of the spectrum, there can be lung units that are ventilated but not perfused (very high ratio mismatch), which wastes the air in those units such that they become alveolar dead space. Ventilation with impaired perfusion, although not very common, may result from pulmonary emboli or loss of capillary beds due to emphysema or vascular injury.[41]

The cardinal features of ventilation-perfusion inequality include hypoxemia (often severe) that is responsive to oxygen therapy, normal or increased CO_2, and a widened alveolar-arterial oxygen difference (see next section).

The third mechanism of hypoxemia, right-to-left shunt, results from perfusion of completely nonventilated lung units.[10,41,45] Because blood flow passes through the lung without exposure to ventilated alveoli, no gas exchange occurs and the right-to-left shunt effect produces arterial hypoxemia. Shunting can be distinguished clinically from the other three types of hypoxemia by failure of 100% inspired oxygen to raise arterial oxygen to expected levels. This is because the shunted blood bypasses ventilated alveoli and thus is never exposed to the increased oxygen.[45] Shunts from unventilated but perfused lung units are caused by collapse of alveoli (atelectasis), fluid-filling of alveoli (edema), or consolidation of alveoli (pneumonia). The same shunt effect also is associated with certain congenital heart defects that cause extrapulmonary right-to-left shunting of blood.

The last mechanism, diffusion impairment, is presumably due to impairment of oxygen transfer across the alveolar-capillary membrane, because either the membrane is thickened (diffuse interstitial disease—fibrosis, inflammation, edema) or there is loss of alveolar-capillary surface area from tissue destruction (emphysema, vascular injury).[10,45] Diffusion hypoxemia is exaggerated during exercise (less contact time for alveolar-capillary gas equilibration) and readily corrected by administering supplemental oxygen. Arterial CO_2 is normal. The importance of diffusion impairment as a mechanism of hypoxemia is uncertain; in most clinical situations it is probably only a minor contributing factor to the hypoxemia of ventilation-perfusion inequality.[10,45]

Blood Gas Analysis in Respiratory Failure

The chief consequences of respiratory failure are hypoxemia, CO_2 retention, and respiratory acidosis. Therefore arterial blood gas analysis can play an important role in diagnosis, management strategy, and monitoring of response to treatment, especially treatment with oxygen or artificial ventilation. Disorders of acid-base homeostasis and blood gas analysis and interpretation are discussed in detail in Chapter 4.

The arterial blood gas values that have been used as guidelines for determining severe (life-threatening) respiratory failure are an oxygen tension (Pa_{O_2}) of less than 60 mm Hg (normal 85–100 mm Hg) and/or a CO_2 tension of greater than 50 mm Hg (normal 35–42 mm Hg). In addition to Pa_{O_2} and Pa_{CO_2} determinations, diagnostic information can be obtained by measuring the response of Pa_{O_2} to supplemental inspired oxygen (up to 100%) and by calculating the alveolar-arterial oxygen difference (A-aD_{O_2}; normal <15 mm Hg), which is a parameter of gas exchange efficiency that makes allowance for over- or under-ventilation[41,45] (Table 3-1).

These blood gas determinations are used to distinguish the four types of hypoxemia described in Table 3-1 as follows: (1) Hypoventilation—always associated with elevated Pa_{CO_2}, but A-aD_{O_2} is normal and the hypoxemia is very

Table 3-1. Pathophysiological Mechanisms of Hypoxemia

Mechanism	Definition	Disease Associations	Arterial Blood Gas Responses			Response to Supplemental O_2
			Pao_2	$Paco_2$	A-aDo_2	
Hypoventilation	Reduced flow of inspired gas to alveoli per unit time	CNS depression Abnormal neural control of respiratory muscles Respiratory muscle fatigue or weakness Chest wall damage or malfunction Pleural space encroachment Upper airway obstruction	Decreased	Increased	Normal	Hypoxemia corrected
Ventilation-perfusion inequality	Mismatching of ventilation and blood flow in areas of lung with uneven ventilation because of nonuniform changes in compliance and airway resistance	Increased resistance (asthma, bronchitis) Decreased compliance (diffuse interstitial disease) Increased compliance (emphysema) Vascular disease (pulmonary embolism)	Decreased	Normal or increased	Increased	Hypoxemia corrected

| Right-to-left shunt | Passage of blood through the lung without exposure to ventilated alveoli | Alveolar collapse (atelectasis) Alveolar fluid-filling (edema) Alveolar consolidation (pneumonia) Extrapulmonary shunting due to congenital heart defect | Decreased | Normal or decreased | Increased | Poor response |
| Diffusion impairment | Failure of pulmonary capillary blood to equilibrate with alveolar gas across the alveolar-capillary interface | Thickened alveolar-capillary membrane (diffuse interstitial disease) Loss of alveolar surface area (emphysema) Loss of capillary surface area (vasculitis) | Decreased | Normal | Increased | Hypoxemia corrected |

Pa_{O_2} = arterial oxygen tension (normal 85–100 mm Hg).
Pa_{CO_2} = arterial carbon dioxide tension (normal 35–42 mm Hg).
$A-aD_{O_2}$ = alveolar-arterial oxygen difference: the measured Pa_{O_2} is subtracted from alveolar oxygen tension (PA_{O_2}) calculated as (barometric pressure minus water vapor pressure) × (fractional inspired oxygen tension) − Pa_{CO_2}. With breathing of room air at sea level, calculation may be simplified to: $A-aD_{O_2} = (150 - Pa_{CO_2}) - Pa_{O_2}$.

responsive to supplemental oxygen. (2) Right-to-left shunting—only form of hypoxemia in which the Pao_2 fails to rise to expected levels during 100% inspired oxygen; the $A\text{-}aDo_2$ is increased whereas hypoxemia-driven hyperventilation usually results in normal or even decreased $Paco_2$. (3) Ventilation-perfusion inequality—only other type that may mimic hypoventilation by sometimes manifesting CO_2 retention; however, there is an increased $A\text{-}aDo_2$ in contrast to hypoventilation, and in distinction from shunting the hypoxemia is abolished by oxygen administration. (4) Diffusion impairment is probably not clinically significant and is usually accompanied and overshadowed by ventilation-perfusion inequality.[45]

CO_2, a product of normal body metabolism, functions as a respiratory acid that must be excreted by the lungs as CO_2. The effect of CO_2 transport in solution in blood on blood pH is defined by the Henderson-Hasselbalch equation (Ch. 4), which can be conceptualized as:

$$pH = constant\ (6.1) + \log \frac{HCO_3\ (\text{what kidney does})}{CO_2\ (\text{what lung does})}$$

Disturbances in acid-base balance are considered to be primarily respiratory when they involve CO_2 (denominator) and primarily metabolic when they involve bicarbonate (numerator).[41]

The two respiratory acid-base derangements, which may be acute or chronic and compensated or uncompensated, are respiratory acidosis (increased CO_2) and respiratory alkalosis (decreased CO_2). The measurement of arterial $Paco_2$ is a sensitive index of alveolar ventilation: An increase indicates hypoventilation and respiratory acidosis, and a decrease indicates hyperventilation and respiratory alkalosis.[41] In addition to primary hypoventilation, ventilation-perfusion inequality may also cause CO_2 retention. However, because of increased ventilatory drive from hypoxemia, most cases of ventilation-perfusion mismatch maintain a normal $Paco_2$.[45] In respiratory acidosis and alkalosis, the kidney responds by conserving or excreting bicarbonate, respectively, resulting in a more normal blood pH by compensation.[45] Respiratory acidosis may be accompanied by metabolic acidosis caused by release of lactic acid from hypoxic tissues.[45]

Recognition of a Respiratory Emergency

The cardinal manifestation of all respiratory emergencies is hypoxemia. Effective therapy often depends on prompt recognition. The clinical signs of hypoxemia are dyspnea and respiratory distress (increased rate, depth, and effort of breathing), restlessness and apprehension, tachycardia, and sometimes cyanosis or collapse. Profound acute hypoxemia (Pao_2 <40–50 mm Hg) with impending respiratory arrest may be indicated by irregular or feeble respirations, bradycardia, hypotension, somnolence, and convulsions.

The diagnosis of a respiratory emergency requires an approach that is efficient and organized, including determination of history, observation of and listening to respirations, auscultation, palpation, and percussion. Table 3-2

Table 3-2. Recognition and Interpretation of Signs of Respiratory Disease

Clinical Sign or Finding	Interpretation or Association
LISTENING	
Voice change	Laryngeal disease
Noisy breathing	
Stridor	Laryngeal/upper airway obstruction
Stertor	Pharyngeal obstruction
Honking/rattling	Tracheal collapse
Expiratory wheeze	Asthma (lower airway obstruction)
OBSERVATION OF BREATHING PATTERN	
Slow, deep, forceful inspiratory effort	Upper airway obstruction
Forceful expiratory effort	Lower airway obstruction (asthma)
Slow, feeble, irregular breathing	CNS respiratory center disturbance
Hyperventilation & periods of apnea	CNS respiratory center disturbance
Paradoxic chest wall motion	Flail chest
Decreased hemithorax expansion	Mainstem bronchus obstruction; diaphragmatic hernia
Rapid, shallow, choppy breathing	Rib fracture (chest wall pain)
Progressive posttraumatic dyspnea	Pneumothorax; pulmonary contusion
Cough: purulent sputum	Bacterial pneumonia
Cough: hemoptysis	Heartworms, trauma, tumor, foreign body
Pink froth expelled from airways	Fulminant pulmonary edema
Kussmaul's hyperventilation	Metabolic acidosis
PALPATION	
Rib cage pain/deformity	Rib fracture; flail chest
Subcutaneous emphysema	Tracheobronchial rupture
Compressable, flaccid, flattened trachea	Tracheal collapse
Decreased thoracic compressibility (feline)	Mediastinal mass (lymphosarcoma)
Edema of head, neck, front limbs	Cranial vena cava obstruction (mediastinal mass)
Displaced cardiac impulse	Diaphragmatic hernia, intrathoracic mass
PERCUSSION	
Hyperresonance (tympanitic)	Pneumothorax
Hyporesonance (dull)	Pleural effusion, diaphragmatic hernia, lung mass or consolidation
AUSCULTATION	
Crackles	Bronchopulmonary disease
Expiratory wheeze	Asthma
Muffled lung sounds	Pleural effusion
Silent lung fields	Atelectasis, consolidation
Distant, hollow lung sounds	Pneumothorax

summarizes the interpretation of respiratory signs. Vital diagnostic information is often also obtained from thoracic radiography, thoracentesis, and arterial blood gas determination.

Management of Respiratory Failure

A respiratory emergency, because of its life-threatening potential, requires prompt detection and immediate therapeutic intervention—the critical first few minutes may determine survival. In general, the following initial steps should be taken: ensure a patent airway (using endotracheal or tracheostomy intubation if necessary), provide ventilatory support, administer supplemental oxygen, support the circulatory system (intravenous fluids, shock therapy), and then investigate and treat the underlying cause. The next phase of management entails following clinical parameters to monitor the response to therapy.

An effort should also be made to anticipate and prevent complications, e.g., bronchospasm, retained respiratory secretions, and bacterial pneumonia. Bronchospasm, which increases airway resistance and the work of breathing, can be controlled with bronchodilator drugs. An additional unforeseen benefit of aminophylline may be its ability to restore contractility to fatigued inspiratory muscles and diaphragm.[1] Retention of airway secretions is another troublesome complication, especially when mucous plugs form in the airways, which can lead to marked deterioration of pulmonary function. This is most effectively prevented by reducing secretion viscosity through patient hydration (fluid therapy) and humidification of all administered gases. In addition, the recumbent animal's position is changed frequently (hourly), cough is encouraged by percussion-vibration, and drugs that depress the cough reflex are avoided. These measures to facilitate clearance of respiratory secretions are also important in protecting against bronchopulmonary infections. When bacterial pneumonia does occur, antibiotics are instituted, preferably based on culture and sensitivity tests of a transtracheal aspirate.

Oxygen Therapy

The administration of supplemental oxygen is indicated for treatment of severe hypoxemia, regardless of the cause. Hypoxemia due to hypoventilation or diffusion impairment is easily reversed with modest oxygen enrichment of inspired gas. Oxygen therapy is usually effective in overcoming the hypoxemia of ventilation-perfusion inequality; however, it may require higher concentrations of oxygen, and it may take many minutes until nitrogen is washed out of all ventilated lung units and the Pa_{O_2} rises to its final level. Right-to-left shunting is the only form of hypoxemia where Pa_{O_2} fails to rise to expected levels with 100% oxygen. This is because blood that completely bypasses ventilated alveoli is never exposed to the added oxygen. Nevertheless, 100% oxygen does raise Pa_{O_2} in a shunt somewhat and thus is beneficial.

For oxygen therapy to be effective, the animal must be breathing spontaneously and have a patent airway and intact chest wall. The animal who is not breathing must be intubated and then ventilated with oxygen or room air by a self-inflating Ambu resuscitation bag, manual compression of the reservoir bag on an anesthetic machine, or a mechanical ventilator (see "Respiratory Arrest"). These methods of endotracheal tube delivery of oxygen may also be used in animals who are severely depressed, unconscious, or anesthetized. Methods for administering oxygen to a conscious, breathing animal include oxygen cage, face mask, or transtracheal catheter. Modern oxygen cages are equipped with controls for oxygen flow, temperature, and humidity, and are the preferred method for continuous delivery of oxygen to animals. The face mask or oxygen cone is not very effective because of difficulty in producing an airtight face-to-mask seal and because animal intolerance of the mask often leads to distressful struggling. A percutaneous transtracheal catheter (large-

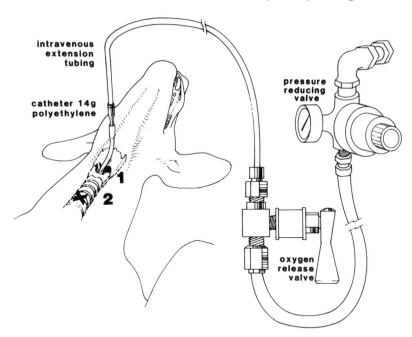

Fig. 3-1. Technique for percutaneous transtracheal catheter delivery of oxygen for management of life-threatening hypoxemia.

bore, through-the-needle, 8–12 inch intravenous catheter unit) can be used for short-term emergency oxygen administration at a flow rate of 3–6 L/min[25] (Fig. 3-1).

The ideal concentration of inspired oxygen is one which satisfies tissue needs but does not produce CO_2 retention (from reduced ventilatory drive) or oxygen toxicity. If arterial blood gas monitoring is available, a practical guide is to use a level of oxygen that maintains the Pao_2 at 60–90 mm Hg. For resuscitation or brief use (<12 hr), it is acceptable to use 100% oxygen. Otherwise, oxygen is usually administered at a concentration of 40–50% or less. In addition, if treatment is to exceed 4 hr, the inspired gas should always be humidified to prevent drying of mucous membranes, which can lead to mucociliary damage and inspissated, viscid mucus that can occlude airways. The oxygen inflow rate for oxygen cages can be adjusted to maintain the oxygen concentration at a desired level between 25 and 40%. Temperature within the cage should be at 72–75°F and the humidity at 45–55%.

Although oxygen is extremely beneficial for the treatment of hypoxemia, there are potential hazards with its use, including pulmonary injury, atelectasis, and CO_2 retention.[45] Exposure to pure oxygen for prolonged periods (24–48 hr or more) damages capillary endothelium and alveolar epithelium leading to interstitial and alveolar edema and hemorrhage, decreased lung compliance, and atelectasis. Chronic lower doses of oxygen (25–60%) have been associated with proliferative changes in alveolar epithelium and diffuse thickening of the alveolar-capillary membrane.

Another complication of oxygen administration is atelectasis and shunt formation. When oxygen washes nitrogen out of the lung, there is accelerated absorption atelectasis of lung units downstream from small airways that are obstructed with mucus or exudate. Also, poorly ventilated lung units may become unstable and collapse when high-oxygen mixtures are inhaled.[45]

Retention of CO_2 may be a dangerous consequence of oxygen overdose in chronically hypoxemic patients with hypercapnia. By relieving hypoxemia, the stimulus for ventilatory drive is removed and the level of ventilation falls dramatically, allowing high arterial CO_2 levels to develop. This can be prevented in decompensated chronic respiratory failure by starting with a low concentration of oxygen and adjusting the dose based on blood gas monitoring.[45]

Mechanical Ventilation

The use of artificial ventilation should be considered in animals who cannot breath adequately without assistance or to augment tidal volume and alveolar ventilation in animals in a severe respiratory crisis. Clinical situations where mechanical ventilation could be helpful include apnea, inability to expand the chest (respiratory muscle fatigue, flail chest), inability to expand the lungs (pleural effusion, restrictive lung disease), or progressive pulmonary insufficiency when severe hypoxemia persists in spite of breathing 100% oxygen.

There are two types of positive-pressure ventilators: volume-cycled and pressure-cycled. A volume-cycled ventilator (e.g., Metomatic) delivers a preset volume of gas by means of a piston or bellows, regardless of the pressure imposed. The advantage is that a known tidal volume is delivered regardless of abnormal compliance or airway resistance. A deleteriously high airway pressure may be generated, although most machines have a blow-off safety valve. A pressure-cycled ventilator (e.g., Bird) delivers an inspiratory flow of gas until a preset pressure is attained, irrespective of inflow volume. Although this type can ensure safe pressure levels, the volume of gas delivered is variable and dependent on airway resistance, pulmonary compliance, and intrathoracic pressure.

Ventilators usually have controls for ventilatory rate (frequency), duration and flow rate of inspiration and expiration, and inspiratory pressure (pressure-cycled) or tidal volume (volume-cycled). An inspiratory trigger setting allows the patient to trigger the ventilatory cycle by initiating an inspiratory effort for an assisted rather than a controlled mode of operation. Most ventilators provide for incorporation of oxygen, humidification, or anesthesia into the circuit. Guidelines for operating a mechanical ventilator are found in Table 3-3.

Mechanical ventilation is delivered through an indwelling endotracheal or tracheostomy tube. In the conscious animal, a tracheostomy tube is often better tolerated; however, the tube may require considerably more care than an endotracheal tube. Tolerance of intubation and mechanical ventilation may be

Table 3-3. Operating Guidelines for Mechanical Ventilation

Parameter	Guidelines
Respiratory rate	6–18/min
Tidal volume	10–20 ml/kg
Inspiratory time	<1.5 sec
Inspiratory/expiratory ratio	1:2–1:3
Peak inspiratory pressure	20–25 cm H_2O
PEEP	3–5 cm H_2O
Sigh (every 5–10 min)	30 cm H_2O
Assessment of ventilatory adequacy	1. Observe chest wall excursions
	2. Monitor blood gases—preferred method (maintain $Paco_2$ at 40 mm Hg)

facilitated by coating the tube with 5% lidocaine cream and sedating the animal with a narcotic, e.g., fentanyl (Innovar-Vet). Other sedatives that can be used are morphine, oxymorphone (Numorphan), pentazocine (Talwin), diazepam (Valium), or phenobarbital. If the animal resists the ventilator even after sedation and oxygen administration, a paralyzing drug, e.g., pancuronium bromide (Pavulon) 0.02–0.04 mg/kg IV, can be used to provide 15–30 min of skeletal muscle paralysis. To wean an animal from a ventilator, narcotics are reversed with naloxone (Narcan) or nalorphine (Nalline) and pancuronium antagonized by atropine (0.02 mg/kg) and neostigmine (0.02–0.04 mg/kg).

The standard mode of operation of a mechanical ventilator is called intermittent positive-pressure ventilation (IPPV). For humans, several other modes have been developed, mostly in an effort to generate pressures that keep small airways open, prevent atelectasis, and increase the functional residual capacity (FRC) of the lung. The most common among these are positive end-expiratory pressure (PEEP) and constant positive airway pressure (CPAP). These techniques of artificial ventilation have not yet been widely adapted to clinical use in animals, although they are available at some of the large referral institutions.

The benefits of mechanical ventilation are reversal of hypoxemia (increased Pao_2) and CO_2 retention (decreased $Paco_2$), although this may be at the expense of reducing cardiac output. During positive-pressure ventilation, the pressure in the airways and lung is transmitted to the thoracic cavity, thus impeding venous return and cardiac output. This means that the artificially ventilated patient is predisposed to hypotension, especially if the animal's fluid needs are not met.[45]

Tracheostomy Intubation

Tracheostomy tube placement is indicated whenever an emergency patent airway is needed and an upper airway obstruction prevents insertion of a standard endotracheal tube. A tracheostomy tube can also be used to deliver mechanical ventilation, especially as, unlike an endotracheal tube, an indwelling tracheostomy tube can be maintained in place without heavy sedation or general anesthesia.

A proper tracheostomy tube should contain a blunt obturator and locking inner cannula which enables periodic cleansing of secretions that accumulate within the lumen of the tube. An inflatable cuff that provides an airtight seal between the tube and the trachea is required for use of the tracheostomy with a mechanical ventilator. Tubes are available in rubber, Silastic, plastic, or metal.

To insert the tracheostomy tube, a ventral midline skin incision is made over the proximal trachea with the animal in dorsal recumbency. General anesthesia as well as aseptic preparation of the skin site are desirable but not always feasible in an emergency situation. The tracheostomy incision is made in the membrane between tracheal rings distal to the site of obstruction, or between the third and fourth ring. A curved hemostat can be used to spread the tracheal incision to allow insertion of the tube. The tube is then fixed in position with umbilical tape around the neck or sutured to adjacent skin, and a sterile dressing may be applied around the stoma. After removal of a tracheostomy tube, the incision heals by granulation within a few days. The technique of tracheostomy tube placement is discussed further in Chapter 1.

A tracheostomy tube can be used to deliver air, oxygen, or positive-pressure ventilation. For the indwelling tracheostomy tube, continuous care is needed to prevent the complications of bronchopulmonary infection or occlusion of the tube with viscid mucus. Tracheostomy bypasses the normal mechanisms for warming, humidifying, and filtering inspired air. The tube also acts as a mechanical irritant and prevents effective cough or airway clearance. For these reasons, tenacious, inspissated mucus tends to accumulate within the tube and airways, and there is increased frequency of infection. Thus frequent suctioning (every 1–2 hr) of the trachea and tube and monitoring for respiratory infection are recommended for animals with an indwelling tracheostomy tube.

RESPIRATORY ARREST

Etiology

Respiratory arrest is the cessation of spontaneous breathing. It may occur suddenly and unpredictably, or it may be the anticipated final stage in the natural progression of chronic severe pulmonary disease. In most cases, respiratory arrest is accompanied by cardiac arrest. The end result is circulation of oxygenated blood that is insufficient for survival of body tissues, especially sensitive tissues, e.g., the brain. Therefore respiratory arrest is a medical emergency that requires immediate correction and takes precedence over all other emergency care.

The numerous etiologies of respiratory arrest (Table 3-4) may be categorized as: (1) medullary respiratory center depression induced by drugs, anesthetics, metabolic derangements, brain injury, or cessation of blood flow (cardiac arrest); (2) respiratory muscle dysfunction associated with neuromuscular

Table 3-4. Etiology of Respiratory Arrest

Medullary respiratory center depression
    Cardiac arrest
        Cessation of CNS respiratory center blood flow
    Drug-induced
        Anesthetics, barbiturates, narcotics, tranquilizers
        Other intoxications
    Brainstem injury
        Acute head trauma
        Elevated intracranial pressure
        Faulty needle puncture of the cisterna magnum
    Metabolic
        Hypoxia
        Acidosis
        Endogenous toxic metabolites

Neuromuscular dysfunction of respiratory muscles
    Paralysis
        Tick paralysis, polyradiculoneuropathy, botulism, myasthenia gravis, etc.
        Phrenic nerve injury
    Spasm (tetanus)
    Respiratory muscle fatigue

Airway obstruction
    Upper airway
        Foreign body, inflammation/edema, laryngospasm, laryngeal paralysis, elongated soft palate,
            tracheal collapse
        Occluded endotracheal tube
    Lower airway
        Asthma (bronchial spasm/inflammation)

End-stage respiratory failure
    Pulmonary disease
        Pneumonia, edema, neoplasia
    Pleural (restrictive) disease
        Pleural effusion, pneumothorax, diaphragmatic hernia

Pulmonary thromboembolism
    Heartworm disease, amyloidosis, sepsis, etc.

disorders; (3) asphyxiation from upper or lower airway obstruction; (4) end stage respiratory failure resulting from severe pulmonary disease or restrictive pleural disease; and (5) pulmonary thromboembolism. Any animal in severe respiratory failure or afflicted with any of the respiratory emergencies discussed in this chapter, regardless of cause, may succumb in respiratory arrest from the stress of restraint and manipulation. Such animals must be handled very carefully to minimize distress, especially as it is easier to prevent cardiopulmonary arrest than to reverse it once it has occurred.

Diagnosis

The diagnosis of respiratory arrest is made by observing the absence of ventilatory attempts, absence of chest movements, cessation of air flow, gray to cyanotic mucous membranes, and dilated pupils.[16] Spasmodic agonal gasps should not be considered true ventilations. Concomitant cardiac arrest is determined by the absence of an auscultatable heartbeat or palpable pulses. Clinical signs of impending respiratory arrest may include either respirations that are slow, irregular, and feeble or respirations that are extremely labored and accompanied by anxiety, restlessness, tachycardia, arrhythmias, vomiting, pupil dilatation, or stupor. The recognition of impending arrest is important because of the possibility that emergency therapeutic intervention may prevent the arrest from occurring.

Pulmonary Resuscitation

The primary goal of cardiopulmonary resuscitation is early reestablishment of oxygenated circulation through the use of emergency maneuvers that restore ventilatory and cardiovascular functions simultaneously.[16] Pulmonary resuscitation is described here, and the details of cardiac resuscitation are provided in Chapter 2. The first priority of resuscitation is to establish and maintain an open airway, usually by means of an endotracheal tube with inflatable cuff. Also, any food, vomitus, secretions, or obstructing foreign objects are cleared from the airway. If endotracheal tube insertion is prevented by an upper airway obstruction, tracheostomy intubation is an alternative method for bypassing the obstruction and providing a patent airway.

Once a patent airway has been established, controlled, artificial positive-pressure ventilation is initiated, assuming that spontaneous breathing is absent. Effective artificial ventilation can be accomplished by means of mouth-to-tube ventilation, self-inflating Ambu resuscitation bag, manual compression of the reservoir bag on a conventional anesthetic machine, or mechanical ventilator. With any of these methods, the ventilatory rate should be approximately 12/min. The procedures for assisted and controlled artificial ventilation are discussed in the first section of this chapter.

If the animal's heart has also arrested and cardiac compression (massage) for circulatory support is being performed at the same time, pulmonary and cardiac resuscitative maneuvers must be coordinated. Artificial ventilations will be effective only between chest compressions. Therefore a useful guide is to perform one deep ventilation every 5 sec (approximately once every fifth chest compression); or when one person is doing both cardiac and ventilatory maneuvers, it may be more feasible to provide two or three deep ventilations in rapid succession for every 15 heart compressions to minimize circulatory interruption.[16]

Mouth-to-nose ventilation can be used for respiratory arrest when endotracheal tubes or other equipment are unavailable. For this procedure, the animal's muzzle is grasped so as to produce an airtight seal of the lips; the head and neck are extended and the larynx pushed dorsally to straighten the upper airway and shut the esophagus; a paper towel or rubber glove is placed over the animal's nose with holes made at the nostril openings—this for sanitary reasons; and then air is blown into the animal's nose to inflate the lungs.

Regardless of resuscitative method used, ventilatory support is continued until the animal is breathing spontaneously and ventilating effectively. Any respiratory depressant drugs, including anesthetics, are discontinued. Narcotics can be reversed with antagonist drugs. If spontaneous respirations fail to occur or are feeble, a respiratory stimulant such as doxapram HCl (Dopram 2–4 mg/kg IV) may be used. Once spontaneous respirations have been reestablished, artificial ventilation can be discontinued, but oxygen supplementation is maintained. Cardiovascular support and continual monitoring of vital signs are essential. It is also important to treat or correct the underlying cause of the arrest.

ACUTE UPPER AIRWAY OBSTRUCTION

Etiology and Pathogenesis

Severe obstruction to the flow of air through the upper airway is a life-threatening emergency that demands immediate therapeutic intervention to prevent suffocation. Airway obstruction may be the result of an acute, sudden occlusion, e.g., a tracheal foreign body, or it may result from the gradual progressive encroachment of the airway by a chronic process which reaches that critical point where physiological reserve is exceeded, e.g., an enlarging airway tumor.[6] In other cases, e.g., laryngeal paralysis or elongated soft palate, the high inspiratory pressures required to overcome the resistance of a chronically obstructed airway, especially during exertion, can lead to acute obstruction from progressive airway edema.[15,36]

For purposes of this discussion, the upper airway is defined as nasal cavity, pharynx, larynx, trachea, and mainstem bronchi. Causes of life-threatening upper airway obstruction are listed in Table 3-5. The most frequently encountered conditions are airway trauma, airway foreign body, and anatomic abnormalities that result in airway blockage or collapse.[15] Tracheobronchial injury is discussed under "Thoracic Trauma."

Airway obstruction increases the work of breathing as greater effort is required to overcome the increased resistance to air flow. Resistance is inversely proportional to the fourth power of the radius of the lumen. This means that if the lumen of an obstructed airway is compromised by one-half there is a 16-fold increase in the resistance to air flow. The pathophysiological response to upper airway obstruction is biphasic.[6] The initial response to a mild or moderate increase in airway resistance is slowing of the respiratory rate and deepening of the tidal volume, accompanied by early failure of CO_2 elimination but an absence of hypoxemia. With more extreme obstruction, the alteration of respiratory mechanics is such that breathing is rapid and shallow, accompanied by CO_2 retention and progressive hypoxemia. This phase is usually accompanied by restlessness, apprehension, and distress. Obstructed respirations are characterized by reduced velocity of air flow, decreased peak flow, lengthened inspiratory and expiratory phases of breathing, and hypoventilation.[6]

Table 3-5. Etiology of Upper Airway Obstruction

Occlusion by foreign material
  Foreign objects
  Food (dysphagia, esophageal disorder)
Occlusion by vomitus, secretions, mucus, blood clots
Airway injury, inflammation, or swelling
  Tracheobronchial rupture
  Severe inflammation (feline viral rhinotracheitis, granulomatous laryngitis)
  Allergic (angioneurotic edema)
Occlusion by intrinsic masses
  Upper airway neoplasia
  Pharyngeal polyp (feline)
  Tracheobronchial granuloma due to *Filaroides osleri*
  Airway edema from elevated inspiratory pressure (complication of other obstructions)
Extrinsic airway compression
  Neoplasms of surrounding tissues (thyroid carcinoma, lymphosarcoma, heart-base tumor)
  Cervical cellulitis, abscess, or hematoma
  Tracheobronchial lymphadenopathy (neoplasia, mycoses)
  Left atrial enlargement (compressed left mainstem bronchus)
Upper airway obstruction of brachycephalic dogs
  Stenotic nares and misshapen nasal cavity
  Redundant pharyngeal folds
  Elongated, thick/edematous soft palate
  Everted laryngeal saccules
  Laryngeal collapse
Laryngeal obstruction—edema, spasm, paralysis, collapse
Tracheobronchial collapse
Tracheal hypoplasia

Clinical Signs

The most consistent signs of upper airway obstruction include increased inspiratory effort, apprehension and restlessness, and intolerance of exercise or exertion.[31,36] Cyanosis and acute collapse (syncope) may be features of severe obstruction. Tracheobronchial disorders are usually accompanied by cough, whereas laryngeal disease is often associated with voice change, and obstructions of the pharynx or larynx usually produce noisy stridorous or stertorous inspiratory sounds. Asymmetry of chest wall excursions and breath sounds may be seen with blockage of one mainstem bronchus. Dogs with chronic upper airway obstruction are predisposed to heat prostration.

Diagnosis

The diagnosis of upper airway obstruction is suspected on the basis of clinical signs, e.g., inspiratory dyspnea, stertor, and stridor. The absence of clinical or radiographic evidence for lower respiratory tract disease in a markedly dyspneic animal is also indicative of upper airway obstruction. In many cases, breed associations are helpful; for example, the brachycephalic breeds are associated with complex upper airway malformations, the Bouvier and sled dogs are associated with congenital laryngeal paralysis,[36,44] and toy and miniature breeds are associated with tracheal collapse.[31] The history may also be important, e.g., a history of recent cervical trauma or the observed aspiration of a foreign body. Chronic history of upper respiratory disease, e.g., tracheal collapse, may suggest that acute upper airway obstruction is due to recent exacerbation or complication of a chronic disorder. Diagnosis includes palpation of the cervical region for: (1) swellings (e.g., abscess, hematoma) or masses (e.g., thyroid neoplasm) that could cause extrinsic airway compression; (2) subcutaneous emphysema that could indicate laryngeal or tracheobronchial rupture; and (3) flaccid, flattened tracheal cartilages that indicate tracheal collapse.

The mainstay of diagnosis is direct visual examination of the pharynx, glottis, larynx, and trachea. Anesthesia may be necessary; a laryngoscope is helpful for visualizing the pharynx and larynx, and a bronchoscope is used for examining the tracheobronchial lumen. The oropharynx is examined for foreign bodies, tumors, and polyps; if the animal is unconscious, any accumulated food, mucus, or blood clots are cleared from the oropharyngeal airway. A light plane of anesthesia is used to observe the larynx for laryngeal abductor dysfunction, an indication of laryngeal paralysis, as evidenced by movements of the larynx and vocal folds that are absent or feeble, asymmetrical, or badly timed with respirations.[36,44] The larynx is also examined for obstructing foreign bodies, tumors, polyps, granulomatous proliferations (chronic laryngitis), everted saccules, or medial collapse of the arytenoids. The upper airway is always evaluated for an elongated soft palate, with or without secondary thickening and inflammation, that may be obstructing the laryngeal opening. Trachea obstruction, including foreign bodies, collapse, injury, tumors, and granulomas due to *Filaroides osleri*, can usually be visualized endoscopically or radiographically.

Radiography is ideal for the diagnosis of certain tracheobronchial obstructions, e.g., tracheobronchial collapse, intraluminal foreign bodies, and extrinsic tracheobronchial compression from mediastinal or heart-base tumors, left atrial enlargement, and neoplastic or mycotic hilar lymphadenopathy. Expiratory radiographs or fluoroscopy may be required for demonstration of expiratory collapse of the distal (intrathoracic) trachea or mainstem bronchi.

Treatment

The initial management of life-threatening upper airway obstruction is aimed toward establishing a patent airway, providing supplemental oxygen, and assisting ventilation if needed. Extreme care must be used in examining, manipulating, and radiographing an animal with a compromised airway; these procedures can precipitate rapid deterioration or even respiratory arrest. As a precaution, resuscitation equipment should be close at hand at all times. If death from asphyxiation appears imminent, a patent airway is established immediately by endotracheal intubation using chemical restraint if necessary. If the obstruction prohibits intubation, a tracheostomy is performed to bypass the blockage. Tracheostomy is particularly appropriate for severe obstruction due to laryngeal disorders. Any debris obstructing the oropharyngeal airway, e.g., food, vomitus, secretions, or clots, must be removed manually or by suctioning if the animal is unconscious.

Foreign objects, e.g., bones, marbles, nuts, pins, wood, or pieces of plastic, are sometimes aspirated into the trachea and may lodge at the bifurcation. These are removed as soon as possible. The animal is suspended with the head down and vigorously shaken to dislodge the foreign body while several quick, forceful compressions of the abdomen against the diaphragm are delivered to expel the object from the airway. If this maneuver is unsuccessful, the foreign body is removed endoscopically or surgically. When the object lodges within the larynx or proximal trachea, a tracheostomy can be used to temporarily bypass the blockage.

Laryngospasm, a tight closure of the glottis, is commonly seen in the cat from manipulation of the larynx, especially during attempted intubation. Acute laryngospasm is treated by pulling the tongue out, spraying the glottis with topical anesthetic, and inserting an endotracheal tube. Also, the glottis can be forced open to allow intubation by briskly compressing the thorax to produce a forceful expiration.[15]

Definitive treatment of many of the disorders listed in Table 3-5 includes surgery and is not discussed here. These include tracheobronchial rupture, tumors, polyps, laryngeal paralysis and collapse, everted laryngeal saccules, and redundant soft palate. However, for most of these, accompanying swelling and inflammation of the airway is a contributing factor to the onset of acute, life-threatening airway obstruction. Therefore in many cases the use of antiinflammatory doses of glucocorticoids and a cooled, humidified oxygen cage may be sufficient to relieve the animal's respiratory distress. Light sedation may help to promote more effective, slow, deep respirations by relieving anxiety, and bronchodilators may improve respirations by reversing reflex bronchoconstriction of lower airways. As mentioned previously, aminophylline may improve the contractility of inspiratory muscles that are fatigued from the increased work of breathing.[1]

LOWER AIRWAY OBSTRUCTION—ASTHMA

Etiology and Pathogenesis of Feline Asthma

Lower airway obstruction due to bronchial asthma, a condition of reversible bronchoconstriction, is one of the most important respiratory emergencies of cats. Feline bronchial asthma is in many ways similar to human asthma and presumably results from an inherent hyperreactivity of bronchial smooth muscle such that a variety of stimuli, including allergies, may trigger bronchospasm.[32] The increased reactivity of the airways in asthma is thought to be related to either the release of bronchoactive chemical mediators (e.g., histamine, kinins, SRS-A, eosinophil chemotactic factor, and prostaglandins) or to an abnormal neuromuscular control of airway caliber because of sympathetic-parasympathetic imbalance.[11] In human asthma there are several known precipitating factors: allergy, respiratory infections, airborne irritants and pollutants, cold air, exercise, certain drugs, and psychological stress. Asthmatic attacks have been precipitated in some cats by exposure to clay kitty litter dust, flea powders, and aerosol sprays; however, in most asthmatic cats a precipitating factor is not found.

The pathogenesis of lower airway obstruction and respiratory distress in asthma is based on three interrelated abnormalities that impinge on the airway: (1) bronchospasm; (2) edema and inflammatory thickening of the bronchial wall; and (3) filling of the lumen with mucus and eosinophil-laden exudate. The resulting narrowing or occlusion of the lower airways increases the resistance to air flow, which in turn leads to increased work of breathing, prolonged forceful expiration, and increased end-expiratory lung volume (air trapping).[11,32] The obstruction of airways in asthma is not uniform, which creates uneven distribution of ventilation and leads to ventilation-perfusion imbalance and hypoxemia.[11] The corresponding histopathologic lesions of asthma include hypertrophy of bronchial smooth muscle, goblet cell and bronchial gland hypertrophy, peribronchial and intraluminal accumulation of eosinophils, and emphysema (trapping of air in alveoli causes overinflation and rupture of alveoli).[9,32]

Clinical Signs of Feline Asthma

A triad of clinical signs characterizes feline asthma: cough, dyspnea, and wheezing.[9,32] These signs may vary in intensity, and they may be acute or chronic, episodic or persistent. Those asthmatic cats who are presented during a so-called asthmatic attack—an episode of severe progressive respiratory distress of sudden onset—are the cases that require immediate emergency management. These animals manifest extreme dyspnea, open-mouth breathing, gasping respirations with forceful expiration and abdominal heave, wheezing sounds, orthopnea, extreme anxiety, and sometimes cyanosis.[9,32] Hyperinflation may be detected by hyperresonant percussion. Cats with asthma are otherwise surprisingly free of malaise and other signs of illness, and many are clinically normal between episodes.

Diagnosis of Feline Asthma

The diagnosis of asthma is based on suggestive clinical signs, increased circulating eosinophils (in about 75% of cases), radiographic findings of bronchial thickening or hyperinflation (increased radiolucency, thoracic overexpansion, flattened diaphragm), and an increased number of eosinophils but absence of parasites in airway cytology specimens taken by tracheobronchial washing or endoscopic brushing.[32] Arterial blood gas analysis consistently shows hypoxemia, whereas CO_2 is normal or mildly reduced, except in the most severe cases in which CO_2 is retained.

Treatment of Feline Asthma

The asthmatic cat in severe respiratory distress must be considered a life-threatening emergency. Therapy includes oxygen administration, bronchodilator drugs, glucocorticoids, and maintenance of patient hydration.[11,32] Oxygen

Table 3-6. Drugs Used in the Treatment of Feline Asthma

Treatment	Trade Name (Manufacturer)	Preparations	Suggested Dosages
Xanthine bronchodilators			
Aminophylline	Many brands	Tab: 100, 200 mg Inj: 25 mg/ml	4–10 mg/kg PO q 6–12 h 2–4 mg/kg IV
Theophylline	Elixophyllin, Elixicon (Berlex), others	Liq: 3, 5, 20 mg/ml	2–8 mg/kg PO q 6–12 h
Oxtriphylline	Choledyl (Parke-Davis)	Tab: 100, 200 mg Liq: 20 mg/ml	4–8 mg/kg PO q 6–12 h
Sympathomimetic bronchodilators			
Epinephrine	Many brands	Inj: 1:1,000	0.1–0.2 ml SC, IM, IV
Terbutaline	Brethine (Geigy), Bricanyl (Astra)	Tab: 2.5, 5 mg	1.25–2.5 mg PO q 8–12 h
Isoproterenol	Isuprel HCl (Breon)	Inj: 1:200	0.5 ml in nebulizer
Combination bronchodilators			
Isoproterenol, ephedrine, theophylline	Isuprel Compound Elixir (Breon)	Liq	0.4 ml/kg PO q 6–8 h
Ephedrine & salts of theophylline	Bronkolixir (Breon), Quadrinal (Knoll), Tedral (Parke-Davis), Marax (Roerig)	Liq and tab	1 mg/kg (ephed.) PO q 8 h
Glucocorticoids			
Prednisolone sodium succinate	Solu-Delta-Cortef (Upjohn)	Inj: 10 mg/ml	5–10 mg/kg IV q 6–12 h
Prednisolone	Many brands	Tab: 5 mg	1–2 mg/kg PO q 12–24 h
Methylprednisolone acetate	Depo-Medrol (Upjohn)	Inj: 20, 40 mg/ml	20 mg IM q 2–4 wk

to alleviate hypoxemia is administered with as little stress to the animal as possible, preferably through an oxygen cage where the inflowing oxygen can be humidified. Bronchodilators are the mainstay of asthma therapy. Commonly used drugs and their dosages are in Table 3-6. Parenteral aminophylline and/or subcutaneous epinephrine along with intravenous prednisolone sodium succinate (Solu-Delta-Cortef) is used for initial management of a severe asthmatic attack. Aerosol delivery of isoproterenol via oxygen cage nebulizer may also provide emergency bronchodilatation. For less severe attacks and for long-term maintenance therapy, oral bronchodilators (methylxanthine, sympathomimetic drugs, or both) are used, with or without glucocorticoids (oral prednisolone or occasional long-acting injections of methylprednisolone acetate used sparingly). Glucocorticoids have a beneficial antiinflammatory effect, they may inhibit some of the chemical mediators of asthma, and they may potentiate bronchial smooth muscle relaxation. Maintenance of systemic hydration, using parenteral fluid therapy if necessary, is important for prevention of inspissation and impaction of mucus in the airways.[11]

Canine Asthma

Bronchoconstriction and pathophysiological features resembling asthma have been produced experimentally in the dog by bronchial antigenic challenge with aerosols of *Toxocara canis* antigens, pollen extracts, and specific hapten-protein conjugates.[13,14,21] However, a naturally occurring form of bronchospastic disease similar to human or feline asthma has not been well documented in the dog. Acute dyspnea and respiratory distress have been associated with a steroid-responsive interstitial lung disease of dogs that is characterized by diffuse pulmonary accumulation of eosinophils.[29] Although primarily interstitial rather than bronchial, this disorder may be another form of respiratory allergy (allergic pneumonitis).

THORACIC TRAUMA

Injury of the thorax and its contents resulting from high-impact trauma is a frequent cause of respiratory emergency. Surveys have shown that approximately 10% of dogs and cats presented as emergencies due to trauma have thoracic injuries.[26,27] This percentage is not likely to reflect the many additional trauma victims with thoracic injury who probably die at the accident scene and are never presented.

The potential seriousness of thoracic trauma should not be underestimated. An injury that is seemingly of minor significance at first glance may be associated with underlying life-threatening consequences requiring immediate diagnosis and treatment. Many trauma victims sustain multiple concomitant thoracic injuries or develop significant posttraumatic respiratory complications. Consequently, intrathoracic injuries and posttraumatic complications must be suspected and systematically searched for as part of the overall evaluation of any trauma victim.

Intrathoracic structures are normally well protected by a strong, resilient, spring-like rib cage.[25] Two forms of high-energy physical trauma are capable of causing significant structural damage to the thorax or its contents: (1) impact from forceful, nonpenetrating compressive or concussive blows (blunt trauma); and (2) penetration by sharp or high-velocity objects (penetrating trauma). Commonly encountered causes of blunt trauma in dogs and cats include motor vehicle accidents, falls from heights, running into stationary objects, kicks or blows inflicted by other animals and humans, and accidental trampling of small puppies or kittens. Penetrating thoracic trauma may result from motor vehicle accidents, running into sharp stationary objects, animal fights (bite wounds), stabbings, and gunshots.

With any type of thoracic injury, there may be damage to the chest wall, lung, tracheobronchial tree, diaphragm, heart, great vessels, thoracic duct, or esophagus. The resulting respiratory consequences may be classified as follows:[28,40]

1. Thoracic wall injury—painful rib fractures, unstable chest wall (flail chest), open chest wound (sucking wound), intercostal tear (lung hernia)
2. Airway injury or obstruction—fractured larynx, tracheal rupture, oropharyngeal occlusion with blood or vomitus
3. Reduced lung volume due to air, fluid, or viscera within the pleural space—pneumothorax, hemothorax, chylothorax, diaphragmatic hernia, mediastinitis/pyothorax (esophageal leakage)
4. Impaired alveolar function—pulmonary contusion and edema
5. Hypovolemic shock—blood loss due to hemothorax

Combinations of injuries are the rule rather than the exception, the number of injuries and their extent often determining the degree of respiratory embarrassment and the animal's chances for survival. The likelihood of the various types of internal injury in a trauma victim may sometimes be anticipated from knowledge of the circumstances surrounding the traumatic event.

Strategy for Initial Management

Emergency management of an injured animal is based on established priorities and following a systematic plan of action. The initial objective is to restore and maintain normal pulmonary and circulatory function. This is accomplished by establishing a patent airway, restoring chest wall integrity, reexpanding the lung, ensuring adequate ventilation and oxygenation, controlling hemorrhage, and supporting circulation and tissue perfusion.[18,25,28,40] After a rapid initial evaluation of the injured animal to determine the extent of the injuries, the following steps are followed as circumstances dictate:

1.   Establish a patent airway—remove obstructions, e.g., blood clots or vomitus, from the oropharynx (suction); intubate the trachea if necessary.

2.   Restore chest wall integrity—seal open ("sucking") chest wounds with an occlusive dressing and stabilize flail segments so the animal can ventilate, or use artificial ventilation.

3.   Reexpand the lung—restore negative intrapleural pressure by removing air or fluid (blood) from the pleural space with needle thoracentesis.

4.   Promote adequate oxygenation—administer oxygen by face mask, oxygen cage, transtracheal catheter, or mechanical ventilation.

5.   Maintain cardiac output and tissue perfusion—control life-threatening hemorrhage and administer intravenous fluids to restore circulatory volume (other measures for treatment of shock are detailed in Chapter 2).

6.   After the animal's cardiopulmonary function is stabilized, perform a more thorough physical examination (as detailed in the next section) and manage other serious injuries, e.g., intracranial injury, spinal injury, urinary tract injury, damage of abdominal organs, bone fractures, and severe external wounds.

7.   Observe and monitor the animal closely for new developments or changes in condition.

Physical Examination

The physical examination of the trauma patient should be methodical, thorough, and efficient, with particular emphasis on: (1) detecting life-threatening injuries that require immediate treatment; and (2) establishing a baseline so that the animal's condition can be monitored for change.[7] The presence of obvious injuries, e.g., fractures, should not distract the emergency clinician from a thorough search for subtle clues to intrathoracic injury. In one survey of dogs injured in motor vehicle accidents, over 50% of animals with intrathoracic injuries also had fractured bones (other than ribs).[26] To save time, the patient's history is obtained while the physical examination is in progress. Simple questions requiring concise answers are used to obtain information concerning the nature of the accident, the animal's condition since the accident, and the presence of any preexisting diseases. If the history or physical examination must be interrupted or curtailed in order to institute treatment for life-threatening conditions, it is completed later when the patient has been stabilized.

The physical examination should begin with an assessment of vital signs: level of consciousness, body temperature, pulse rate and quality, oral mucous membrane color and perfusion, and respirations (rate, depth, and effort).[7] An impaired or deteriorating level of consciousness may suggest severe intracranial (brainstem) injury, which could lead to feeble respirations or even apnea. A decreasing body temperature in the trauma victim is frequently associated with shock. Weak pulses accompanied by pallor and hypoperfusion of oral mucous membranes are also indicative of shock. Intrathoracic injuries commonly associated with shock include tension pneumothorax, hemothorax, intrapulmonary hemorrhage, and cardiac injury. Cyanosis of mucous membranes, although uncommon, indicates severe hypoxemia and respiratory failure.

Examination of the respiratory system itself for detection of traumatic injury is accomplished by: (1) inspection; (2) palpation; (3) percussion; (4) auscultation; and (5) radiography.[7,18,25] The entire chest wall is inspected for open ("sucking") wounds that freely communicate with the pleural space, so they can be sealed immediately. Other external signs of thoracic trauma are noted, as the location of cutaneous abrasions, bruises, hematomas, and wounds may pinpoint likely sites for intrathoracic injury. The oropharynx is inspected for accumulations of fluid, clots, or vomitus that could cause asphyxiation. This is especially important in unconscious animals or cases of severe epistaxis with postnasal drainage of blood into the pharynx.

Observation of respirations can yield valuable information. A significant increase in the rate, depth, and effort of respirations usually indicates impaired ventilation or gas exchange due to injury of the thorax or its contents. Dyspnea, especially if developing rapidly, is often the result of pneumothorax, pulmonary contusion, or both. Recognition of an abnormal breathing pattern is also important. For example, restricted movement of the chest wall because of painful rib fractures may give rise to a rapid, shallow, choppy breathing pattern; and periods of apnea or respirations that are abnormally slow, feeble, or irregular may be seen with brainstem injury.[7]

The symmetry of chest wall movements are also observed.[7,18] Paradoxical motion, caused by collapse of a portion of the thoracic wall on inspiration, occurs when multiple rib fractures create an unstable or flail chest wall. Decreased hemithorax movement (fixation) can be seen on the side into which abdominal viscera have herniated through a ruptured diaphragm. With tears of the intercostal muscles where overlying skin remains intact, a bulge under the skin at the intercostal space is created by countercurrent protrusion of the lung through the defect (lung hernia) during each respiration.[40]

Physical examination should include palpation of the chest wall for rib fractures, unstable (flail) segments, hematomas (usually adjacent to rib fractures), and intercostal muscle defects (tears) under intact skin. The entire chest wall and cervical region are palpated for the crepitus of subcutaneous emphysema, which, if developing rapidly, may indicate tracheobronchial rupture. The larynx and cervical trachea are palpated for pain or damage. Palpation of the cardiac impulse may reveal its point of maximum intensity on the chest wall to be at an abnormal location if the heart has been displaced by abdominal viscera herniated through a ruptured diaphragm.[7]

Percussion of each hemithorax is performed to detect abnormalities of resonance.[7,18] Hyperresonance (tympany) is an indication of pneumothorax. Hyporesonance (dullness) is associated with the presence of fluid (hemothorax, chylothorax) or abdominal viscera (diaphragmatic hernia) within the pleural space, or with lobes of lung that are nonaerated because of atelectasis, hemorrhage, or consolidation.

Auscultation of the thoracic trauma patient may reveal pulmonary fluid sounds (crackles or rales) from hemorrhage or edema in the lung, or dampening of the normal heart and breath sounds due to the presence of air (pneumo-thorax), fluid (hemothorax, etc.), or viscera (diaphragmatic hernia) within the pleural space. In addition, the heart and lung sounds in pneumothorax may seem distant and hollow. Areas of lung that are relatively silent may also be found with atelectasis or large areas of consolidation. The cardiac rhythm is also evaluated during auscultation. The onset of posttraumatic arrhythmia from myocardial contusion, however, is usually delayed until 12–48 hr after the injury.

Radiography

Thoracic radiography can be extremely helpful for the accurate diagnosis and assessment of thoracic injury.[23,24,38,40] The potential benefits, however, must be weighed against the risks of distressful patient restraint and positioning during the procedure. It is sometimes advisable to delay radiography of the injured animal until after emergency treatment measures have stabilized the patient's condition.

When evaluating thoracic radiographs for traumatic injury, systematic evaluation of all anatomic structures is essential.[38] Rib fractures are identified and a determination made of the position (displacement and distraction) of their fractured ends. Subcutaneous emphysema is recognized by air accumulation within the subcutis and fascial planes of the thoracic wall or cervical region, and pneumomediastinum by air contrast outlining the mediastinal contents, both of which indicate tracheobronchial rupture. Also with rupture of the trachea, a defect or interruption may be seen in the luminal air column at the injury site. Detection of fluid accumulation within the mediastinum suggests hemorrhage or esophageal rupture. The pleural space is evaluated for the presence of abdominal viscera or abnormal accumulation of air or fluid. Free air within the pleural space, seen as radiolucency surrounding the margins of collapsed lung lobes, indicates pneumothorax. Free pleural fluid, which causes opacification of interlobar fissures and blunting of the costophrenic angles, suggests hemothorax or chylothorax. The displacement of abdominal viscera into the thorax with discontinuity of the diaphragm indicates diaphragmatic hernia. The most frequent posttraumatic radiographic finding is pulmonary contusion, a condition of intrapulmonary hemorrhage and edema that causes patchy areas of opacity, and, if extensive, air bronchograms.

Monitoring

Laboratory data are of secondary importance in the initial resuscitation and management of thoracic trauma. After initial lifesaving emergency care, however, the monitoring of laboratory parameters, e.g., hematocrit, arterial blood gas, and electrocardiogram (ECG), may facilitate early detection of developing problems, especially bleeding, shock, respiratory failure, and cardiac arrhythmias.[18] Laboratory monitoring is especially effective when combined with monitoring of physiological parameters, e.g., temperature-pulse-respirations (TPR), urine output, and central venous pressure (CVP) or pulmonary capillary wedge pressure (via Swan-Ganz catheter) to assess circulatory status and guide fluid volume replacement.

Serial repetition of thoracic radiographs can be beneficial in monitoring the results of therapy and in detecting progressive accumulations of air or blood in the pleural space.

Large Airway Injury (Tracheobronchial Rupture)

Penetrating or nonpenetrating traumatic rupture of a large airway, e.g., larynx, trachea, or bronchus, often leads to severe dyspnea and rapidly developing pneumothorax, pneumomediastinum, or subcutaneous emphysema.[15,25,28,40] The impact of a forceful, nonpenetrating blow to the thorax while the glottis is closed can produce a blowout rupture of the tracheobronchial airway.[25] In humans, a higher incidence of blowout rupture in children has been attributed to the more flexible, resilient rib cage of young age. Airway injury in the dog or cat due to penetrating trauma occurs most frequently in the neck region as is associated with bite wounds or gunshot wounds that sever or damage the cervical trachea or larynx.[15,28,40] In the cat, a complete separation of the trachea within the cranial mediastinum has been attributed to a whiplash effect from fight injury.[28]

The consequence of rupture, laceration, or severance of a large airway is rapid escape of air into the surrounding tissues. Therefore this diagnosis should be suspected whenever a trauma victim has rapidly developing pneumothorax or subcutaneous and mediastinal emphysema. Suspicion of airway injury is increased with a history of deep trauma to the neck or a finding of penetrating external wounds around the cervical region. Dyspnea is also a common feature of large airway injury and in some cases is severe and life-threatening. Dyspnea may be the result of pneumothorax, loss of airway continuity when the airway has been severed, obstruction of the airway by displaced or damaged tissue at the injury site creating a flap-valve effect within the lumen, or external compression of the airway by hematoma and posttraumatic soft tissue swelling.[15,28]

Confirmation of tracheobronchial rupture is by radiography or bronchoscopy.[25,28,40] The radiographic defect is an airway lumen that is distorted, attenuated, or discontinuous at the damage site. When the injury site is not seen radiographically, bronchoscopic examination can be used to demonstrate the injury.

Treatment of large-airway injury may or may not require emergency measures or surgery.[25,28,40] In some cases, conservative medical therapy is successful, consisting of oxygen administration, cage confinement for activity restriction, and needle thoracentesis for removal of intrapleural air if pneumothorax is present. Severe obstruction or discontinuity of the larynx or trachea at the site of injury may require emergency intubation with passage of the tube past the injury site into the distal segment or tracheostomy below the injury. Pneumothorax in some animals can be severe, requiring immediate thoracentesis as a lifesaving procedure. If intrapleural air reaccumulates after aspiration, the thorax is continuously evacuated by a chest tube and one-way valve drainage system. Surgical repair of the defect is performed if it does not heal spontaneously within a few days. In cases where the trachea is severed, surgery is done as soon as possible rather than delayed. Cicatricial stenosis of the injured airway can be a sequela.[25]

Rib Fracture

Fractured ribs are a common result of blunt thoracic trauma. Single rib fractures are often asymptomatic and of minor clinical significance unless complicated by concomitant injury of thoracic soft tissues. The potentially serious complications of rib fracture are: (1) hemothorax due to bleeding from torn intercostal vessels, lacerated lung, or the exposed marrow cavity of the fractured rib; (2) pneumothorax from laceration of underlying lung by the jagged end of a displaced fractured rib; and (3) pulmonary contusion.[19,20,28,40] In addition, damage to adjacent intercostal soft tissues may cause swelling, hematoma, and subcutaneous and fascial emphysema of the thoracic wall.[40]

Because respirations are painful with rib fracture, many animals adopt a shallow, choppy breathing pattern in order to restrict motion of the thoracic wall.[28] The diagnosis of rib fracture is suspected by palpation of the deformity, pain, or crepitation (emphysema) of the thoracic wall and is confirmed by radiography.

Treatment of simple rib fracture is conservative in most cases. The intact adjacent ribs usually maintain alignment of the fractured rib.[28] Therefore isolated rib fractures that are minimally displaced and do not impair the integrity of the thoracic wall do not require surgery and should be permitted to heal without interference.[20] Cage rest and exercise restriction are adequate therapy for most cases. A light, padded support bandage may help reduce pain from fracture movement. Analgesics and intercostal nerve blocks can also be used to control pain, thereby promoting uninhibited cough and deeper, less-restricted breathing that will help prevent hypoventilation, atelectasis, retained airway secretions, and pneumonia.[19,20] Surgical reduction and stabilization using pins and wires is indicated in rib fracture cases where fragments are severely displaced, especially when laceration of the lung is likely.

Flail Chest

Fractures of several adjacent ribs in at least two places or proximal fracture of consecutive ribs in young animals with pliable costal cartilages result in an unstable, flail segment of chest wall that exhibits paradoxical motions during respiration.[19,20,25,28,33,37] During inspiration, negative intrapleural pressure draws the flail segment inward while the remainder of the rib cage is expanding; then during expiration the flail segment moves outward. This abnormal wall motion increases the work of breathing, causes ineffectual respirations, and results in hypoventilation and hypoxemia. Not only does the flailing side fail to expand properly and remain underventilated, but the higher intrapleural pressure during inspiration on the injured side shifts the mediastinum toward the uninjured side, restricting lung expansion in that hemithorax as well. Accompanying pneumothorax and contusion of underlying lung on the affected side are also common, further adding to the respiratory insufficiency of flail chest.[25] Flail chest occurs most often after motor vehicle accidents or "big dog/little dog" interactions when a small dog is attacked and has its rib cage entrapped and crushed within the jaws of a large dog.

The diagnosis of flail chest is made by observation of paradoxical respirations, palpation of the chest wall defect, and radiography.[25,28] Initial treatment to temporarily stabilize the flail segment can include positioning the animal in lateral recumbency with the flail side down, applying a padded elastic support bandage, or using lateral traction with towel clamps placed around the fractured ribs to pull the flail segment outward.[20,33,37] One author has recommended that the fractured ribs be attached by means of sutures to an aluminum rod frame or other orthopedic external support device for 14–21 days.[25] In severe flail chest cases, the animal can be intubated and positive-pressure ventilated to mechanically inflate the lungs and expand the unstable chest wall outward, in effect serving as an internal balloon splint.[19] As soon as the animal is able to tolerate surgery, severe flails are reduced and stabilized by internal fixation using pins and wires.

Intercostal Tears With Lung Hernia

With thoracic wall trauma, especially when a large dog seizes a small dog's rib cage in its jaws during a dog fight, the intercostal musculature is sometimes torn with the overlying skin remaining intact.[40] This allows the lung to protrude (herniate) through the intercostal defect into the subcutis, causing a visible bulge under the intercostal skin with each respiration. By itself, intercostal lung hernia does not significantly disturb respiratory function. Small intercostal tears may heal spontaneously, whereas large defects may eventually require surgical closure.

Pneumothorax

Pneumothorax, the accumulation of free air in the pleural space, is a frequent consequence of thoracic trauma in the dog and cat. Injuries that commonly result in pneumothorax are penetrating wounds of the chest wall or ruptures, tears, and lacerations of tracheobronchial airways or lung parenchyma.[20,25,28,40] It has been proposed that the pathogenesis of lung rupture from nonpenetrating trauma (e.g., motor vehicle accidents) involves closure of the glottis and tensing of the diaphragm at the moment of impact so that the transmission of the force of impact to the thorax compresses the air within the lung and airways, producing rupture.[20] In addition, shearing forces created by the abrupt change in velocity and different rates of acceleration/deceleration between fluid-filled and air-filled hilar structures may stretch and tear the airways.[20] Pneumothorax can also occur atraumatically from spontaneous rupture of pulmonary cysts, e.g., pneumatocysts of the lung fluke *Paragonimus kellicotti*, or pulmonary blebs and emphysematous bullae.[3,48] Iatrogenic pneumothorax may be a consequence of intrathoracic surgery, thoracostomy tube placement, thoracentesis, or overinflation of the lungs during overzealous artificial positive-pressure ventilation.[33]

The primary deleterious effect of pneumothorax is the loss of negative intrapleural pressure, which causes the lungs to collapse due to elastic recoil.[20] The resulting atelectasis leads to reduced lung volume, impaired ventilation, ventilation-perfusion mismatching, and decreased systemic venous return to the heart. The end result is hypoxemia.

There are three categories of pneumothorax: simple, open, and tension.[20,25,28,40] Simple pneumothorax is usually associated with nonpenetrating trauma that injures the lung or airways and allows escape of air into the pleural space, but shortly thereafter the defect seals itself so that no further air leakage occurs. Open pneumothorax is created by an open, sucking chest wound that allows communication of the pleural space with atmospheric air so that air enters the pleural space with each respiration. The usual causes are penetrating bite wounds, knife wounds, and projectile wounds. Tension pneumothorax is the most severe and potentially life-threatening type of intrapleural air accumulation. Air enters and is trapped in the pleural space during each inspiration but is not expelled during expiration because the torn edges of lung come together to form a flap that has one-way valve action. The consequence of this is a progressive increase in intrathoracic pressure above atmospheric pressure, which leads to severe compression atelectasis of the lung and impaired cardiac venous return. The resulting ventilatory impairment, hypoxemia, and circulatory collapse can be rapidly fatal.[25]

The diagnosis of pneumothorax is suspected on the basis of clinical signs and confirmed by radiography or emergency diagnostic thoracentesis. The physical features of severe pneumothorax may include: apprehension and restlessness; "gasping" dyspnea, orthopnea, open-mouth breathing, and cyanosis; reduced tidal volume and a fixed, hyperexpanded thorax with reduced range of ventilatory movement; heart and lung sounds that are diminished or distant and hollow-sounding; hyperresonance on percussion; and sometimes associated subcutaneous emphysema.[20,25,28,33] Clinical features of shock are also frequently present. The radiographic abnormalities of pneumothorax are lungs that are decreased in size and air content, causing them to appear relatively radiopaque with retracted lung margins surrounded by a widened, air-filled pleural space.[35] Shifting of the mediastinum when the animal is in lateral recumbency results in an apparent elevation of the heart off the sternum.

Simple, closed pneumothorax is often well tolerated by the animal and can be successfully managed by cage rest and careful observation in many cases, especially if clinical signs are mild or absent.[19,20,25,28,33] The air leak usually seals itself within hours, and the residual intrapleural air is resorbed over a few days. In general, dogs have a high tolerance for the effects of pneumothorax; experimental studies have shown that dogs are able to compensate through hyperventilation and chest expansion for intrapleural air volumes equal to twice the FRC without distress or hypoxemia.[17,22]

On the other hand, lifesaving emergency treatment may be necessary in animals with open pneumothorax or with closed pneumothorax in which considerable forceful ventilatory effort is required for breathing at rest, indicating severe or tension pneumothorax.[19,20,25,28,33] Open, sucking chest wounds are occluded with any dressing that quickly produces an airtight seal, e.g., a gauze pad or padded bandage covered with petroleum jelly.[37] Surgical débridement and closure of the wound can be performed later.

Severe pneumothorax, especially tension pneumothorax, is treated by immediate evacuation of air from the pleural space via thoracentesis to reestablish negative intrapleural pressure and allow lung reexpansion.[20,25,28] If dyspnea is severe, oxygen can be administered by face mask while preparing for thoracentesis. Air can be aspirated with a large syringe, three-way stopcock, and 18- or 20-gauge needle (or butterfly needle). After the penetration site has been clipped, surgically prepared, and infiltrated with lidocaine, the puncture is made at the dorsolateral aspect of the 7th, 8th, or 9th intercostal space, avoiding the caudal border of the rib where the intercostal vessels are located. Enough air is evacuated to stabilize repiration, and if necessary thoracentesis can be performed bilaterally.

If air reaccumulates rapidly during or after thoracentesis, the leak is considered serious and an indwelling chest tube is inserted for continuous or intermittent pleural evacuation.[18,20,28,33,37] Two basic types of tube can be used: (1) commercially available chest tubes with metal trocars; or (2) soft rubber Brunswick feeding tubcs that lack a trocar so they must be inserted using a curved hemostat. For cats and small dogs, 10–16 Fr. tube size is appropriate, and up to 28–38 Fr. can be used in large dogs. An area of skin over the lateral thorax, usually at the 7th–10th interspaces, is clipped and surgically prepared, and the thoracostomy site infiltrated with lidocaine. The chest tube is inserted through a stab incision in the skin at the junction of the dorsal and middle third of the 9th or 10th interspace; then it is advanced cranially for one or two interspaces through a subcutaneous tunnel to the 7th or 8th interspace, where it is punched through into the pleural cavity; finally, the tube is fed into the pleural cavity such that the fenestrated portion lies entirely within the thorax. The free end of the tube must be kept clamped or attached to an evacuation system. To secure the tube and prevent it from dislodging, a purse-string skin suture is placed and a nonrestrictive chest bandage applied. Chest tube placement is discussed further in Chapter 1.

The intrapleural drainage tube is then attached to a closed-chest evacuation system.[18,20] Simple intermittent manual aspiration using a syringe and three-way stopcock is adequate in many cases. The tube may be removed once negligible amounts of air are obtained, which is usually within 2–3 days. When intrapleural air reaccumulates rapidly, air is evacuated continuously using either a unidirectional flutter (Heimlich) valve or a system of underwater chest drainage bottles with controlled suction. Continuous drainage systems such as these should be closely supervised and therefore are more suitable for use in

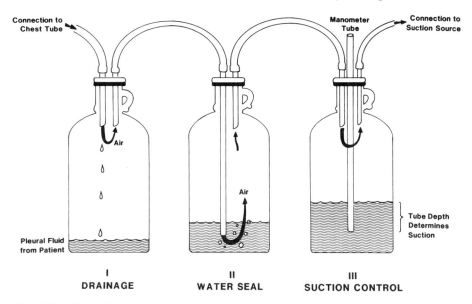

Fig. 3-2. Three-bottle system for suction drainage of the pleural cavity. Bottle I, a reservoir for blood or fluid draining from the pleural space, is optional and may be omitted in cases of pure pneumothorax (two-bottle system). In bottle II, the underwater seal provides for unidirectional flow of air evacuated from the pleural space. Continuous suction is applied to bottle III, and the depth to which the manometer tube is submerged regulates the suction pressure (centimeters of H_2O).

an emergency/critical care facility. Mismanagement of the chest tube or drainage apparatus can cause serious complications and even death.

The one-way flutter valve is a simple, relatively inexpensive means of continuous drainage of intrapleural air that at the same time allows maximal patient mobility.[8,18] It is most effective in large dogs. Small dogs, cats, and animals with shallow breathing due to chest pain may not generate enough pressure for effective drainage through the flutter valve. The most frequent malfunction is when blood and serum enter the valve and cause it to stick.

The underwater bottle drainage apparatus is considerably more complicated and confining to the animal, yet has greater versatility and reliability.[18] Tubing attaches the patient's chest tube to a bottle which contains sterile water and two built-in tubes that enter through an airtight cap (Fig. 3-2). Air from the pleural cavity vents into the bottle through the open end of the tubing, which is under water. This creates a water trap that acts as a one-way valve. With modifications, controlled suction can be applied to the system or a reservoir can be added for simultaneous collection of blood or fluid from the pleural space (Fig. 3-2).

Thoracotomy may be required in cases of pneumothorax where massive volumes of air accumulate more rapidly than drainage methods can accomodate or where severe air leakage continues beyond 2–3 days.

Hemothorax

Hemothorax, the accumulation of blood within the pleural space, may occur with any form of chest trauma that lacerates the lung parenchyma or ruptures intrathoracic vessels.[19,20,28,40] The seriousness depends on the rate and volume of blood loss. Bleeding from the venous circulation or the low-pressure pulmonary arterial circulation is usually self-limiting, whereas hemorrhage may be more severe from high-pressure systemic arteries, e.g., the intercostal or bronchoesophageal arteries.[19,20] Hemorrhage due to injury of the heart or great vessels results in massive hemothorax that is rapidly fatal.[28]

The two major consequences of hemothorax are shock due to loss of circulating blood volume into the pleural space and ventilatory impairment due to fluid compression of the lung.[19,20,28,40] As a general rule, in rapidly developing hemothorax fatal circulatory failure (exsanguination) occurs before the volume of pleural fluid that accumulates is sufficient to cause respiratory compromise. However, blood or fluid replacement therapy in the presence of continued bleeding may allow a larger intrapleural fluid accumulation, resulting in severe lung compression and ventilatory failure.

Clinical signs of hemothorax are attributed to shock and pleural effusion: dyspnea, tachypnea, weakness, pallor, and thready pulses.[19,20,28,40] The heart and lung sounds are usually muffled, and percussion of the ventral thorax may be hyporesonant. The presence of pleural effusion can be confirmed radiographically, and definitive diagnosis is made by aspiration of blood from the pleural space via needle thoracentesis.[19,20,28,40]

The treatment of hemothorax depends on the severity of bleeding and the patient's condition. The initial priority is rapid intravenous infusion of blood or fluid to correct hypovolemic shock. The pleural space is then drained by thoracentesis followed by cage rest (preferably in an oxygen cage), close observation of vital signs, and monitoring of serial hematocrits and total plasma proteins.[19,28] Sequential radiographs are also helpful for detecting progressive hemorrhage. Some clinicians prefer to place an indwelling chest tube to monitor for further bleeding.[20] Most cases of hemothorax respond to conservative management. In those few animals where significant bleeding continues, emergency exploratory thoracotomy is indicated in order to control the bleeding and prevent exsanguination.[19,20,28] If thoracotomy is necessary, the likely sites of bleeding may be determined from prior evaluation of radiographs for rib fractures and telltale areas of pulmonary contusion.[20]

Chylothorax

Chylothorax is characterized by the leakage of intestinal lymph (chyle) into the pleural space from a ruptured, obstructed, or anomalous thoracic duct or one of its collateral branches.[4,40] After traumatic injury of the thoracic duct, it often takes several days for a clinically significant volume of chylous effusion to accumulate. Thus there is usually a delayed onset of progressive dyspnea, which is the most frequent clinical sign of chylothorax.[19,20,40]

The diagnosis of chylothorax is based on radiographic detection of pleural effusion and aspiration of a characteristic milky, chylous fluid by thoracentesis.[4,40] Laboratory analysis of the fluid can confirm that it is true chyle.

Spontaneous healing of the injured lymphatic and resolution of effusion may occur with medical management.[19,40] This consists of: (1) pleural drainage by either periodic thoracentesis or continuous chest tube drainage; and (2) decreasing thoracic duct flow by exercise restriction (cage rest) and a low-fat diet supplemented with medium-chain triglycerides. If medical management fails, thoracotomy is recommended for surgical ligation of the thoracic duct (and any branches) at the point where it enters the thorax through the diaphragm. A higher success rate for the ligation procedure can be obtained by using pre- and immediate postligation lymphangiography to define anatomic abnormalities and to confirm that all branches of the duct were adequately occluded.[4]

Diaphragmatic Hernia

Diaphragmatic rupture with displacement of abdominal viscera into the thorax occurs when blunt trauma or falling from a height creates a transdiaphragmatic pressure gradient; this is caused by abruptly increased pressure on the abdominal side of the diaphragm, and an open glottis allows the lungs to deflate so that there is no counterbalancing force on the thoracic side.[28,40,42] This is in contrast with the situation when a forceful blow occurs against a closed glottis, which elevates intrapulmonary airway pressure causing pneumothorax.[19]

The severity of the clinical signs associated with diaphragmatic hernia depends on the size of the tear and the content and volume of the herniated viscera, most commonly liver, intestine, stomach, spleen, and omentum.[20,28,40,42,47] Animals generally tolerate the injury well, and many cases go unrecognized initially unless respiratory compromise results from displacement and compression of lung, or the entrapped viscera become incarcerated. Ventilatory impairment is caused by reduced lung volume (from displacement and compression by the herniated viscera), loss of diaphragm function, and a vicious cycle that as respiratory efforts are increased more bowel is sucked into the chest cavity. The clinical manifestations of diaphragmatic hernia may include dyspnea, tachypnea, abdominal respirations that are accentuated or paradoxical, reluctance to lie down (orthopnea), asymmetry of chest wall motion due to less mobility on the affected side, and an empty, tucked-up abdomen.[19,40,42,47] The heart and lung sounds may be muffled and the apex beat of the heart displaced; percussion often reveals a localized area of dullness. A life-threatening emergency situation is created by the acute intrathoracic dilatation of a herniated stomach or strangulation of herniated bowel.

Many diaphragmatic hernias are chronic, remaining undetected for months or even years after the traumatic event before causing clinical signs.[47] Some of the most frequent signs such patients eventually develop are pleural effusion, chronic gastrointestinal disturbances (anorexia, weight loss, and intermittent vomiting and diarrhea), and icterus due to liver entrapment.

Radiography is the most reliable method for diagnosing diaphragmatic hernia.[19,25,28,40,42] Radiographic features include loss of continuity of the diaphragm outline, increased soft tissue density in the caudal thorax, displacement of identifiable abdominal organs into the thorax (e.g., gas-filled stomach or loops of bowel), and forward displacement of abdominal viscera. If necessary, a barium contrast study can be used to demonstrate gastrointestinal tract displacement.

The treatment for diaphragmatic hernia is surgical repair. However, surgery should be postponed until the animal has been treated for shock and stabilized.[20,28,42] Surgery should not be delayed when the hernia is causing severe respiratory or liver failure, or when there is an enlarging gas accumulation in herniated stomach or intestine suggesting incarceration or obstruction. Acute intrathoracic gastric dilatation requires immediate decompression.

Pulmonary Contusion

Pulmonary contusion, a common bruise-like injury of the lung, occurs when a sudden forceful concussive blow to the thorax damages capillaries and small vessels within the lung leading to intrapulmonary hemorrhage and edema.[19,20,25,28,40] Blood and edema fluid leak into the interstitial space, flood the alveoli, and may even enter and obstruct adjacent small airways. Rupture and collapse of alveoli and decreased compliance in affected lobes may contribute to ineffective gas exchange. With extensive pulmonary contusion, the consequences are ventilation-perfusion mismatching and hypoxemia.[34]

The clinical signs of pulmonary contusion are dyspnea, tachypnea, pallor, and occasionally hemoptysis.[25,28,40] Whereas animals with only small areas of contusion may show minimal signs, those with extensive contusion or concomitant injuries (e.g., flail chest or pneumothorax) may present in life-threatening respiratory distress. Auscultation may reveal areas of pulmonary crackles along with areas of diminished breath sounds.[25]

The consequences of pulmonary contusion are usually fully developed, and the radiographic abnormalities become apparent within a few hours after the injury.[25,28,40] The diagnosis is made radiographically by finding patchy areas of alveolar density and air bronchograms. In severe cases diffuse consolidation of an entire lobe may be seen.

The treatment of pulmonary contusion is mostly supportive. Small contusions with mild to moderate respiratory distress may require no specific treatment, although enforced rest and oxygen therapy are often helpful. Follow-up radiographs usually show improvement within 24–48 hr and resolution within 3–10 days.[40] Antiinflammatory doses of glucocorticoids may be beneficial for reducing inflammation and preventing further edema, and bronchodilators, e.g., aminophylline, may improve ventilation by keeping airways open.[25] Diuretics (e.g., furosemide) have also been advocated for preventing or reducing pulmonary edema,[19,25,28] but their use should be restricted until circulatory status has been stabilized.

Fluid therapy during resuscitative efforts or treatment of shock must be carefully regulated in an animal with pulmonary contusion in order to prevent further edema in damaged lung.[25,28] Rapid administration of crystalloid fluids (>30 ml/kg/hr) has been shown to aggravate pulmonary contusion.[12] This is less of a problem with administration of colloids, e.g., blood or plasma. In the proper setting, e.g., an intensive care unit, Swan-Ganz catheter monitoring of pulmonary capillary pressure is ideal for precise control of fluid replacement.

Because contused areas of lung are likely sites for infection, the animal is monitored for pneumonia. Antibiotics are instituted at the first indication of pulmonary infection. In animals who are recumbent, frequent repositioning may help prevent hypostatic congestion, atelectasis, and pneumonia.[25]

When pulmonary contusion is extensive and ventilatory impairment is severe, mechanical positive-pressure ventilation via endotracheal or tracheostomy tube may be necessary, especially if respiratory function is deteriorating rapidly.[19,20,25]

PULMONARY EDEMA

Etiology and Pathogenesis

Pulmonary edema, the excessive accumulation of fluid within the lung, is an important medical emergency of the respiratory system. Rational therapy requires an understanding of the mechanisms that cause it. In the normal lung there is a constant transcapillary fluid exchange due to Starling hydrostatic and oncotic forces. The major force tending to push fluid out of the capillary into the lung interstitium is the capillary hydrostatic pressure. This transfer is facilitated by interstitial oncotic and negative hydrostatic forces but is opposed by plasma oncotic pressure. Under normal conditions, this extravasated fluid, which amounts to only a few milliliters per hour, is readily removed from the lung interstitium by pulmonary lymphatics, thereby preventing any fluid accumulation (edema). Fluid exchange is also influenced by the permeability of the alveolar-capillary membrane.

Pulmonary edema occurs when excessive transcapillary leakage of fluid into the lung interstitium overloads lymphatic drainage capacity. The causes of pulmonary edema are classified by pathophysiological mechanism in Table 3-7: (1) elevated capillary hydrostatic pressure, as occurs in left heart failure or overinfusion of fluids (see Chapter 2 for discussion of cardiogenic pulmonary edema); (2) decreased plasma oncotic pressure as occurs in hypoalbuminemic conditions; (3) altered alveolar-capillary permeability caused by a diversity of lung insults; and (4) lymphatic insufficiency due to obstructing neoplastic or inflammatory diseases of intrathoracic lymphatic tissues.[5] In addition, some forms of pulmonary edema are due to complex or poorly understood mechanisms, e.g., electrocution pulmonary edema, neurogenic pulmonary edema (sei-

Table 3-7. Mechanisms and Etiologies of Pulmonary Edema

I.   Increased pulmonary capillary hydrostatic pressure
   A. Cardiogenic (left-sided congestive heart failure)
   B. Fluid overload (overinfusion of fluids or blood)
II. Decreased plasma oncotic pressure (hypoproteinemia)
   A. Liver failure
   B. Protein-losing renal disease
   C. Protein-losing enteropathy
   D. Starvation/malnutrition
   E. Blood loss
III. Altered alveolar-capillary permeability
   A. Pulmonary infections (viral, bacterial)
   B. Toxic injury
      1. Inhaled toxins
         a. Smoke inhalation
         b. Aspiration of vomitus (gastric HCl)
         c. Toxic gases (>50% oxygen, chlorine, ammonia, etc.)
      2. Circulating exogenous toxins
         a. Snake venom, ANTU, paraquat, monocrotaline
         b. Endotoxins (endotoxemia, sepsis)
      3. Circulating endogenous toxins
         a. Uremia (''uremic pneumonitis'')
         b. Toxins released due to shock, thrombosis, or damaged tissue (pancreatitis)
   C. Osmotic injury from near-drowning (saltwater vs. freshwater)
   D. Disseminated intravascular coagulation (microembolic damage to capillary endothelium)
   E. Immunologic reactions (anaphylaxis, drug reactions, transfusion reactions)
   F. Pulmonary contusion (lung trauma)
   G. Shock and nonpulmonary trauma (''shock lung'')
   H. Fat embolism (after bone trauma)
IV. Lymphatic insufficiency (inflammatory or neoplastic lymphatic disease)
V.   Causes of pulmonary edema with multiple or undetermined mechanisms
   A. Electrocution (electric cord shock, cardioversion)
      1. Redistribution of blood from systemic to pulmonary circulation, acute left heart failure, neurogenic effects, and increased pulmonary capillary permeability
   B. Neurogenic (following seizures or head trauma)
      1. Adrenergic-mediated pulmonary capillary hypertension from pulmonary overcirculation and venoconstriction
   C. Drug-induced (?): ketamine HCl, anesthetics
   D. Rapid pleural drainage/lung reexpansion

Adapted from Bonagura JD: Pulmonary edema. p. 243. In Kirk RW (ed): Current Veterinary Therapy VII. W. B. Saunders, Philadelphia, 1980.

zures, head trauma), the edema occasionally seen after ketamine anesthesia in cats, and the edema triggered by pleural drainage and rapid lung reexpansion.[2,5]

The sequence of fluid accumulation is predictable for all types of pulmonary edema. The earliest accumulation is within the peribronchial and perivascular interstitium, followed by generalized interstitial edema. In the later stages, edema fluid crosses the alveolar epithelium and floods the alveolar spaces, which is more serious than interstitial edema because of interference with pulmonary gas exchange. Flooding of the airways with frothy edema fluid is rapidly fatal. Pulmonary edema adversely affects several aspects of respiratory function. Mechanical compression of small airways by the fluid and impairment of the surfactant system cause atelectasis. The lung interstitium, expanded by edema fluid, is less compliant, which makes breathing more difficult and alveolar ventilation less uniform. Alveoli filled with fluid are under-ventilated, and oxygen does not reach the alveolar membrane for diffusion. Thus the end result of pulmonary edema is ventilation-perfusion inequality and hypoxemia.

Clinical Signs

The major clinical signs of pulmonary edema are cough, hyperpnea-dyspnea, and moist rales (crackles). The animal may open-mouth breathe, appear anxious, and be reluctant to lie down. Severely impaired oxygenation may manifest as cyanosis. In fulminant edema, pink froth may be expelled from the nose and mouth.[5]

Diagnosis

The animal's recent medical history may provide the first clue to the diagnosis of pulmonary edema. Noncardiogenic pulmonary edema should be suspected when delayed-onset respiratory distress follows such clinical situations as electric shock, seizures, head trauma, thoracic trauma, circulatory shock, smoke inhalation, near-drowning, aspiration of gastric contents, heat stroke, sepsis, uremia, or rapid infusion of intravenous fluids.[5]

Physical examination is the initial step in determining whether pulmonary edema is cardiogenic or noncardiogenic, murmurs, gallops, or arrhythmias indicating heart disease. Physical examination may also reveal necrotic oral burns in victims of electric cord shock. Animals with decreased plasma oncotic pressure due to hypoalbuminemia usually manifest ascites, pleural effusion, or subcutaneous pitting edema.

Thoracic radiography is the most reliable means of clinically detecting pulmonary edema. Interstitital pulmonary edema initially results in linear interstitial densities with blurring of vascular margins. As edema becomes alveolar, a pattern of coalescing densities and air bronchograms becomes apparent. The distribution of edema may be of diagnostic significance: Cardiogenic edema is characterized by a bilateral perihilar-dorsal distribution (in dogs), often accompanied by venous congestion and left heart enlargement; noncardiogenic edema is characterized by a dorsocaudal (peripheral) distribution; and aspiration or bacterial pneumonia results in a ventral distribution within the cranial and middle lobe regions.[5]

Electrocardiography may also help differentiate cardiogenic from noncardiogenic pulmonary edema. In the critical care unit setting, a flow-directed, balloon-tipped, Swan-Ganz catheter (5–7 Fr.) can be used to determine pulmonary capillary-wedge pressure; and increased level (above 25–30 mm Hg) indicates a likely role for elevated pulmonary capillary hydrostatic pressure in the pathogenesis of the patient's pulmonary edema.[5] An arterial blood gas determination can be used to assess the severity of hypoxemia and establish a baseline for measuring response to treatment.

Table 3-8. Therapy of Pulmonary Edema

I.   Measures to improve ventilation/gas exchange
    A. Reduction of activity (cage rest): to decrease oxygen demand
    B. Sedation/relief of anxiety
        1. Morphine (dogs): 0.2–0.5 mg/kg SC, IM, IV
        2. Acepromazine (cats): 0.1–0.2 mg/kg SC, IM
        3. Valium (cats): 2–5 mg IV
    C. Oxygen therapy (40–50%)
    D. Ethyl alcohol nebulization (40%) into O_2 (prevents foaming in airways)
    E. Bronchodilator (e.g., aminophylline 6–10 mg/kg PO, SC, IV q 6 h)
    F. Endotracheal suctioning in severe cases to clear foam from airways
    G. Positive-pressure ventilation via endotracheal tube
        1. Manual or mechanical (PEEP, CPAP)
        2. Use only as a last resort when life-threatening respiratory failure persists despite other measures
        3. Criteria: $Pao_2 < 60$ mm Hg, $Paco_2 > 50$ mm Hg, persistent cyanosis, dyspnea, or tachypnea (all while breathing 60% O_2)
II. Measures to reduce capillary hydrostatic pressure
    A. Decrease circulating blood volume
        1. Diuretics (furosemide 2–4 mg/kg IV, IM, SC, PO q 6–8 h)
        2. Phlebotomy (remove 6–10 ml/kg, rarely used)
    B. Redistribute pulmonary blood flow to other circulatory beds
        1. Morphine (in addition to sedative effects, increases systemic venous capacitance)
        2. Furosemide (Lasix) (in addition to diuresis, redistributes pulmonary blood flow by increasing systemic venous capacitance)
        3. Vasodilators
            a. Na nitroprusside, nitroglycerin, hydralazine, prazosin, etc.
            b. Peripheral vasodilatation redistributes circulation away from pulmonary beds (noncardiogenic) and decreases resistance to outflow (afterload; cardiogenic)
    C. By improving cardiac function (cardiac output): Mostly used in cardiogenic edema
        1. Digitalis and other positive inotropes (dopamine, dobutamine)
        2. Antiarrhythmics to control arrhythmias, if present
III. Other therapy: corticosteroids
    A. To stabilize capillary permeability and microcirculation in permeability types of edema (efficacy is questionable)
    B. Prednisone 1 mg/kg q 12–24 h (or other glucocorticoid at comparable dose)
IV. Monitoring of response to therapy
    A. Physical examination (rate and depth of breathing, auscultation, mucous membrane color, etc.)
    B. Sequential arterial blood gas analyses
    C. Thoracic radiography
    D. Pressure data (pulmonary capillary wedge pressure)

Adapted from Bonagura JD: Pulmonary edema. p. 243. In Kirk RW (ed): Current Veterinary Therapy VII. W. B. Saunders, Philadelphia, 1980.

Treatment

The goals of therapy of pulmonary edema (Table 3-8) are to: (1) decrease oxygen demand (activity restriction); (2) improve ventilation and gas exchange; (3) reduce capillary hydrostatic pressure by decreasing circulating blood volume, redistributing pulmonary blood flow, and improving cardiac output; (4) stabilize capillaries that are abnormally permeable; and (5) control precipitating or complicating factors.[2,5]

The management of fulminant cardiogenic pulmonary edema, discussed in Chapter 2, usually encompasses oxygen therapy, activity restriction, morphine, intravenous furosemide, aminophylline, vasodilator drugs, and inotropic support with digitalis or infusion of catecholamine precursors (dopamine, dobutamine).

For noncardiogenic edema, the animal is placed at rest in a cooled oxygen cage (at a concentration that maintains the Pao_2 at >60 mm Hg) and treated with aminophylline, furosemide, and morphine. Aminophylline alleviates bronchospasm, improves contractility of fatigued inspiratory muscles, and induces a mild diuresis. Both furosemide and morphine may be beneficial because they redistribute pulmonary blood flow to other vascular beds; however, furosemide should be avoided in hypovolemic-hypotensive animals, and morphine is contraindicated in neurogenic edema because it augments intracranial pressure.[5] Vasodilator drugs (nitroglycerin ointment, hydralazine, etc.) may be used to counter the adrenergic-mediated systemic vasoconstriction associated with neurogenic pulmonary edema, thereby relieving the relatively overloaded pulmonary circulation. Corticosteroids may have a stabilizing effect on membrane permeability and microcirculation, although their efficacy in noncardiogenic pulmonary edema is controversial.[2,5]

Artificial ventilation is the treatment of choice for severe progressive pulmonary edema and hypoxemia unresponsive to these other measures, especially if Pao_2 remains <50–60 mm Hg and $Paco_2$ >50 mm Hg in spite of 60–100% inspired oxygen. Because edematous lungs tend to be stiff and noncompliant, pressures of 25–30 cm H_2O or more will likely be required to inflate the lungs. PEEP may be used to reduce atelectasis and improve oxygenation.[2,5]

An essential part of the management of noncardiogenic pulmonary edema is specific therapy directed toward any underlying condition that can be identified. Therefore disorders such as shock, sepsis, disseminated intravascular coagulation (DIC), uremia, pancreatitis, heat stroke, pulmonary infection, smoke inhalation, and CNS disease should be managed as discussed elsewhere in this book.

ACUTE BACTERIAL BRONCHOPNEUMONIA

Acute, fulminating bacterial bronchopneumonia in the dog and cat can be rapidly fatal if not promptly diagnosed and treated. Common isolates include *Klebsiella*, *Escherichia coli*, *Brodetella*, *Streptococcus*, *Pasteurella*, *Pseudomonas*, and *Mycoplasma*. Such pulmonary infections may be primary or secondary. Predisposing factors may include viral respiratory infection, aspiration of food or vomitus, thoracic surgery or trauma, chronic tracheobronchial disease, septicemia, prolonged recumbency, and compromised host defense mechanisms associated with many debilitating conditions.[30,39]

Bacterial pneumonia may be suspected on the basis of clinical findings, e.g., moist cough, dyspnea, fever, malaise, nasal discharge, and abnormal lung sounds (crackles, wheezes, silent areas). The diagnosis can usually be established by the results of a hemogram, thoracic radiography, and culture/cytology of a transtracheal or pulmonary aspirate.[30,39] A neutrophilic leukocytosis with left shift is typically found on the white blood cell count, and radiographs usually demonstrate pronounced alveolar pulmonary infiltrates with air bronchograms distributed in particular to ventral regions of the cranial and middle lung lobes. A specimen for culture and cytology is obtained by transtracheal aspiration/washing or by fine-needle pulmonary aspiration. Septic, mucopurulent inflammation is indicative of bacterial pneumonia.

Antibiotics are the foundation of therapy. The initial choice of an antibiotic may be guided by a gram stain of the transtracheal or lung aspirate; however, a culture and sensitivity test is recommended. Some antibiotics that are frequently effective in bacterial lung infections are cephalosporins, ampicillin-aminoglycoside combination, trimethoprim-sulfa, chloramphenicol, and tetracycline.

In addition to antibacterial therapy, measures to facilitate clearance of exudate and secretions from the lungs are essential. Such measures include: (1) fluid therapy to maintain systemic hydration, thereby preventing inspissation and retention of secretions; (2) airway humidification (vaporizer, nebulizer) to reduce viscosity of airway secretions; (3) mild exercise and chest percussion/vibration to promote cough and mobilization of exudate and secretions; and (4) use of bronchodilator drugs.[30,39]

For relief of hypoxemia, the animal with pneumonia should receive supplemental oxygen guided by arterial blood gas monitoring if possible. This initial phase of treatment is monitored very closely; the success of therapy is indicated by resolution of hypoxemia, fever, neutrophilia, and radiographic pulmonary infiltrates. Following the response to therapy by serial radiographs is very useful. Antibiotics are continued for a minimum of 1 week beyond remission.

REFERENCES

1. Aubier M, Detroyer A, Sampson M, et al: Aminophylline improves diaphragm contractility in man. N Engl J Med 305:249, 1981
2. Bauer TG, Thomas WP: Pulmonary edema. In Kirk RW (ed): Current Veterinary Therapy VIII. p. 252. Saunders, Philadelphia, 1983
3. Berzon JL, Rendano VT, Hoffer RE: Recurrent pneumothorax secondary to ruptured pulmonary blebs: a case report. J Am Anim Hosp Assoc 15:707, 1979
4. Birchard SJ, Cantwell HD, Bright RM: Lymphangiography and ligation of the canine thoracic duct: a study in normal dogs and three dogs with chylothorax. J Am Anim Hosp Assoc 18:769, 1982
5. Bonagura JD: Pulmonary edema. In Kirk RW (ed): Current Veterinary Therapy VII. p. 243. Saunders, Philadelphia, 1980
6. Bone RC, Nahum AM: Acute upper airway obstruction. In Moser KM, Spragg RD (ed): Respiratory Emergencies. p. 123. Mosby, St. Louis, 1982
7. Brace JJ, Bellhorn T: The history and physical examination of the trauma patient. Vet Clin North Am 10:533, 1980
8. Butler WB: Use of a flutter valve in treatment of pneumothorax in dogs and cats. J Am Vet Med Assoc 166:473, 1975
9. Carpenter JL: Bronchial asthma in cats. In Kirk RW (ed): Current Veterinary Therapy V. p. 208. Saunders, Philadelphia, 1974

10. D'Alonzo GE, Dantzker DR: Respiratory failure, mechanisms of abnormal gas exchange, and oxygen delivery. Med Clin North Am 67:557, 1983
11. Fish JE, Summer WR: Acute lower airway obstruction: asthma. In Moser KM, Spragg RG (eds): Respiratory Emergencies. p. 144. Mosby, St. Louis, 1982
12. Fulton RL, Peter ET: Compositional and histologic effects of fluid therapy following pulmonary contusion. J Trauma 14:783, 1974
13. Gold WM, Kessler GF, Yu DYC, Frick OL: Pulmonary physiologic abnormalities in experimental asthma in dogs. J Appl Physiol 33:496, 1972
14. Gold WM, Meyers GL, Daln DS, et al: Changes in airway mast cells and histamine caused by antigen aerosol in allergic dogs. J Appl Physiol 43:27, 1977
15. Harvey CE, O'Brien JA: Management of respiratory emergencies in small animals. Vet Clin North Am 2:243, 1972
16. Haskins SC: Cardiopulmonary resuscitation. Compend Contin Educ 4:170, 1982
17. Hemingway A, Simmons DH: Respiratory response to acute progressive pneumothorax. J Appl Physiol 13:165, 1958
18. Hunt CA: Chest trauma—the approach to the patient with chest injuries. Compend Contin Educ 1:537, 1979
19. Hunt CA: Chest trauma—specific injuries. Compend Contin Educ 1:624, 1979
20. Kagan KG: Thoracic trauma. Vet Clin North Am 10:641, 1980
21. Kepron W. James JM, Kirk B, et al: A canine model for reaginic hypersensitivity and allergic bronchoconstriction. J Allergy Clin Immunol 59:64, 1977
22. Kilburn KH: Cardiorespiratory effects of large pneumothorax in conscious and anesthetized dogs. J Appl Physiol 18:279, 1963
23. Kleine LJ: Radiologic aspects of thoracic trauma in the dog and cat. Part I. Compend Contin Educ 1:199, 1979
24. Kleine LJ: Radiologic aspects of thoracic trauma in the dog and cat. Part II. Compend Contin Educ 1:287, 1979
25. Kolata RJ: Management of thoracic trauma. Vet Clin North Am 11:103, 1981
26. Kolata RJ, Johnston DE: Motor vehicle accidents in urban dogs: a study of 600 cases. J Am Vet Med Assoc 167:938, 1975
27. Kolata RJ, Kraut NH, Johnston DE: Patterns of trauma in urban dogs and cats: a study of 1,000 cases. J Am Vet Med Assoc 164:499, 1974
28. Krahwinkel DJ Jr: Thoracic trauma. In Kirk RW (ed): Current Veterinary Therapy VII. p. 268. Saunders, Philadelphia, 1980
29. Lord PF, Schaer M. Tilley L: Pulmonary infiltrates with eosinophilia in the dog. J Am Vet Radiol Soc 26:115, 1975
30. McKiernan B: Canine and feline pneumonia. In Kirk RW (ed): Current Veterinary Therapy VII. p. 235. Saunders, Philadelphia, 1980
31. McKiernan B: Diseases of the canine and feline tracheobronchial tree. In Kirk RW (ed): Current Veterinary Therapy VII. p. 229. Saunders, Philadelphia, 1980
32. Moise NS, Spaulding GL: Feline bronchial asthma: pathogenesis, pathophysiology, diagnostics, and therapeutic considerations. Compend Contin Educ 3:1091, 1981
33. Morgan RV: Respiratory emergencies. Part II. Compend Contin Educ 5:305, 1983
34. Mosely RV, Vernick JJ, Doty DB: Response to blunt chest injury: a new experimental model. J Trauma 10:673, 1970
35. Myer W: Pneumothorax: a radiography review. J Am Vet Radiol Soc 19:12, 1978
36. O'Brien JA, Harvey CE: Diseases of the upper airway. In Ettinger SJ (ed): Textbook of Veterinary Internal Medicine. p. 692. Saunders, Philadelphia, 1983
37. Rodkey WG: Initial assessment, resuscitation, and management of the critically traumatized small animal patient. Vet Clin North Am 10:561, 1980

38. Spencer CP, Ackerman N: Thoracic and abdominal radiography of the trauma patient. Vet Clin North Am 10:541, 1980
39. Thayer GW: Pneumonia. In Kirk RW (ed): Current Veterinary Therapy VIII. p. 247. Saunders, Philadelphia, 1983
40. Ticer JW, Brown SG: Thoracic trauma. In Ettinger SJ (ed): Textbook of Veterinary Internal Medicine. p. 269. Saunders, Philadelphia, 1975
41. Tisi GM: Clinical pulmonary physiology. In Moser KM, Spragg RG (eds) Respiratory Emergencies. p. 27. Mosby, St. Louis, 1982
42. Toomey A, Bojrab MJ: Traumatic diaphragmatic hernias. Compend Contin Educ 11:866, 1980
43. Trinkle JK, Richardson JD, Franz JL, et al: Management of flail chest without mechanical ventilation. Ann Thorac Surg 19:4, 1975
44. Venker-van Haagen AJ: Laryngeal paralysis in young Bouviers. In Kirk RW (ed): Current Veterinary Therapy VII. p. 290. Saunders, Philadelphia, 1980
45. West JB: Pulmonary Pathophysiology—The Essentials. 2nd Ed. Williams & Wilkins, Baltimore, 1982
46. Williams JR, Stembridge VA: Pulmonary contusion secondary to nonpenetrating chest trauma. Am J Roentgen 91:284, 1964
47. Wilson GP, Newton CD, Burt JK: A review of 116 diaphragmatic hernias in dogs and cats. J Am Vet Med Assoc 159:1142, 1971
48. Yoshioka MM: Management of spontaneous pneumothorax in twelve dogs. J Am Anim Hosp Assoc 18:57, 1982

4 | Disorders of Fluid, Acid-Base, and Electrolyte Balance

Stephen P. DiBartola

Disturbances of fluid, electrolyte, and acid-base balance occur in a wide variety of medical emergencies, and their treatment is an essential part of the management of the patient. Often fluid therapy must be started before the diagnosis has been established, requiring the clinician to make therapeutic decisions based on a careful history and physical examination. Recognition of the fluid and electrolyte disturbances likely to be present in a given disease state depends on an understanding of the pathophysiology of the disease in question.

DISTURBANCES OF FLUID BALANCE

Total body water represents approximately 60% of body weight in the adult animal and is divided into intracellular water (30% of body weight) and extracellular water (30% of body weight). Extracellular water is divided into plasma volume (5% of body weight) and interstitial volume (25% of body weight). Variations in total body water are due to differences in body fat, sex, and age. Obese animals have less total body water than lean animals of the same weight, and male animals have slightly more than females. The total body water of neonates may be as great as 70–80% of body weight.

Maintenance of normal fluid balance depends on regulation of fluid influx via the gastrointestinal tract and efflux via the gastrointestinal tract, lungs, skin, and kidneys. Dehydration occurs when water and electrolyte efflux ex-

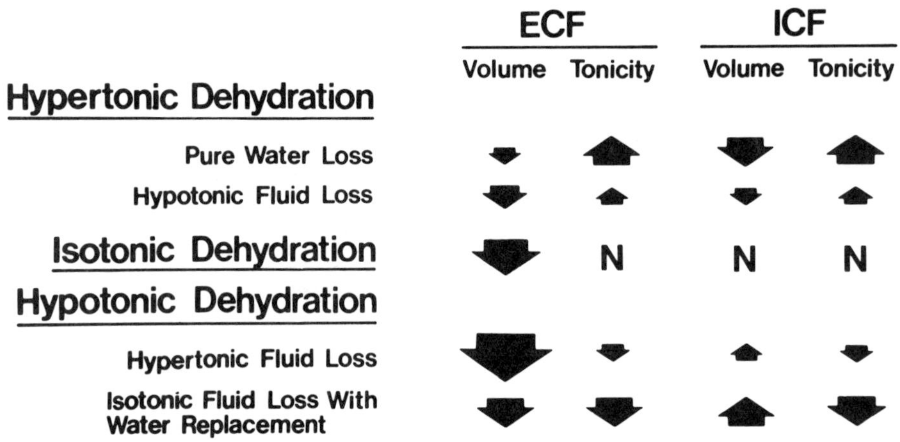

	ECF Volume	ECF Tonicity	ICF Volume	ICF Tonicity
Hypertonic Dehydration				
Pure Water Loss	↓	↑	↓	↑
Hypotonic Fluid Loss	↓	↑	↓	↑
Isotonic Dehydration	↓	N	N	N
Hypotonic Dehydration				
Hypertonic Fluid Loss	↓↓	↓	↑	↓
Isotonic Fluid Loss With Water Replacement	↓	↓	↑	↓

Fig. 4-1. Changes in volume and tonicity of body fluid compartments with different types of dehydration. (ECF) extracellular fluid. (ICF) intracellular fluid. (N) normal. (Reproduced by permission from Muir WW, DiBartola SP: Fluid therapy. In Kirk RW (ed): Current Veterinary Therapy VIII. Saunders, Philadelphia, 1983.)

ceeds influx. Dehydration is classified according to the type of fluid lost and the tonicity of the fluid remaining in the body (Fig. 4-1). Pure water loss and hypotonic fluid loss result in hypertonic dehydration with an increase in the tonicity of the remaining body fluids. Loss of hypertonic fluid or isotonic fluid with water replacement results in hypotonic dehydration wherein the remaining body fluids are hypotonic. In isotonic dehydration, there is no osmotic stimulus for water movement between body compartments, and the remaining body fluids are unchanged in tonicity. In hypotonic dehydration, the intracellular compartment is actually overhydrated.

The distribution of fluids among body fluid compartments depends on the ionic composition of the fluid and its osmolality. Osmolality reflects only the number of osmotically active particles without regard to their permeability across biologic membranes. On the other hand, tonicity reflects also the permeability of particles and may be thought of as effective osmolality.[7] For example, a 0.6 M glucose solution would be considered hyperosmotic and hypertonic because the solute in question is relatively impermeant. However, a 0.6 M urea solution is hyperosmotic but not hypertonic because urea is freely permeant across plasma membranes.

The osmolal gap[8] is defined as the difference between the measured serum osmolality and that derived from the following calculation:

$$P_{osm} = 1.86\,(Na^+ + K^+) + \frac{glucose}{18} + \frac{BUN}{2.8}$$

The osmolal gap increases when unmeasured osmotically active solutes are present in plasma. Examples include ethylene glycol and its metabolites, lactate, mannitol, and radiographic dyes.

Evaluation of Hydration

A decision regarding the need for fluid therapy is based on an assessment of hydration which is made by evaluating the history, physical examination, and simple laboratory tests. A carefully obtained history aids in the determination of the time period over which fluid losses have occurred and their magnitude. The route of fluid loss often suggests the patient's likely electrolyte and acid-base derangements. Information about food and water intake, gastrointestinal losses (vomiting, diarrhea), urinary losses (polyuria), and traumatic losses (blood loss, burns) is obtained from the owner. Excessive insensible losses (increased panting, fever) and third space losses (effusions, sequestration of fluid in an obstructed bowel segment) can be determined from a careful physical examination. The clinician's knowledge of a suspected disease process aids in predicting the composition of the fluid lost. For example, chronic vomiting of stomach contents would be expected to result in sodium, potassium, hydrogen ion, and chloride losses and metabolic alkalosis, whereas uncontrolled diabetes mellitus would be expected to result in sodium and potassium losses and metabolic acidosis.

The physical findings associated with fluid losses of 5–15% of body weight vary from subtle changes (5%) to signs of hypovolemic shock and impending death (15%).[4] The hydration deficit is estimated by evaluating skin turgor, moistness of mucous membranes, position of the eyes in their orbits, the heart rate, and the character of the peripheral pulses. The clinical assessment of hydration may be quite inaccurate. Detection of dehydration by skin turgor depends on the animal's skin turgor prior to dehydration, the position of the animal when the skin is checked, the site of evaluation, and the amount of subcutaneous fat.[12] Skin turgor is checked over the lumbar region with the animal in a standing position. Obese animals may appear well hydrated due to excessive subcutaneous fat despite the presence of dehydration. Emaciated animals often appear more dehydrated than they actually are due to lack of subcutaneous and retrobulbar fat. Persistent panting can dry oral mucous membranes and further confuse the evaluation. When dehydration becomes severe (12–15% body weight), signs of hypovolemic shock appear. These include depression, cool extremities, tachycardia, rapid and weak pulses, and prolonged capillary refill time.

Body weight recorded serially is an excellent indicator of hydration status, especially when fluid loss has been acute and the previous body weight has been recorded. Loss of 1 kg body weight indicates a fluid deficit of 1 L. An anorexic animal may lose 0.1–0.3 kg/day/1,000 calories energy requirement.[9] Losses in excess of this amount indicate fluid loss.

The hematocrit (PCV), total plasma proteins (TPP), and urine specific gravity are simple laboratory tools which can aid in the assessment of hydration, but it is essential to obtain these parameters before initiating fluid therapy. PCV and TPP are evaluated together to minimize errors of interpretation. Urine specific gravity before fluid therapy is helpful in the preliminary evaluation of renal function. Providing diuretics have not been given and medullary washout

Table 4-1. Components of Fluid Therapy

Hydration deficit (replacement requirement)
  Body weight (lb) × % dehydration (as a decimal) × 500^a = deficit (ml)
  Body weight (kg) × % dehydration (as a decimal) = deficit (L)
Maintenance requirement (40–60 ml/kg/day)
  Sensible losses (urine output): 27–40 ml/kg/day
  Insensible losses (fecal, cutaneous, respiratory): 13–20 ml/kg/day
Contemporary (ongoing) losses (e.g., vomiting, diarrhea, polyuria)

^{a} 500 ml = 1 lb fluid
Reproduced by permission from Muir WW, DiBartola SP: Fluid therapy. In Kirk RW (ed): Current Veterinary Therapy VIII, Saunders, Philadelphia, 1983.

of solute is not present, urine specific gravity should be high (>1.048) in a markedly dehydrated dog if renal function is normal.[12] After fluid therapy has begun and hydration is restored, the urine specific gravity should fall into the isosthenuric range.

Administering Fluid Therapy

Most animals requiring fluid therapy can be managed with one of three parenteral fluids: lactated Ringer's solution, normal saline (0.9%), or 5% dextrose in water. Supplementation with KCl may be necessary when losses include large amounts of potassium. The clinician should attempt to replace fluid losses with a fluid which is similar in volume and composition to that which has been lost. Knowledge of the route of fluid loss and the underlying disease process aids in the selection of fluid type.

The route of fluid therapy depends on the nature of the clinical disorder, its severity, and its duration. When fluid loss has been sudden or extensive, the intravenous route is preferred. The subcutaneous route is convenient for maintenance fluid therapy in cats and small dogs. This route is not recommended in extremely dehydrated animals because absorption may be erratic. The volume of fluid which may be given subcutaneously is limited by skin elasticity, and only isotonic fluids should be used.

The rate of fluid administration is determined by the magnitude and rapidity of fluid loss. Rapid or extensive losses require rapid replacement. When necessary, fluids can be given safely at a rate of one blood volume per hour (100 ml/kg/hr).[5] When fluids are given rapidly, it is essential to monitor cardiovascular function. It is not usually necessary to replace the hydration deficit rapidly in chronic diseases. Instead, the hydration deficit is calculated, the daily maintenance requirement added to this, and the total amount given over 24 hr. An alternative is to replace the hydration deficit over the first few hours followed by maintenance therapy.

The initial assessment of hydration determines the volume of fluid needed to replace the hydration deficit (replacement requirement) (Table 4-1). This calculation underestimates the fluid requirement in hypovolemic shock, wherein the volume of fluid required for treatment may be two to four times the volume of blood lost due to vasodilation and increased volume of distribution of fluid.[2] Maintenance fluid requirements are calculated on the basis of 40–60 ml/kg/day with large dogs requiring the lower limit and small dogs and cats the upper limit.[4] Approximately 67% of the maintenance requirement represents sensible fluid losses (urine output) and 33% insensible losses (fecal, cutaneous, and respiratory losses).

In addition to the hydration deficit and maintenance needs, contemporary or ongoing losses must be estimated and added to the daily fluid requirements. These may include fluid lost through vomiting, diarrhea, polyuria, large wounds or burns, peritoneal or pleural losses, panting, fever, and blood loss. During surgery, careful attention is given to the amount of blood lost, drying of exposed tissues, and effusions removed by suction. Blood lost at surgery is estimated, and 3 ml crystalloid solution is administered for each milliliter of blood lost.

Monitoring Fluid Therapy

Repeated assessment of the patient by observation of clinical signs and determination of weight, urine output, PCV, TPP, and urine specific gravity is necessary for making appropriate readjustments of fluid needs. Reasons for failure to achieve rehydration include calculation errors, underestimation of the original hydration deficit, contemporary losses greater than appreciated, infusion of fluid at an excessively rapid rate with consequent diuresis and obligatory urine loss, technical problems with the intravenous catheter, sensible losses larger than appreciated (e.g., polyuria), and insensible losses larger than appreciated (e.g., fever, panting). Failure to achieve rehydration is an indication to increase the volume of fluid administered if renal and cardiovascular function are adequate. As a rule, the daily fluid volume may be increased by an amount equal to 5% of body weight if the initial infusion fails to restore hydration.

Fluid therapy is monitored by performing physical examinations daily on patients receiving fluids. The animal is weighed at least once a day using the same scale. A gain or loss of 1 kg may be considered an excess or deficit of 1 L of fluid.

When fluids are administered intravenously at a rapid rate and renal function is in question, urine output must be monitored. Normal urine output is 1–2 ml/kg/hr. After the hydration deficit has been replaced, the daily fluid requirement may be divided into six 4-hr aliquots if the status of renal function is uncertain. The calculated 4-hr insensible volume plus a volume equal to the urine output of the previous 4 hr is admiinistered over each 4-hr period. The risk of overhydration is minimized, and fluid therapy will keep pace with urine output even if oliguria is present. If oliguria persists, an increase in the daily fluid volume by an amount equal to 5% of body weight may be justified on the assumption that the initial clinical estimation of hydration was inaccurate. If oliguria does not respond to mild volume expansion, administration of increased volumes of fluid may be detrimental.

Measurement of central venous pressure (CVP) with a jugular catheter positioned at the level of the right atrium allows cardiac function to be monitored. Normal CVP is 0–5 cm H_2O. A progressive increase in CVP during fluid therapy is an indication to decrease the rate of fluid administration. Sudden increases in CVP may indicate a failure of the cardiovascular system to effectively handle the fluid load and could result in pulmonary edema due to left heart failure. In addition to the volume of fluid administered, heart rate, vascular capacity, and cardiac contractility may affect CVP. A reduction in any of these three parameters may cause an increase in CVP. An even more accurate indication of impending pulmonary edema is measurement of pulmonary capillary wedge pressure using a Swan-Ganz catheter, but this technique is more cumbersome to perform.

Signs of overhydration occur when fluid is administered too rapidly. These include serous nasal discharge, chemosis, restlessness, cough, dyspnea, pulmonary edema, ascites, polyuria, exophthalmos, diarrhea, and vomiting.[5] The expected laboratory abnormalities are a reduction in PCV and TPP and an increase in body weight.

DISTURBANCES OF ACID-BASE BALANCE

Acid-Base Balance

Acid-base balance is evaluated by determining the following blood parameters:

pH
Partial pressure of carbon dioxide (P_{CO_2})
Total CO_2 content
Bicarbonate concentration (HCO_3)
Base deficit (or excess)

Each of these parameters is defined in the following discussion because they form the basis for understanding and treating disturbances of acid-base balance.

Most electrolytes in the extracellular fluid are present in milliequivalent amounts: 10^{-3} equivalent (Eq). Hydrogen ions are present in nanoequivalent amounts (10^{-9} Eq) however; and so to facilitate discussion of hydrogen ion activity the term pH has become established. The pH of a solution is the negative logarithm of its hydrogen ion concentration, and thus pH and [H^+] are inversely related.

$$pH = -\log [H^+]$$

In the normal animal, [H^+] is 40 nEq/L, or 4×10^{-8} Eq/L, and

$$pH = -\log 4 \times 10^{-8} = 7.4$$

The relationship between hydrogen ion concentration and pH is not linear.

However, in the pH range of 7.2–7.5 the relationship is approximately linear, and a 0.01 unit pH change corresponds to an inverse 1 nEq/L change in hydrogen ion concentration.[19]

The terms acidemia and alkalemia refer to the pH of the patient's blood, and the terms acidosis and alkalosis refer to the processes which cause acid or alkali to accumulate in the body. The distinction here, for example, is that a mild metabolic acidosis may exist with a pH which is lower than normal for the individual but not outside the established normal range. Such a patient would be acidotic but not acidemic.

Buffers are substances which can absorb or donate protons and thus mitigate but not eliminate pH changes when acids or alkali are added to a system. Weak acids behave as buffers. Because of its central importance in the body's defense against acid-base disturbances, the bicarbonate-carbonic acid buffer system is routinely studied in the clinical evaluation of acid-base disorders. The ability of alveolar ventilation to regulate P_{CO_2} (and thus pH) increases the efficiency of this system. Changes in alveolar ventilation occur within minutes, and respiratory compensation for an acid load is complete within 12–24 hr.

Carbon dioxide produced in tissues undergoes hydration to H_2CO_3 in the presence of carbonic anhydrase (CA) in erythrocytes and renal tubular cells. Carbonic acid then dissociates to H^+ and HCO_3^-.

Lungs

$$CO_2 + H_2O \overset{CA}{\rightleftharpoons} H_2CO_3 \rightleftharpoons H^+ + HCO_3^-$$

Tissues

metabolic processes

Carbon dioxide produced in the tissues is carried in the blood to the lungs in three ways. The majority enters erythrocytes and is hydrated in the presence of carbonic anhydrase to H_2CO_3, which dissociates to H^+ and HCO_3^-. The H^+ is buffered by hemoglobin, and HCO_3^- leaves the erythrocyte and enters plasma in exchange for chloride. A small amount of CO_2 combines with amino groups on hemoglobin, and a small amount is dissolved in plasma. The amount of CO_2 dissolved in plasma is proportional to the partial pressure of CO_2 in the blood (P_{CO_2}). Therefore, based on a solubility coefficient of 0.03 for CO_2

$$0.03 \ P_{CO_2} \ (mm \ Hg) = \text{dissolved } CO_2 \ (mEq/L)$$

Total CO_2 is determined by adding a strong acid to blood and measuring the amount of CO_2 released. Thus total CO_2 = dissolved CO_2 + H_2CO_3 + HCO_3^-. Because the amount of H_2CO_3 is negligible (500 molecules of dissolved CO_2 for each molecule of H_2CO_3), HCO_3^- can be estimated by subtracting $0.03 \ P_{CO_2}$ from total CO_2. The term base deficit or excess refers to the number of milliequivalents of acid or base required to titrate blood back to pH 7.4 under standard conditions.

The Henderson-Hasselbalch equation defines the relationship between pH, P_{CO_2}, and HCO_3^- based on a pKa of 6.1 and emphasizes that pH is determined by the bicarbonate/dissolved CO_2 ratio:

$$pH = 6.1 + \log \frac{[HCO_3^-]}{0.03\ P_{CO_2}}$$

This equation may be rearranged to reflect the actual H^+ concentration:

$$[H^+] = 24 \frac{P_{CO_2}}{[HCO_3^-]}$$

In most instances the laboratory measures pH and P_{CO_2}, and then HCO_3^- is calculated from the Henderson-Hasselbalch equation.

The normal endogenous acid load comes from the metabolism of proteins, which releases sulfates and phosphates, and from the incomplete oxidation of energy stores, which produces organic acids. The normal rate of endogenous acid production in man is 1 mEq/kg/day.[19] Approximately half of this acid load is buffered by HCO_3^- and the remainder by HPO_4^{2-}, hemoglobin, and other proteins. Over periods of long-term acid loading, calcium carbonate from bone becomes an important source of buffer. Through these buffers, the acid load is accommodated and pH changes minimized; however, eventually the depleted buffers must be restored by regeneration of bicarbonate and excretion of hydrogen ions. This work is done by the kidneys. Bicarbonate is the only buffer which can be consumed during buffering and then be regenerated and returned to the body by the kidney.

The kidneys reabsorb filtered bicarbonate and excrete the daily endogenous acid load as titratable acidity (phosphate) and ammonium through the process of H^+ secretion. If secreted H^+ titrates filtered bicarbonate, the net effect is reclamation of filtered bicarbonate. This process occurs largely in the proximal tubule where 90% of filtered bicarbonate is reabsorbed. If secreted H^+ combines with phosphate or ammonia, there is net acid excretion and regeneration of bicarbonate stores which were depleted through buffering. These processes occur mainly in the distal tubule and collecting ducts. The amount of H^+ excreted with phosphate is relatively constant and dependent on the amount of phosphate excreted.

Enzymatic release of NH_3 from glutamine can be increased by the kidney under conditions of acidosis wherein an increased acid load necessitates increased H^+ excretion. This adaptive mechanism takes 3–5 days to reach maximal effect. The ability of the kidney to augment ammonia excretion is the main adaptive response of the kidney to an acid load, and ammonia excretion can be increased up to five-fold in metabolic acidosis.[23] Ammonia is a strong base and very effectively binds H^+ in tubular fluid. The resulting ammonium ion (NH_4^+) is a charged particle and cannot easily diffuse back into the renal tubular cell. Hence total H^+ secretion by the kidney includes that required for bicarbonate reabsorption as well as that required for titratable acidity and ammonium excretion.

Several factors affect renal H^+ excretion. A major function of the kidney is to protect the extracellular fluid volume, and this is accomplished by conservation of sodium and water. The kidney reabsorbs sodium along with a resorbable anion (chloride or bicarbonate) or in exchange for another cation (hydrogen or potassium). Normally, chloride is quantitatively most important in this process, and in states of relative chloride depletion the kidney's attempt to conserve sodium may result in excessive reclamation of bicarbonate as well as excretion of hydrogen and potassium ions. Arterial pH affects acid secretion with lowered pH causing increased H^+ excretion. When plasma K^+ is lowered K^+ leaves cells and H^+ enters them, and increased H^+ in renal tubular cells results in increased H^+ excretion and HCO_3^- regeneration.

Sampling for Acid-Base Evaluation

Samples for blood gas evaluation are taken from the femoral artery in the dog and cat. The site should be clipped and surgically prepared. A 3-cc syringe with a 23- to 25-gauge $\frac{1}{2}$–$\frac{5}{8}$ inch needle is coated with a small amount of heparin (less than 0.1 cc or 100 units). The artery is located by palpating the femoral pulse and is immobilized beneath the first and second fingers of the operator's hand. Needle puncture is made with the syringe directed perpendicular to the course of the vessel. At least 1 cc of blood is withdrawn, and the vessel is compressed for 5 min after removing the needle to prevent hematoma formation. All air bubbles are dislodged by tapping the barrel and expelling any air from the hub of the needle. The needle is inserted into a rubber stopper to prevent exposure to room air. If the sample cannot be evaluated immediately, the syringe is placed in crushed ice. Samples are stable for up to 2 hr at 4°C, but P_{CO_2} values begin to increase and the pH to decrease after 20–30 min at room temperature due to leukocyte metabolism.[18] Air bubbles cause elevations of P_{O_2}. P_{O_2} values begin to decrease after 30 min of storage at either 4° or 25°C.

Arterial samples are preferred over venous ones because there is less variability in values. The most conspicuous difference between arterial and venous samples is the difference in P_{O_2}, which reflects oxygenation of blood in the lungs and utilization in the tissues. The P_{CO_2} and HCO_3^- values are slightly higher and the pH slightly lower in venous samples because of local tissue effects. Normal arterial blood gas values for dogs have recently been described as: pH 7.45 (7.39–7.51); P_{CO_2} 31.0 (23.9–38.3) mm Hg; P_{O_2} 90.7 (73.1–108.3) mm Hg; and HCO_3^- 20.9 (16.3–25.5) mEq/L.[6] Normal arterial blood gas values for cats have recently been reported as: pH 7.344 ± 0.1038; P_{CO_2} 33.6 ± 7.06 mm Hg; P_{O_2} 102.9 ± 15.22 mm Hg; and HCO_3^- 17.5 ± 2.98 mEq/L.[21] Values may vary slightly from one laboratory to another, and normal canine and feline values should be established by the individual laboratory.

Interpretation of Acid-Base Data

When interpreting acid-base values, the following questions should be considered by the clinician:

1. What is the pH? Natural compensatory mechanisms rarely overcompensate, and so in most cases the pH is altered in the direction of the primary disturbance.

Table 4-2. Primary and Compensatory Acid-Base Alterations in Various Disorders

Primary disorder	pH	$[H^+]$	Primary disturbance	Compensatory response
Metabolic acidosis	↓	↑	↓ HCO_3^-	↓ P_{CO_2}
Metabolic alkalosis	↑	↓	↑ HCO_3^-	↑ P_{CO_2}
Respiratory acidosis	↓	↑	↑ P_{CO_2}	↑ HCO_3^-
Respiratory alkalosis	↑	↓	↓ P_{CO_2}	↓ HCO_3^-

From Rose, BD: Clinical Physiology of Acid-Base and Electrolyte Disorders. Copyright © 1977, McGraw-Hill Book Company, New York. By permission.

2.   What are the metabolic (HCO_3^-) and respiratory (P_{CO_2}) components of the disorder? In most cases this evaluation allows the clinician to determine which disorder is primary and which is secondary.

3.   Is the degree of compensation as expected? This allows detection of mixed acid-base disorders.

A simple acid-base disorder refers to a single initiating abnormality with its accompanying secondary physiological compensatory response. A mixed acid-base disorder indicates the presence of two or more independent abnormalities. To correctly diagnose mixed disorders, the normal limits of the compensatory response must be known. The simple acid-base disorders are defined as follows:

Metabolic acidosis: increased H^+ activity (decreased pH) and decreased plasma HCO_3^-. It may arise from loss of HCO_3^- or buffering of noncarbonic acids (e.g., lactate, ketoacids).

Metabolic alkalosis: decreased H^+ activity (increased pH) and elevated plasma HCO_3^-. It may arise from loss of H^+ or addition of HCO_3^-.

Respiratory acidosis: impaired pulmonary excretion of CO_2 resulting in elevated P_{CO_2} (hypercapnia).

Respiratory alkalosis: hyperventilation resulting in a decrease in P_{CO_2} (hypocapnia).

The primary and compensatory acid-base alterations in these disorders are shown in Table 4-2.

Metabolic Acidosis

Metabolic acidosis due to loss of bicarbonate or an added acid load is the most commonly encountered acid-base disturbance in small animal practice. The response to an acid load includes immediate extracellular buffering by HCO_3^-, which lowers plasma HCO_3^-. Intracellular buffering by phosphates and proteins occurs when H^+ enters the cell in exchange for K^+. This H^+-K^+ exchange causes roughly a 0.4–0.6 mEq/L increase in serum K^+ for every 0.1 unit decrease in pH.[17] These extra- and intracellular events take 2–4 hr for completion.

Metabolic acidosis stimulates chemoreceptors controlling alveolar ventilation so that there is increased removal of CO_2 from the body. The normal

Table 4-3.   Causes of Metabolic Acidosis

Normal Anion Gap	Increased Anion Gap
Diarrhea	Diabetic ketoacidosis
Renal tubular acidosis	Uremia
Proximal	Acute renal failure
Distal	Chronic renal failure
Carbonic anhydrase inhibitors (e.g.,	Lactic acidosis (e.g., shock)
acetazolamide)	Intoxications
NH$_4$Cl administration	Ethylene glycol
	Methanol
	Salicylate
	Paraldehyde

compensatory response is complete within 12–24 hrs and causes a 1.2 mm Hg decrease in P_{CO_2} for every 1.0 mEq/L decrease in plasma HCO_3^-.[23] If the patient's P_{CO_2} is higher or lower than predicted, a mixed disorder with concurrent respiratory acidosis or respiratory alkalosis, respectively, must be considered. Finally, the kidney increases its acid excretion to eliminate the H^+ and regenerate titrated HCO_3^-.

The causes of metabolic acidosis are usually classified by the presence or absence of an anion gap.[19] The anion gap[8] is defined as the difference between the commonly measured cations ($Na^+ + K^+$) and anions ($Cl^- + HCO_3^-$). The normal anion gap is 10–25 mEq/L in the dog and 15–35 mEq/L in the cat. In the normal animal it is accounted for by the difference between unmeasured anions (phosphate, sulfate, and negatively charged proteins) and cations (calcium and magnesium), which are fewer in number. This relationship is expressed as follows:

$(Na^+ + K^+)$ + unmeasured cations

$$= (Cl^- + HCO_3^-) + \text{unmeasured anions}$$

$(Na^+ + K^+) - (Cl^- + HCO_3^-)$

$$= \text{unmeasured anions} - \text{unmeasured cations} = \text{anion gap}$$

In metabolic acidosis due to renal or gastrointestinal loss of bicarbonate, there is renal retention of NaCl to conserve extracellular fluid volume. Hence chloride levels rise in proportion to the decrease in plasma bicarbonate levels, and the anion gap is normal. This is called hyperchloremic metabolic acidosis. If H^+ accumulates along with any anion other than Cl^-, the titrated HCO_3^- is replaced by an unmeasured anion, and the anion gap is increased. This is called normochloremic metabolic acidosis. Examples of such unmeasured anions are ketones in diabetic ketoacidosis, sulfates and phosphates in renal failure, lactate in lactic acidosis (e.g., shock), and anionic metabolites of ingested poisons. Table 4-3 lists the causes of metabolic acidosis.

The most important principle in the treatment of metabolic acidosis and all other acid-base disorders is diagnosis and treatment of the underlying disease process. This alone is often adequate to restore the acid-base balance. However, when metabolic acidosis is severe (pH < 7.1–7.2) treatment with parenteral alkali should be considered. Sodium bicarbonate ($NaHCO_3$) is most readily available to the body.[14] Lactate, gluconate, and acetate must be metabolized in the liver and muscles to produce bicarbonate. When the pH is <7.1, the metabolism of lactate by the liver is impaired. In man, complete distribution of HCO_3^- to the interstitial space requires approximately 30 min, whereas distribution to intracellular water takes 18 hrs for completion.[15] For these reasons, the following formula is recommended for calculating the dosage of bicarbonate:

$$\underset{\text{(mEq)}}{HCO_3^-\text{ needed}} = \underset{\text{(mEq/L)}}{\text{base deficit}} \times 0.3 \times \underset{\text{(kg)}}{\text{body weight}}$$

The factor 0.3 represents the extracellular fluid volume and hence the acute volume of distribution for bicarbonate. It is recommended that 25–50% of the calculated dose be given intravenously over 30 min and serial blood gas values be used to determine the need for further therapy. Rapid and complete correction of metabolic acidosis with $NaHCO_3$ is neither necessary nor desirable. Appropriate treatment of the underlying disease process may eliminate further need for alkali therapy. When blood gas values are not known, an $NaHCO_3$ dosage of 1–2 mEq/kg may be used as a guideline. Complications[14] associated with alkali therapy include: tetany due to lowering of serum ionized calcium levels by pH-induced changes in plasma protein charge; volume overload due to sodium content of administered bicarbonate (e.g., congestive heart failure patient or oliguric acute renal failure patient); hyperosmolality due to sodium load in cats and small dogs; paradoxical cerebrospinal fluid (CSF) acidosis; decreased oxygen delivery to tissues due to left shift of the hemoglobin-oxygen saturation curve; and hypokalemia due to induced shift of potassium into cells and hydrogen ions out of cells. For these reasons, bicarbonate therapy must be approached with careful consideration. Also, $NaHCO_3$ must not be combined with calcium-containing solutions because $CaCO_3$ may precipitate.

Metabolic Alkalosis

Metabolic alkalosis is the second most common acid-base disturbance encountered in small animal medicine. Metabolic alkalosis can result from the administration of alkali, loss of acid from the stomach, excess renal excretion of acid, or disproportionate loss of chloride wherein there is a compensatory increase in renal bicarbonate reclamation to maintain electroneutrality. For every milliequivalent of H^+ lost there will be an equal amount of HCO_3^- generated in the extracellular fluid. The causes of metabolic alkalosis are listed in Table 4-4.

Metabolic alkalosis results in hypoventilation and a compensatory increase in P_{CO_2} which decreases pH toward normal. This response is not nearly as effective as the hyperventilatory response to metabolic acidosis. There is an approximately 0.6–0.7 mm Hg increase in blood P_{CO_2} for every 1.0 mEq increase in plasma HCO_3^-.[23]

Once generated, metabolic alkalosis tends to be perpetuated by the kidney. When metabolic alkalosis is associated with excessive loss of chloride (e.g.,

Table 4-4. Causes of Metabolic Alkalosis

Chloride-Responsive (urine chloride <10 mEq/L)	Chloride-Resistant (urine chloride >10 mEq/L)
Vomiting (gastric contents)	Hyperaldosteronism
Diuretics (e.g., furosemide, thiazides)	Primary (not yet reported in dogs and cats)
Other	Secondary
Excessive administration of alkali	Nephrotic syndrome
	Cirrhosis
	Congestive heart failure
	Hyperadrenocorticism
	Potassium depletion

gastric losses, diuretics) the volume contraction and relative lack of chloride for reabsorption cause the kidney to increase sodium-cation exchange to conserve sodium. When sodium is reabsorbed in exchange for H^+, equal amounts of HCO_3^- are generated, thus perpetuating the metabolic alkalosis in the extracellular fluid and causing paradoxical aciduria. Thus the body maintains extracellular fluid volume at the expense of extracellular pH. Increased sodium-potassium exchange results in the potassium depletion which frequently develops in the face of metabolic alkalosis. Urinary potassium losses are aggravated if the cause of H^+ loss also causes K^+ loss (e.g., gastric losses, diuretics) or if volume depletion severe enough to cause aldosterone release occurs, thus augmenting K^+ depletion. These relationships are shown in Figure 4-2.

Metabolic alkalosis may be classified as chloride-responsive or chloride-resistant.[19] In chloride-responsive metabolic alkalosis, there is very little chloride in the urine (<10 mEq/L) because of volume contraction and a maximal attempt by the kidneys to conserve NaCl. Administration of 0.9% NaCl restores volume and provides the appropriate resorbable anion (chloride), thus allowing HCO_3^- to be excreted in the urine. In chloride-resistant metabolic alkalosis there is either severe K^+ depletion, causing increased renal sodium-hydrogen ion exchange, or a factor is present that causes increased sodium-potassium exchange (e.g., mineralocorticoid effect) and the urine contains chloride at a concentration of >10 mEq/L. Eventual K^+ depletion in the latter instance results in increased sodium-hydrogen ion exchange and enhanced HCO_3^- reabsorption. Therapy for chloride-resistant metabolic alkalosis necessitates 0.9% NaCl along with adequate KCl administration to restore the K^+ deficit. When metabolic alkalosis is due to excessive alkali administration ($NaHCO_3$), the excess sodium allows the HCO_3^- to be easily excreted in the urine.

Respiratory Acidosis

Respiratory acidosis is the third most frequent acid-base disorder in small animal medicine. The causes of respiratory acidosis (Table 4-5) include those diseases which lead to decreased alveolar ventilation and consequent retention of CO_2 (hypercapnia). The causes of hypoventilation are discussed in Chapter 3. In the course of progressive respiratory disease, hypoxemia often precedes

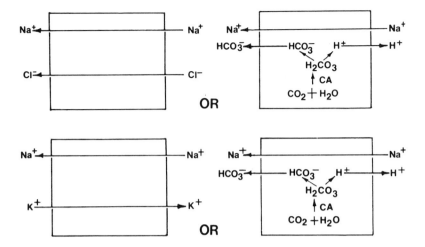

Effects of Cl⁻ and K⁺ Depletion on Acid—Base Balance

Fig. 4.2. Conceptually, reabsorption of sodium by the kidney may be represented as occurring in conjunction with chloride reabsorption, in exchange for potassium, or in exchange for hydrogen ions with concurrent reabsorption of bicarbonate. The squares represent renal tubular cells, the space to the right of the cell represents tubular fluid, and that to the left the extracellular fluid. It can be seen that in states of chloride depletion there is enhanced reabsorption of bicarbonate and excretion of hydrogen ions and potassium, predisposing to metabolic alkalosis and hypokalemia. If potassium depletion is superimposed, the metabolic alkalosis is aggravated further. In the former situation, 0.9% saline is the therapy of choice. In the latter, the metabolic alkalosis will be saline-resistant and therapy will require KCl supplementation in addition to 0.9% saline. (CA) carbonic anhydrase.

the development of hypercapnia, and the initial response to hypoxemia is increased alveolar ventilation and respiratory alkalosis.

The body responds to respiratory acidosis by the hydration of CO_2 to H_2CO_3 and conversion to H^+ and HCO_3^-. The H^+ is buffered by intracellular buffers (including hemoglobin). If respiratory acidosis persists, there will be increased renal H^+ excretion, which further elevates plasma HCO_3^-. In acute respiratory acidosis, there is approximately a 1 mEq/L increase in plasma HCO_3^- for every 10 mm Hg increase in blood P_{CO_2}.[23] This is due largely to intracellular buffering. In chronic respiratory acidosis, there is an approximately 3.5 mEq/L increase in plasma HCO_3^- for every 10 mm Hg increase in blood P_{CO_2}.[23] This enhancement of the compensatory response is due to increased renal excretion of H^+, which takes 3–5 days to reach maximum effect. Therapy of respiratory acidosis is directed at removing retained CO_2 by improving ventilation. Intubation and mechanical ventilation may be required until the underlying cause can be corrected. In chronic respiratory acidosis, the primary drive for ventilation may be hypoxemia. Hence oxygen must be

Table 4-5. Causes of Respiratory Acidosis

Respiratory center
  CNS lesions
Drugs
  Narcotics
  Barbiturates
  Sedatives
  Inhalation anesthetics
Respiratory muscle dysfunction
  Myasthenia gravis
  Tick paralysis
  Polyradiculoneuritis
  Botulism
Chest wall trauma
Pneumothorax
Pleural effusion
Pulmonary disease
  Pneumonia
  Pulmonary edema
  Chronic obstructive pulmonary disease
  Diffuse metastatic disease
Airway obstruction
Cardiopulmonary arrest

given with great caution in this situation as overzealous correction of low Pa_{O_2} by oxygen administration may diminish ventilatory drive, thereby worsening CO_2 retention and respiratory acidosis.

Respiratory Alkalosis

Respiratory alkalosis is the least common acid-base disorder in small animal medicine, and its causes are listed in Table 4-6. When present in small animals, respiratory alkalosis is usually a compensatory response to primary metabolic acidosis. Diseases which lead to alveolar hyperventilation can cause primary respiratory alkalosis. The initial response to reduction in P_{CO_2} is a

Table 4-6. Causes of Respiratory Alkalosis

Hypermetabolic states
  Fever
  Thyrotoxicosis
  Anemia
Salicylate ingestion
Gram-negative sepsis
Assisted ventilation
CNS disease
Cirrhosis
Hypoxemia
  Reduced inspired oxygenation concentration (high altitude)
  Ventilation/perfusion mismatch
  Right-to-left shunting of blood
  Congestive heart failure
  Pulmonary embolism

lowering of plasma HCO_3^-. Initially this decrease is mediated by intracellular buffers through the release of H^+, which moves to the extracellular fluid to combine with HCO_3^-. Later, reduced renal reclamation of HCO_3^- further contributes to lowering of plasma HCO_3^-. In acute respiratory alkalosis the plasma HCO_3^- falls 2 mEq/L for each 10 mm Hg decrease in blood P_{CO_2}. In chronic respiratory alkalosis, the added effect of renal compensation results in a 5 mEq/L decrease in plasma HCO_3^- for each 10 mm Hg reduction in blood P_{CO_2}.[23] Treatment of respiratory alkalosis is aimed at diagnosis and treatment of the underlying cause.

DISTURBANCES OF ELECTROLYTE BALANCE

Disorders of Potassium Balance

Potassium is the major intracellular cation of the body. Over 95% of the body's potassium stores are intracellular, whereas only 2–5% are in the extracellular fluid. In the animal with potassium balance, the kidneys are responsible for excreting excess ingested potassium. Unlike the case of sodium depletion, wherein the kidney can reduce its excretion of sodium to very low levels, there is a daily obligatory loss of potassium. The daily requirement of potassium in dogs varies between 2 and 40 mEq depending on the size of the dog.[13]

Potassium is essential for the maintenance of electrical excitability in many tissues, notably the heart, skeletal muscles, and gastrointestinal tract. The resting potential of cells is directly related to the intracellular/extracellular potassium ratio. Hyperkalemia reduces the resting membrane potential, making the tissues more excitable, whereas hypokalemia increases the resting potential, hyperpolarizing the tissue and making it less excitable.[23]

Acid-base balance influences the translocation of potassium between the intra- and extracellular compartments. In acidosis, potassium leaves cells and hydrogen ions enter them to be buffered there. Conversely, in alkalosis potassium enters cells and hydrogen ions leave them. In general, for every 0.1 unit change in arterial pH there is a reciprocal 0.4–0.6 mEq/L change in serum potassium.[17] Because of its intracellular location and the effects of acid-base balance on the translocation of potassium, serum potassium values are not a good indication of total body stores. In chronic muscle wasting, 3 mEq potassium may be lost per gram of protein nitrogen, but serum potassium values may remain normal.[1] The patient with diabetic ketoacidosis is a good example of the effects of chronic disease and acidosis on potassium balance. In such patients total body stores of potassium are decreased because of urinary losses, vomiting, anorexia, and loss of muscle mass, but serum potassium values may be normal or even elevated owing to metabolic acidosis.

When hypokalemia is observed and there is a chronic disease process present, depletion of potassium stores is expected. On the other hand, hyperkalemia is usually due to decreased renal excretion or translocation from intracellular to extracellular sites. The causes of hypokalemia (Table 4-7) are

Table 4-7. Causes of Hyperkalemia and Hypokalemia

Hyperkalemia	Hypokalemia
1. Increased intake	1. Decreased intake
a. High doses of potassium penicillin G intravenously	a. Aberrant diet
b. Excessively rapid infusion of KCl	b. Anorexia
c. Inadequate mixing of KCl in flexible infusion bags	c. Potassium-poor fluid infusion
d. KCl as a salt substitute during sodium restriction	2. Translocation
2. Decreased renal elimination	a. Glucose and insulin
a. Oliguric acute renal failure	b. Metabolic alkalosis
b. Terminal oliguric chronic renal failure	3. Excessive gastrointestinal losses
c. Hypoadrenocorticism	a. Chronic vomiting
d. Use of potassium-sparing diuretics	b. Overuse of laxatives, enemas, or exchange resins
e. Urethral obstruction	4. Excessive urinary losses
f. Uroabdomen	a. Secondary hyperaldosteronism
3. Translocation	Liver failure
a. Metabolic acidosis	Nephrotic syndrome
b. Tissue injury	Congestive heart failure
	b. Renal disease
	Renal tubular acidosis
	Postobstructive diuresis
	Chronic pyelonephritis
	c. Drugs (diuretics, amphotericin B)

decreased intake, increased urinary losses, increased gastrointestinal losses, and translocation from extracellular to intracellular sites. The clinical signs of hypokalemia and potassium depletion are those of muscle weakness (decreased excitability), defective urinary concentrating ability, impaired gastrointestinal motility (paralytic ileus), and electrocardiographic (ECG) changes. The ECG changes associated with hypokalemia in man are attributed to delayed ventricular repolarization and include ST segment depression, decreased amplitude T waves, and the appearance of U waves. The ECG changes in the dog, except for tachycardia, are quite variable and inconsistent. Severe hypokalemia may cause ventricular arrhythmias.

The treatment of hypokalemia involves potassium supplementation and treatment of the underlying predisposing disease process. There is no clear correlation between the level of serum potassium and the magnitude of the total potassium deficit. For this reason, potassium supplementation is approached empirically. Normal saline supplemented with KCl is used for parenteral administration. The NaCl helps restore the extracellular fluid volume deficit, and the resorbable anion (chloride) allows excretion of bicarbonate and correction of the metabolic alkalosis that often accompanies potassium depletion. The following guidelines[11] are used for intravenous potassium supplementation:

Serum potassium (mEq/L)	Potassium (mEq) to add to 250 ml fluids
<2.0	20
2.1–2.5	15
2.6–3.0	10
3.1–3.5	7

do NOT exceed 0.5 mEq/kg/hr

Infusion fluids containing KCl up to 30 mEq/L may be used by the subcutaneous route. In many cases, marked dehydration or vomiting necessitates parenteral fluid administration, but in patients taking oral medication liquid oral potassium supplements containing 20 mEq KCl/15 ml may be used (e.g., Kaon, Kay Ciel). Such preparations may cause vomiting, and dilution with water may be necessary. Enteric-coated potassium tablets are to be avoided because of the risk of gastrointestinal ulceration or stenosis. Return of oral alimentation as well as correct diagnosis and treatment of the underlying disease responsible for the hypokalemia usually resolve the potassium deficit.

The causes of hyperkalemia are increased intake, decreased renal excretion, and translocation from intracellular to extracellular stores. The causes of hyperkalemia are listed in Table 4-7. It is unlikely that increased intake of potassium would result in hyperkalemia in the presence of normal renal function. The signs of hyperkalemia are weakness and cardiac conduction abnormalities. The ECG changes associated with hyperkalemia are very helpful in the diagnosis and management of this electrolyte disorder. The changes include peaked T waves, decreased QT interval, widening of the QRS complex, and decreased amplitude and eventual disappearance of the P waves. The result is a slow sinoventricular rhythm which may terminate in ventricular fibrillation or asystole. Monitoring the ECG aids in assessing the response of hyperkalemia to treatment.

Treatment of hyperkalemia includes attempts to antagonize the effects of potassium, promote its intracellular movement, and remove it from the body. A slow intravenous infusion (0.5 ml/kg) of a 10% solution of calcium gluconate may be used to antagonize the detrimental effects of potassium on the heart. The heart is auscultated and the ECG monitored during calcium gluconate administration. The intravenous administration of $NaHCO_3$ 1–2 mEq/kg promotes the intracellular movement of potassium and the extracellular movement of hydrogen ions by its alkalinizing effect. The risks of hypervolemia and hyperosmolality must be considered in cats and small dogs. Also, tetany may occur during bicarbonate infusion by lowering serum ionized calcium levels (e.g., in cats with urethral obstruction). Regular insulin and glucose-containing solutions may be used to promote the intracellular movement of potassium and glucose, thereby decreasing extracellular potassium levels.

These treatments are transient, and a conscientious effort must be made to diagnose and treat the underlying disease responsible for the hyperkalemia. If hyperkalemia is persistent (e.g., oliguric acute renal failure), additional steps must be taken to maintain a sustained reduction in serum potassium levels. Sodium polystyrene sulfonate (Kayexalate) is an ion-exchange resin which may be given orally or by retention enema using a large Foley catheter to bind potassium in the gastrointestinal tract. One gram of the resin removes approximately 1 mEq potassium in exchange for 1 mEq sodium.[16] Kayexalate is given in combination with sorbitol to cause osmotic diarrhea and further enhance potassium loss. If this therapy is unsuccessful, peritoneal dialysis or hemodialysis must be considered.

Disorders of Sodium Balance

Sodium is the major cation of the extracellular fluid, and the amount of sodium and its anions largely determines the volume of the extracellular fluid compartment. Sodium balance is regulated by renal conservation of sodium and water. The kidneys have a remarkable ability to conserve sodium, and it is unlikely that a deficit of sodium could be created by dietary restriction alone. The daily requirement for sodium in the dog ranges from 2 to 50 mEq/day depending on the size of the dog.[13]

There are several mechanisms by which the kidneys regulate sodium balance. Glomerulotubular balance refers to the ability of the kidneys to increase sodium reabsorption when the filtered load of sodium is increased and to decrease sodium reabsorption when the filtered load is decreased. Aldosterone plays an important role in the conservation of sodium in the distal nephron in exchange for other cations. Other factors which contribute to sodium conservation in the kidneys include the effects of Starling forces in the peritubular capillaries, shifting of renal blood flow from cortical to juxtamedullary nephrons, and the probable existence of a natriuretic hormone released in response to volume expansion.

Serum sodium values indicate the amount of sodium present relative to the amount of water present in the extracellular fluid. Thus the serum sodium value is determined more by water balance than by the absolute amount of sodium present. Hyponatremia indicates retention of water relative to sodium in the extracellular fluid, and hypernatremia reflects the loss of water relative to sodium. In fact, serum sodium values may be decreased, normal, or increased in a dehydrated patient depending on the composition and tonicity of the fluid which has been lost from the body. Hence serum sodium values do not necessarily reflect the status of total body stores of sodium.

The clinical signs of hyponatremia are dependent on the rapidity of onset and include weakness, depression, anorexia, vomiting, abdominal pain, paralytic ileus, muscular twitching, and signs of hypovolemic shock. Sudden development of hyponatremia could lead to loss of water from the extracellular fluid into the central nervous system (CNS) and development of cerebral edema. The causes of hyponatremia are those associated with loss of salt, gain of water, or a combination of these (Table 4-8).

The clinical signs of hypernatremia are weakness, thirst, muscular twitching, depression, coma, and seizures. When hypernatremia develops rapidly, loss of water from the CNS can result in shrinkage of the brain and associated neurologic signs. The causes of hypernatremia are gain of salt, loss of water, or both (Table 4-8).

Pseudohyponatremia develops when certain plasma solutes (lipids or proteins) are increased to the extent that they contribute a substantial amount to plasma volume. Serum sodium is measured using whole serum, and although the concentration of sodium present in the aqueous phase is normal, the concentration in the total volume of serum is low because sodium is absent in the nonaqueous phase. Whenever hyponatremia occurs in conjunction with grossly

Table 4-8. Causes of Hypernatremia and Hyponatremia

Hypernatremia
  Lack of water intake
  Pure water loss
  Salt poisoning
  Infusion of hypertonic sodium-containing fluids
  Advanced chronic renal failure with GFR <5% normal
  Hypotonic fluid loss
  Primary hyperaldosteronism (not reported in dogs or cats)
Hyponatremia
  In the OVERHYDRATED patient
    Secondary hyperaldosteronism (liver failure, nephrotic syndrome, congestive heart failure)
    Psychogenic polydipsia
    Iatrogenic water load
    Syndrome of inappropriate ADH secretion (CNS disease, pulmonary disease, drugs, neoplasia)
  In the DEHYDRATED patient
    Gastrointestinal losses
    Isotonic losses with water replacement
    Hypoadrenocorticism
    Sodium-losing renal disease
    Diuretic therapy
    Hypertonic fluid loss (burns, large wounds, body cavity lavage)
Pseudohyponatremia
  Hyperlipidemia
  Multiple myeloma
Physiological hyponatremia
  Hyperglycemia

lipemic plasma or in the presence of severe hyperproteinemia, pseudohyponatremia should be suspected. Physiological hyponatremia occurs when a small aqueous solute draws water into plasma diluting the amount of sodium present (e.g., hyperglycemia, mannitol infusion).

The treatment of hyponatremia consists of infusing sodium-containing solutions and terminating any infusion of sodium-poor fluid (e.g., 5% dextrose). In most cases, isotonic saline (0.9% NaCl) is adequate. In cases where sodium has been lowered suddenly, 3% saline solution should be considered. Therapy for hypernatremia consists of infusion of a sodium-poor fluid (5% dextrose or 2.5% dextrose in 0.45% saline) and termination of any sodium-rich infusion. Diuretic therapy (e.g., furosemide) may be indicated to remove excess sodium if a known sodium load was ingested or given iatrogenically. Rapid lowering of extracellular tonicity in animals with chronic hypertonicity may result in development of an unfavorable osmotic gradient and overhydration of the brain. Therefore therapy to lower serum sodium levels must be carried out slowly. In both hypo- and hypernatremia, the underlying disease process must be identified and treated appropriately.

Disorders of Calcium and Phosphorus Balance

Calcium is an important structural component of the skeleton and an essential cofactor in blood coagulation. It plays an important role in the cellular secretion of hormones. One of its most important roles is in the maintenance of normal neuromuscular contractility in the heart, gastrointestinal tract, and skeletal muscles. Hypocalcemia increases the threshold potential of the cellular membranes, making the tissue more excitable. Hypercalcemia, on the other hand, reduces the threshold potential, making the tissue less excitable.[23] Most of the body's calcium and phosphorus are in bone. The calcium that is not in bone is largely extracellular, whereas the phosphorus that is not in bone is largely intracellular.

Serum calcium and phosphorus levels are regulated by the effects of parathyroid hormone, vitamin D, and calcitonin acting on the kidney, gastrointestinal tract, and bone. Parathyroid hormone increases calcium and phosphorus resorption from bone, renal calcium reabsorption, and renal phosphorus excretion. Parathyroid hormone also enhances the conversion of vitamin D to its most active form, 1,25-dihydroxycholecalciferol. Activated vitamin D stimulates gastrointestinal absorption of calcium and phosphorus and increases mobilization of calcium from bone. Calcitonin decreases calcium mobilization from bone by inhibiting osteoclastic bone resorption.

Calcium in the blood is present in three forms: protein-bound (50%), free ionized (40%), and complexed (10%). Free ionized calcium is the biologically active form. Standard laboratory techniques measure total calcium, and such values are affected by the serum protein level. In the presence of hypoproteinemia, total serum calcium values may be low although ionized calcium values remain normal. The following formula[20] may be used to correct serum calcium values for the effects of protein:

$$\text{Corrected calcium} = \text{measured calcium} - \text{albumin} + 3.5$$

Acid-base balance affects the fraction of calcium which is ionized. Acidosis increases the ionized calcium fraction by decreasing protein binding of calcium. Alkalosis decreases ionized calcium through opposite effects.

The causes of hypercalcemia are listed in Table 4-9. The consequences of hypercalcemia may be apparent in several organ systems. Because of decreased excitability of smooth muscle in the gastrointestinal tract there may be anorexia, vomiting, and constipation. Effects on nervous tissue may result in depression, coma, seizures, or muscular twitching. Skeletal muscle weakness may be observed, and the effects on the heart may result in ECG changes, e.g., prolongation of the PR interval and shortening of the QT interval. One of the earliest effects of hypercalcemia on the kidney is impaired urinary concentrating ability due to interference with the generation of cyclic adenosine monophosphate (cAMP) in response to antidiuretic hormone (ADH) at the level of the distal nephron. The vasoconstrictive effects of hypercalcemia lead to a reduction in renal blood flow and glomerular filtration rate. Calcium precipitation in the kidney may lead to tubular necrosis, interstitial inflammation, and fibrosis.

Therapy for hypercalcemia involves rapid lowering of the serum calcium level to prevent renal damage while an attempt is made to diagnose and treat the inciting disease. The first approach to managing hypercalcemia is volume expansion with 0.9% saline. Sodium competes with calcium for reabsorption

Table 4-9. Causes of Hypercalcemia and Hypocalcemia

Hypercalcemia	Hypocalcemia
1. Physiological (young growing animal)	1. Hypoproteinemia (hypoalbuminemia)
2. Malignancy	2. Eclampsia
a. Lymphosarcoma	3. Renal failure
b. Apocrine gland adenocarcinoma of anal	a. Chronic
sac	b. Acute
c. Primary bone tumor or metastatic bone	4. Urethral obstruction in the cat
tumor	5. Pancreatitis
d. Multiple myeloma	6. Hypoparathyroidism
e. Others	7. Intestinal malabsorption
3. Hypoadrenocorticism	8. Ethylene glycol intoxication
4. Renal failure	9. Phosphate enema
a. Chronic	10. Intravenous phosphates
b. Acute (diuretic phase)	11. Administration of EDTA
5. Hypervitaminosis D	12. Hypovitaminosis D
6. Primary hyperparathyroidism	13. Postoperative after thyroidectomy in cats
7. Fungal osteomyelitis	with hyperthyroidism
8. Hemoconcentration	
9. Laboratory error	

and enhances calciuresis. Furosemide (4 mg/kg) is given to further promote diuresis and calciuresis. Glucocorticoids impair gastrointestinal absorption of calcium, inhibit osteoclastic bone resorption of calcium, and increase renal excretion of calcium. Corticosteroids may be helpful in cases of hypercalcemia due to vitamin D intoxication and hypoadrenocorticism. Their cytolytic effect on tumor cells in lymphosarcoma makes them very useful in this situation.

Other therapy to lower serum calcium includes sodium sulfate infusion to promote diuresis. The nonresorbable anion (sulfate) enhances calcium loss in the urine. Intravenous phosphates may lower serum calcium by inhibiting bone resorption and accelerating mineralization of bone, by inhibiting calcium absorption from the gut, and by promoting the formation of colloidal calcium phosphate complexes, which can be removed by phagocytosis. Intravenous phosphates also promote soft tissue mineralization, and this is a major detriment to their usefulness. Sodium EDTA chelates calcium but is short-acting and potentially nephrotoxic. Mithramycin effectively inhibits osteoclastic bone resorption but is associated with many serious side effects. Indomethacin may be effective in the hypercalcemia of malignancy if the cause of the hypercalcemia is production of a prostaglandin-like substance. Calcitonin also inhibits osteoclastic bone resorption and is safe but fairly expensive. Diphosphonates decrease osteoclastic bone resorption and inhibit deposition of hydroxyapatite crystals on bone collagen. Dialysis may be necessary if hypercalcemia is refractory to conservative therapy.

The most common cause of hypocalcemia is hypoproteinemia. This situation, however, does not require therapy because ionized calcium levels are presumably normal. The consequences of hypocalcemia are those of increased neuromuscular excitability and include tremors, muscular twitching, muscle spasms, behavioral changes, and seizures. Because of the increased muscular activity, hyperthermia is frequently present. The ECG changes include tachycardia and prolongation of the QT interval.

Table 4-10. Causes of Hyperphosphatemia and Hypophosphatemia

Hyperphosphatemia	Hypophosphatemia
1. Physiological (young growing animal)	1. Diabetes mellitus
2. Renal failure	2. Translocation
a. Chronic	a. Glucose
b. Acute	b. Insulin
3. Urethral obstruction/uroabdomen	c. Alkalosis
4. Tissue trauma	d. Hyperalimentation
5. Hypoparathyroidism	3. Eclampsia
6. Hypervitaminosis D	4. Hyperparathyroidism
7. Phosphate enema	5. Intestinal binding agents
8. Intravenous phosphates	6. Malabsorption
9. Hemolysis	7. Hypovitaminosis D
10. Laboratory error	8. Renal tubular defects
	9. Dialysis
	10. Laboratory error

Treatment of hypocalcemia is indicated only if clinical signs are present. Alkali therapy is to be avoided because such treatment may lower ionized calcium levels and precipitate tetany. Parenteral calcium therapy must be used with caution in the presence of hyperphosphatemia because of the risk of soft tissue mineralization (especially if the Ca × P product is greater than 70). Calcium chloride or calcium gluconate may be used for parenteral therapy. Ten milliliters of 10% calcium chloride provides 272 mg of calcium, whereas the same amount of 10% calcium gluconate provides 96 mg calcium.[3] In many instances, an empirical dosage of 3–10 ml 10% calcium gluconate is used intravenously. Cardiac function must be monitored during the administration of calcium solutions. Diagnosis and treatment of the underlying disease is important in the further management of hypocalcemia. Longstanding therapy for hypocalcemia (e.g., hypoparathyroidism) necessitates the use of oral calcium lactate or calcium gluconate in conjunction with oral vitamin D products to enhance gastrointestinal absorption of calcium.[22]

Like calcium, phosphorus has diverse roles in the body. Phospholipids are important structural components of cell membranes, and phosphate is an integral component of nucleic acids. Adenosine triphosphate (ATP) is a ubiquitous energy storage compound in cells, and 2,3-diphosphoglyceric acid plays an important modulatory role in oxygen transport by hemoglobin. Phosphorylated glycolytic intermediates are essential in the utilization of carbohydrates for energy.

Mild to moderate hypophosphatemia is not associated with clinical signs. The consequences of severe hypophosphatemia include impairment of energy utilization and oxygen delivery to tissues as well as hematologic effects, e.g., hemolytic anemia due to spherocytosis, platelet dysfunction, and disturbances of leukocyte function.[10] The causes of hypophosphatemia are listed in Table 4-10. With many causes of hypophosphatemia, the problem is intracellular shifting of extracellular phosphorus. When treatment of diabetic ketoacidosis causes severe lowering of serum phosphorus by intracellular translocation of phosphate, the use of parenteral KH_2PO_4 may be indicated.

The causes of hyperphosphatemia are listed in Table 4-10. The most common cause is decreased renal excretion. This may be due to primary renal failure, prerenal azotemia, or postrenal azotemia. Therapy is directed at diagnosis and treatment of the underlying disease. Intravenous fluid therapy and administration of phosphorus binding agents, e.g., Amphojel or Basaljel, may help lower serum phosphorus. Dietary phosphorus restriction may also be beneficial in long-term management of hyperhosphatemia.

REFERENCES

1. Black DAK: Potassium metabolism. In Maxwell MH, Kleeman CR (eds): Clinical Disorders of Fluid and Electrolyte Metabolism. 2nd Ed. p. 121. McGraw-Hill, New York, 1972
2. Brasmer TH: Fluid therapy in shock. J Am Vet Med Assoc 174:475, 1979
3. Chew DJ, Meuten DJ: Disorders of calcium and phosphorous metabolism. Vet Clin North Am 12:411, 1982
4. Cornelius LM: Fluid therapy in small animal practice. J Am Vet Med Assoc 176:110, 1980
5. Cornelius LM, Finco DR, Culver DH: Physiologic effects of rapid infusion of Ringer's lactate solution in dogs. Am J Vet Res 39:1185, 1978
6. Cornelius LM, Rawlings CA: Arterial blood gas and acid-base values in dogs with various diseases and signs of disease. J Am Vet Med Assoc 178:992, 1981
7. Feig PU, McCurdy DK: The hypertonic state. N Engl J Med 297:1444, 1977
8. Feldman BF, Rosenberg DP: Clinical use of anion and osmolal gaps in veterinary medicine. J Am Vet Med Assoc 178:396, 1981
9. Finco DR: Fluid therapy. In Kirk RW (ed): Current Veterinary Therapy VI. p. 3. Saunders, Philadelphia, 1977
10. Fitzgerald F: Clinical hypophosphatemia. Annu Rev Med 29:177, 1978
11. Greene RW, Scott RC: Lower urinary tract disease. In Ettinger SJ (ed): Textbook of Veterinary Internal Medicine. p. 1572. Saunders, Philadelphia, 1975
12. Hardy RM, Osborne CA: Water deprivation test in the dog: maximal normal values. J Am Vet Med Assoc 174:479, 1979
13. Harrison JB, Sussman HH, Pickering DE: Fluid and electrolyte therapy in small animals. J Am Vet Med Assoc 137:637, 1960
14. Hartsfield SM, Thurmon JC, Benson GJ: Sodium bicarbonate and bicarbonate precursors for treatment of metabolic acidosis. J Am Vet Med Assoc 179:914, 1981
15. Haskins SC: An overview of acid-base physiology. J Am Vet Med Assoc 170:423, 1977
16. Katsikas JL, Goldsmith C: Disorders of potassium metabolism. Med Clin North Am 55:123, 1975
17. MacLeod SM: The rational use of potassium supplements. Postgrad Med 57:123, 1975
18. Madiedo G, Sciacca R, Hause L: Air bubbles and temperature effect on blood gas analysis. J Clin Pathol 33:864, 1980
19. Maxwell MH, Kleeman CR: Clinical Disorders of Fluid and Electrolyte Metabolism. 3rd Ed. McGraw-Hill, New York, 1980
20. Meuten DJ, Chew DJ, Capen CC, et al: Relationship of serum total calcium to albumin and total protein in dogs. J Am Vet Med Assoc 180:63, 1982

21. Middleton DJ, Ilkiw JE, and Watson ADJ: Arterial and venous blood gas tensions in clinically healthy cats. Am J Vet Res 42:1609, 1981
22. Peterson ME: Treatment of canine and feline hypoparathyroidism. J Am Vet Med Assoc 181:1434, 1982
23. Rose BD: Clinical Physiology of Acid-Base and Electrolyte Disorders. McGraw-Hill, New York, 1977

5 | Endocrine Emergencies

Michael Schaer
Janice M. Bright

There are five endocrine disorders that qualify as creating an emergency situation. These are acute adrenocortical insufficiency, diabetic ketoacidosis, nonketotic hyperosmolar diabetic syndrome, hypoglycemia, and thyrotoxicosis. Each of these is discussed in this chapter.

ACUTE ADRENOCORTICAL INSUFFICIENCY

Etiology

Adrenocortical insufficiency can result from the following causes: iatrogenic adrenocortical atrophy from glucocorticoid administration, *o,p'*-DDD-induced adrenocortical destruction, hemorrhage or infarction of the adrenal glands, mycotic or neoplastic involvement, surgical adrenalectomy, anterior pituitary gland insufficiency, and primary hypoadrenocorticism. The latter disorder typifies canine Addison's syndrome and is pathologically characterized as a bilateral adrenocortical atrophy. Most of the veterinary literature applies an idiopathic cause for canine Addison's disease; however, in man this disorder is associated with an autoimmune destruction of the adrenal cortices.[54]

Pathophysiology

The pathophysiological consequences of primary adrenocortical insufficiency are a direct result of glucocorticoid and aldosterone deficiencies. Glucocorticoid depletion causes impaired gluconeogenesis and glycogenolysis, decreased sensitization of blood vessels to catecholamines, impaired renal water excretion, and decreased vitality characterized by poor appetite, lethargy, and impaired cerebration.

163

Aldosterone is a mineralocorticoid hormone which plays an important role in sodium and potassium homeostasis. Hypoaldosteronism causes renal sodium and chloride ion wasting and potassium and hydrogen ion retention. The clinical and pathophysiological effects of hyponatremia include lethargy, mental depression, nausea, hypotension, impaired cardiac output and renal perfusion, and hypovolemic shock. Hyperkalemia causes muscle weakness, hyporeflexia, and impaired cardiac conduction. The addisonian crisis most often occurs in the setting of moderate to marked hyponatremia (serum sodium < 132 mEq/L) and hyperkalemia (serum potassium > 7.0 mEq/L).

Diagnosis

A tentative diagnosis of acute adrenocortical insufficiency can be made on the basis of the history and physical examination findings. Historically, the dog might have had a chronic phase characterized by an inability to gain weight, weight loss, periodic vomiting and/or diarrhea, and lethargy.[85] Polydipsia and polyuria are also present in some patients.[85] The chronicity might vary from weeks' to months' duration and then suddenly culminate in an acute hypotensive state of collapse. On the other hand, the addisonian crisis can occur acutely with or without an associated stress trigger.

On physical examination the acutely decompensated patient is usually either hypo- or normothermic. Hydration varies from normal to varying degrees of dehydration. The mentation is dull, and muscle weakness is usually profound. The respiratory rate can be normal or rapid, the latter due to either shock and/or compensation for metabolic acidosis. The mucous membranes are usually pink, but the capillary refill time is prolonged. Cardiac auscultation might depict a normal sinus rhythm or arrhythmias, especially bradyarrhythmias. The pulse quality is weak, and the rate varies from normal to slow.

The electrocardiogram (ECG) is a useful tool for detecting the various electrophysiological abnormalities of the heart associated with hyperkalemia. The most common abnormalities include flattened P waves, increased positive or negative deflection in the T waves, broadened QRS complexes, bradycardia, sinoventricular complexes, and atrial standstill.[83]

The definitive diagnosis of Addison's disease is based on clinicopathologic test results. The hallmark findings include hyperkalemia and hyponatremia (Na/K < 20:1). Additional associated abnormalities include mild to moderate hypochloremia, azotemia, hyperphosphatemia, and metabolic acidosis.[71] Mild hypercalcemia is often present,[57,85] but hypoglycemia is rarely seen.[85]

Although the above historical, physical, clinicopathologic, and ECG abnormalities are strongly suggestive of acute hypoadrenocorticism and usually constitute the basis for the clinical diagnosis and the need for immediate therapy, the absolute diagnosis depends on the demonstration of absent or minimal adrenocortical response to an injection of corticotropin (ACTH).[23,57,85] To avoid an unnecessary delay of therapy for the sake of performing a diagnostic test, the following procedure is recommended soon after the patient's admission:

1. Obtain blood for hemogram, serum biochemistry, and basal cortisol determinations, and perform a baseline urinalysis.
2. Begin intravenous fluids and give dexamethasone 2–5 mg/kg IV.
3. Immediately give 0.25 mg of $\alpha^{1\text{-}24}$-corticotropin [Cortrosyn (cosyntropin), Organon Inc, West Orange, NJ 07052] IM or IV.
4. One hour later obtain a second blood sample for plasma cortisol determination.[29]

With this technique the patient derives the benefit of undelayed treatment while confirmatory diagnostic tests are performed simultaneously. In the addisonian patients the post-ACTH injection cortisol blood level is barely increased above the basal value.[23,29,57,85]

Treatment

Whenever the index of suspicion is strong toward a diagnosis of addisonian crisis, treatment is begun without delay. The therapeutic objectives include: (1) intravascular volume resuscitation; (2) reversal of the hyponatremia and hyperkalemia; (3) provision of glucocorticoids; and (4) recognition and reversal of any life-threatening cardiac arrhythmias.

Sodium chloride (0.9%) is the fluid of choice and is delivered through an indwelling intravenous catheter. If the dog is markedly hypotensive, the saline is infused at a rate of 20–40 ml/kg body weight during the first 1–2 hr of treatment. Because of the addisonian patient's intolerance to acute water loading, care must be taken to avoid iatrogenic intravascular fluid overload.[29] Where facilities permit, central venous pressure (CVP) determinations provide a safeguard against this complication. For the remaining 24-hr period, the isotonic saline is evenly infused at a maintenance rate of approximately 60 ml/kg. The intravenous fluids are discontinued when hydration, urine output, serum electrolyes, and BUN levels are restored to normal (usually after 48–72 hr of treatment).

Although intravenous saline helps counter the hyponatremia and hyperkalemia, the patient must also receive desoxycorticosterone acetate (DOCA). This mineralocorticoid hormone enhances renal distal tubular sodium reabsorption and potassium excretion. The dose ranges from 1.0 mg for a small dog to 5.0 mg for a large dog and is given once daily intramuscularly. In many patients the subsequent daily doses of DOCA can be decreased to approximately one-half of the initial dose due to the synergistic effects of fluids, DOCA, and glucocorticoid medications. Reassessment of the serum electrolyte levels serves as a helpful treatment guide.

The glucocorticoid deficiency is best corrected with rapid-acting drugs, e.g., prednisolone sodium succinate (Solu-Delta-Cortef, Upjohn Company, Kalamazoo, MI 49001) or dexamethasone. These glucocorticoid drugs are given intravenously initially. The initial doses of prednisolone sodium succinate and dexamethasone are 5–10 mg/kg and 2–5 mg/kg, respectively. Subsequent glucocorticoid requirements are fulfilled by administering prednisolone 1 mg/kg PO, IM, or IV every 12 hr through the second day and then reducing the dose to 0.25–0.5 mg/kg every 12 hr for the remaining duration of hospitalization.

Serum potassium concentrations greater than 7.0 mEq/L cause progressive depressions of the excitability and conduction velocity of the myocardium.[19] The degree of hyperkalemic myocardial toxicity ranges from mild to severe, and only in the latter situation is special therapy warranted. ECG signs of life-threatening myocardial toxicity include widened QRS complexes, sinoventricular complexes, atrial standstill, and other bradyarrhythmias. Treatment entails the administration of 10% calcium gluconate solution at a dose of 0.5–1.0 ml/kg IV. This is given slowly over a 10- to 20-min period, accompanied by continuous ECG monitoring. Calcium gluconate directly antagonizes the myocardial toxic effect of hyperkalemia but does not lower the serum potassium level. To accomplish the latter effect, sodium bicarbonate solution can be given at a dose of 1–2 mEq/kg IV over a 5- to 15-min period. An intravenous injection of regular crystalline insulin at a dose of 0.25 unit/kg also lowers the serum potassium level. To avoid the anticipated hypoglycemic side effects of insulin, 2–3 g of dextrose per unit of insulin is also given by intravenous push. The above emergency measures for the treatment of myocardial toxicity usually are required once and need not be repeated.[69]

Complications

The majority of dogs with Addison's disease have an excellent prognosis for a normal quality of life. Early complications which might alter an optimistic outcome include irreversible renal failure resulting from renal ischemia associated with protracted hypotension and cardiac dysfunction. If the patient is oliguric or anuric following the initial period of intravascular volume expansion, mannitol is given intravenously at a dose of 0.5 g/kg in order to promote an osmotic diuresis. The therapy of oliguric renal failure is discussed further in Chapter 6. An indwelling urethral catheter is inserted to quantitate the urine output. The treatment of hyperkalemic myocardial toxicity has been discussed in the preceding section.

Iatrogenic complications include pulmonary edema resulting from excess parenteral fluid administration during the initial phase of intravascular volume resuscitation and hypokalemia as a consequence of excess DOCA treatment. Pulmonary edema can be avoided by closely observing the patient for signs of respiratory distress and by not exceeding the recommended volume of fluid delivery (20–40 ml/kg) during the first 2 hr of therapy. Hypokalemia can occur on the second or third day of therapy and is mostly due to the combined effects of the saline infusion and excess amounts of DOCA. Daily monitoring of the patient's serum sodium and potassium levels provide objective criteria for providing any necessary treatment adjustments.

DIABETIC KETOACIDOSIS

Etiology

A detailed description of the recent advances in human medicine which explain the causes of the primary forms of diabetes mellitus is beyond the scope of this text. However, compelling evidence in man has provided evidence for the heterogeneity of this syndrome in which genetic, viral, environmental, and immunologic factors play an important role.[2]

Secondary factors known to induce diabetes in the dog and cat include pancreatitis, diffuse pancreatic carcinoma, and total pancreatectomy. Endocrinologic abnormalities, e.g., hypercortisolism[60] and hyperprogestinism,[58] can also induce diabetes mellitus as a result of increased peripheral insulin inhibition.

Pathophysiology

Hyperglycemia and ketoacidosis occur when there is an absolute or relative deficiency of insulin. Recent evidence provides a bihormonal hypothesis for the development of diabetic ketoacidosis where absolute or relative hypoinsulinemia and hyperglucagonemia each play important biochemical roles.[42,48] Insulin deficiency results in decreased glucose use and an increased release of glucose precursors and free fatty acids by peripheral tissues. Hepatic gluconeogenic pathways are activated, and the extraction of glucogenic substrates becomes more efficient. In addition to increased hepatic glucose production, insulin deficiency promotes a significant increase in hepatic glucose output. The resulting hyperglycemia can raise the plasma osmolality, which causes cellular dehydration owing to the shift of water along the osmotic gradient. When the blood glucose level exceeds the maximal renal tubular threshold for glucose reabsorption, glucosuria occurs along with the excretion of water and electrolytes (Na^+, K^+, Cl^-, HPO_4^{2-}, $H_2PO_4^-$).

In the past, increased hepatic ketone body production was primarily attributed to the increased free fatty acid flux from adipose tissue as a result of insulin lack. Although this event strongly contributes to ketogenesis, intrahepatic processes and the disposition of incoming fatty acids are now recognized as equally important.[42,48] Within the liver, increased carnitine levels resulting from insulin deficiency and activation of the enzyme acylcarnitine transferase (resulting from glucagon excess) stimulate the mitochondrial β-oxidative pathway and augmented ketogenesis. The ketones released by the liver cannot be metabolized at normal rates by muscle tissue and thus accumulate within the blood. The ketone acids acetoacetate and β-hydroxybutyrate neutralize blood bicarbonate, resulting in a metabolic acidosis with an elevated anion gap. [The anion gap represents unmeasured anions associated with the acidic cation H^+. It is calculated according to the following formula: (Na^+ + K^+) − (Cl^- + HCO_3^-), where a result in excess of 30 mEq/L is generally significant.[25]]

Diagnosis

Diabetic ketoacidosis can be suspected when the patient's history is characterized by polydipsia, polyuria, weight loss, and polyphagia of several weeks' or months' duration which progresses to include the signs of lethargy, anorexia, and vomiting during the several days prior to examination. Some patients present with an acute history exemplified by a recent onset of polydipsia, polyuria, vomiting, weakness, and depression.

The physical examination abnormalities vary from minimal to extreme debilitation. The decompensated patient is often dehydrated, weak, and depressed, and has palpable hepatomegaly. The presence of cataracts of recent onset alert the clinician to suspect diabetes. A thorough history is taken and a complete physical examination is done to detect any coexisting disease processes, e.g., acute pancreatitis, Cushing's syndrome, pyometra, and sepsis.

The absolute diagnosis depends on the clinicopathological demonstration of hyperglycemia, glucosuria, hyperketonemia, and ketonuria. Other commonly associated serum biochemical abnormalities include azotemia, hypobicarbonatemia, hypokalemia, hyponatremia, hypophosphatemia, and elevated serum liver enzyme levels.[45,67] The hemogram results can be normal or show varying degrees of anemia and leukocytosis, the latter associated with a stress response or a coexisting inflammatory process. The urine microscopic examination often reveals white blood cells and bacteria indicative of a lower urinary tract infection.[45]

Treatment

The therapeutic principles for treating the depressed, anorectic, dehydrated ketoacidotic diabetic include: (1) restoration of hydration with isotonic intravenous fluids; (2) correction of any electrolyte deficiencies, especially hypokalemia and hyponatremia; (3) correction of severe metabolic acidosis (arterial pH < 7.1) with sodium bicarbonate solution; (4) use of regular crystalline insulin; and (5) provision of a carbohydrate substrate when the blood glucose falls below 250 mg/dl.

Fluid Replacement. The estimated total 24-hr fluid requirement amounts to the sum of the patient's dehydration deficit, the 24-hr maintenance needs, and the extra losses incurred from vomiting and diarrhea. The dehydration status is approximated on a scale ranging from mild (5%) to extreme (10%), and the needed volume of isotonic replacement solution is calculated with either of the following formulas:

Dehydration volume deficit (ml) = % dehydration × body weight (kg) × 1,000

Dehydration volume deficit (ml) = % dehydration × body weight (1b) × 500

The 24-hr maintenance volume is roughly estimated (assuming adequate urine output) at 60 ml/kg body weight. If the patient is oliguric, the amount of maintenance solution equals the volumes of urine output and the estimated insensible water loss (15 ml/kg/day). If the patient is 8–10% dehydrated, one-half of the estimated dehydration deficit is administered intravenously over the first 2–4-hr of hospitalization, with the remaining replacement and maintenance volumes given over the following 20–22 hr.

Lactated Ringer's solution is usually the initial fluid of choice. The lactate is not associated with an H^+ and therefore does not promote the onset of a lactic acidosis.[31] Saline (0.9%) can also be used as the initial rehydrating solution and is the fluid of choice when the patient is significantly hyponatremic (serum sodium < 132 mEq/L). Principles of fluid therapy are discussed further in Chapter 4.

Sodium Replacement. Hyponatremia can be factitious (due to hypertriglyceridemia) or real (due to urinary sodium ion loss).[28] Factitious hyponatremia or pseudohyponatremia is suspected when the plasma sample is grossly lipemic, although this does not always rule out a true sodium deficit.

In the past, true hyponatremia associated with diabetes mellitus was attributed to the osmotic diuresis induced by glucosuria and the renal excretion of ketone salts. Recent evidence suggests that insulin deficiency may directly contribute to the renal sodium loss because experiments have shown that insulin promotes the tubular reabsorption of sodium.[17] Hyponatremia is corrected with intravenous 0.9% saline solution in order to avoid any plasma hyposmolality which might occur when the hyperglycemia is reduced with insulin treatment. Plasma hyposmolality causes a reversal of osmotic gradients and overexpansion of the intracellular compartment, particularly the nervous system, with resultant cerebral edema.[3,14]

Potassium Replacement. Hypokalemia is the most important electrolyte disturbance in diabetic ketoacidosis and reflects a substantial reduction in the total body potassium stores.[40] The major causes of potassium depletion include: (1) lean tissue breakdown; (2) hypoinsulinemia, allowing cellular potassium to enter the plasma and be lost in the urine; (3) secondary hyperaldosteronism, in response to hypovolemia; and (4) gastrointestinal loss from vomiting.[40] After the commencement of therapy, a further decline in serum potassium levels occurs owing to: (1) serum dilution from rehydration; (2) continued urinary losses brought about by sodium ion delivery to the distal renal tubule; (3) correction of acidosis and the accompanying cellular influx of potassium ions; and (4) increased cellular uptake of potassium due to insulin.[42]

Most ketoacidotic, dehydrated diabetics with normokalemia actually have a considerable total body potassium deficit.[41] Potassium supplementation is best provided with potassium chloride (KCl) solution, which is added to the parenteral fluids. If concurrent hypophosphatemia is present, potassium phosphate solution can be added as well. Potassium supplementation is best begun after the first 2 hr of fluid replacement when hydration, blood pressure, and urine output are improved. If the patient is initially hypokalemic, KCl can be added to the hydrating solution, but the infusion is slowed down to where one-half of the dehydration replacement volume is delivered over an additional 1- to 3-hr period. The recommended amount of potassium supplementation to be administered *over a 24-hr period* is as follows:

1. Mild hypokalemia (serum K^+ = 3.0–3.5 mEq/L): give 2–3 mEq KCl/kg.
2. Moderate hypokalemia (serum K^+ = 2.5–3.0 mEq/L): give 3–5 mEq KCl/kg.
3. Severe hypokalemia (serum K^+ = < 2.5 mEq/L): give 5–10 mEq KCl/kg.

Daily serum electrolyte determinations and the necessary treatment adjustments are made until normal values are obtained. The intravenous fluids are discontinued when serum biochemistries are normal, euhydration is present, and the patient is able to eat.

Acidosis. The metabolic acidosis results from the accumulation of acid organic anions (acetoacetate and β-hydroxybutyrate), which buffer and thereby lower the plasma bicarbonate level. In most patients the use of lactated Ringer's solution and insulin effectively counteract the acidosis.[1,41] Restoration of a normal blood pH is also significantly aided by the patient's own physiological response mechanisms, which include tissue and blood protein buffering, increased ventilation, renal regeneration and absorption of bicarbonate ions, and metabolic conversion of the ketone acids to bicarbonate.

The use of sodium bicarbonate solution is reserved for those patients with a blood pH of less than 7.1.[16,53] The amount (milliequivalents) of bicarbonate required for extracellular replacement = 0.3 × kg body weight × base deficit. To avoid complications (see Table 5-2, below), the sodium bicarbonate supplementation is discontinued when the blood pH is restored to a level of 7.25. The management of metabolic acidosis is detailed in Chapter 4.

Insulin. Regular crystalline insulin is used when the patient has signs of depression, dehydration, anorexia, and vomiting. The advantages of regular insulin include: (1) various routes of administration (IV, IM, and SQ); (2) rapid onset of action; and (3) short duration of action. These properties allow adequate insulin titration throughout the day according to the animal's needs. The clinician must acknowledge that blood glucose levels decline much earlier than ketone levels and so anticipate the persistence of some ketonemia and ketonuria for the first 48–72 hr.

Bolus intravenous doses of insulin offer the advantage of an immediate onset of action for the critically hypotensive patient. The recommended dose for a medium-sized to large dog is 1–2 units/kg.[45,50,74] In the small dog and cat the dose is reduced to 0.5 units/kg.[50] Subsequent doses are given at the same amount every 2–3 hr until the blood glucose levels decrease to less than 250 mg/dl, at which time the patient is switched over to subcutaneous insulin injections given approximately every 6 hr. The disadvantages of this technique include the need for intensive care monitoring with frequent (every 1–2 hr) blood glucose determinations, the likelihood of hypoglycemia and hypokalemia, and the possibility of cerebral edema resulting from a too-rapid fall in blood glucose levels. When laboratory facilities are unavailable, blood glucose reagent strips (Chemstrip bG reagent strips, Biodynamics, Inc., Indianapolis IN 46250; or Dextrostix reagent strips, Ames Division, Miles Laboratories,

Inc., Elkart, IN 46515) can be used for approximate blood glucose determinations, although their accuracy is questionable. Several reflectance colorimeters are now commercially available to enhance the accuracy of these reagent strips.

To circumvent the occurrence of the aforementioned side effects, a continuous low-dose insulin infusion can be used. One successfully applied technique in the dog involves the addition of 5 units of regular insulin to a 500 ml bottle of lactated Ringer's solution after the first 2 hr of rehydration and adjusting the *pediatric* infusion set whereby 0.5–1.0 unit/hr is delivered to the patient.[74] Care must be taken to avoid intravascular fluid overload in the small animal which might result from this technique. Blood glucose determinations should be made every 1–2 hr.

Low-doses of regular insulin can also be given intramuscularly.[11,12] Initially 2 units are given into the thigh muscles of cats and dogs weighing less than 10 kg. For dogs weighing more than 10 kg, the initial dose is 0.25 unit/kg. Subsequent hourly injections of 1 unit for cats and small dogs and 0.1 unit/kg for larger dogs are given until the blood glucose level is less than 250 mg/dl, at which time the subcutaneous route can be used every 6 hr. The low doses used in this technique can be accurately measured with low-dose syringes (Lodose Insulin Syringe, Becton Dickinson, Rutherford, NJ 07070).

Subcutaneous regular insulin treatment is a suitable alternative to the intravenous and intramuscular methods when intensive care monitoring is unavailable.[70,72] The initial dose is 0.5 unit/kg followed by subsequent doses every 6 hr (Table 5-1).

The patient is regarded as stable and able to receive intermediate-acting (NPH, Lente) or ultralong-acting (PZI, Ultralente) insulin when normal hydration is restored, blood glucose levels are below 350 mg/dl, serum or urine ketones are minimal to absent, and oral feedings are accepted.

Complications

A list of complications, causative factors, and corrective measures (when possible) is provided in Table 5-2.

NONKETOTIC HYPEROSMOLAR DIABETIC SYNDROME

Etiology

The nonketotic hyperosmolar diabetic syndrome (NKHDS) is a serious metabolic emergency characterized by extreme dehydration, abnormal brain function, marked hyperglycemia, and the lack of significant ketoacidosis.[41] The incidence of this disorder in the dog and cat has not been reported; however, isolated case reports can be found in the veterinary literature.[68,73] In man, the NKHDS has been well described, with the majority of patients being middle-

Table 5-1. Sliding Scale Technique for Subcutaneous Regular Insulin Administration in the Ketoacidotic Cat and Dog after the Initial Injection

Urine Glucose[a]	Urine Ketones	Regular Insulin Every 6 hr (units)	IV Drip Supplement
2% (4+) *or* 1% (3+)	Large-small	Increase 1–2 units (cat and small dog) Increase 2–4 units (medium to large dog)	—
0.5% (2+)	Large-small	Repeat previous dose	Dextrose 2.5% or force feed[b]
2% (4+) *or* 1% (3+)	Trace-negative	Increase 1–2 units (cat and small dog) Increase 2–4 units (medium to large dog)	—
0.25% (1+), 0.1% (trace), negative	Large-negative	Omit insulin and reassess in 4 hr	Dextrose 2.5% or force feed
2% (4+) *or* 1% (3+)	Negative	Increase 1 unit (cat and small dog) Increase 2–4 units (medium or large dog)	—
0.5% (2+) *or* 0.25% (1+)[c]	Negative	Decrease 1–2 units	—
Negative	Negative	Decrease 2–4 units	Dextrose 2.5% or force feed

[a] Because simultaneous measurements of urine and blood glucose levels can differ, the clinician should determine the blood glucose concentration whenever an exact assessment is deemed necessary.[51]

[b] Forced feeding is not attempted if the animal is vomiting.

[c] When the animal is minimally or negative ketonuric, one of the longer-acting insulins is given at a dose amounting to two-thirds of the average total 24 hr requirement of regular insulin or 0.5 unit/kg body weight.

aged or elderly with mild adult-onset diabetes.[62] Several cases have been associated with glucocorticoid[8] and/or thiazide diuretic therapy.[75] Underlying renal disease, hypertension, and congestive heart failure are common. In most instances a precipitating condition, e.g., pneumonia and pancreatitis, can be implicated.[27]

Pathophysiology

Two concepts have been advanced to reasonably explain the pathophysiology of the NKHDS.[37] The first suggests that an insulinized liver (reflecting residual β-cell secretory activity) coexists with a diabetic periphery, thereby inactivating intrahepatic oxidation of incoming free fatty acids, which are directed largely along nonketogenic metabolic pathways, e.g., triglyceride synthesis. This could account for the absence of hyperketonemia. The second hypothesis provides that enhanced gluconeogenesis occurs in the liver due to the prevailing portal vein glucagon/insulin ratio. This effect is mainly responsible for the development of massive hyperglycemia.

The marked decreased in consciousness and the onset of associated neurologic abnormalities characterize this syndrome. Experiments have shown that marked hyperosmolality can cause restlessness, ataxia, nystagmus, irreg-

Table 5-2. Complications During Treatment of Diabetic Ketoacidosis

Complication	Causative Factors	Prophylaxis and/or Treatment
Hypoglycemia	Insulin overdose Failure to accurately measure blood glucose levels Failure to provide dextrose when the blood glucose level falls below 250 mg/dl	Give 50% dextrose 1 ml/kg by IV push followed by maintaining the patient with a 2.5–5% dextrose infusion
Hypokalemia	Failure to determine and monitor serum potassium levels Insulin overdose Inadequate potassium supplementation Excess bicarbonate administration	Monitor serum potassium levels at least once daily Provide potassium chloride supplementation as described in the text Use sodium bicarbonate only when metabolic acidosis is severe
Cerebral edema	Too rapid decline of the blood glucose level, causing an osmotic gradient shift of water into the brain parenchyma	Lower the blood glucose level gradually over a 6- to 12-hr period
Metabolic alkalosis	Excess bicarbonate use Continuous vomiting Hypokalemia	Avoid excess bicarbonate use Correct the hypokalemia Stop the lactated Ringer's and switch to 0.9% saline solution Given antemetics if necessary
Paradoxical CSF acidosis	Excess bicarbonate administration	Avoid excess bicarbonate use No treatment because sudden death ensues
Sepsis	Urinary or intravenous catheter contamination Failure to thoroughly assess patient	Maintain strict catheter aseptic techniques Culture any body fluid or site of suspected infection Use bactericidal antibiotics according to results of sensitivity testing

ular twitchings, convulsions, hyperthermia, and eventually death from respiratory failure.[46] Hyperglycemia of sufficient degree can establish an osmotic gradient between the extra- and intracellular compartments of the brain resulting in neuronal cellular dehydration and subsequent dysfunction. The brain attempts to counteract this osmotic gradient by forming "idiogenic osmols."[3] However, as the surrounding hyperosmolality increases, water eventually leaves the cells. The resulting cellular changes include shrinking of the oligodendroglial cytoplasm, decreased oligodendroglial processes about the vessels, vacuolation of endothelial cells, and increased neuronal density.[46]

Diagnosis

Historically, many patients have earlier signs of polydipsia, polyuria, weakness, and vomiting. Thirst can eventually diminish despite the mounting levels of hyperglycemia.[62]

On physical examination there is marked dehydration, hypotension, and depression. In addition to the altered state of consciousness, humans often present with a variety of neurologic signs, including grand mal seizures, hemiparesis, Babinski reflexes, muscle fasciculations, and nystagmus suggestive of diffuse cortical or subcortical damage.[62]

Several clinicopathologic abnormalities characterize the NKHDS. The blood glucose levels are often elevated above 800 mg/dl. Serum osmolality is elevated (normal serum osmolality = 290–310 mOsm/kg H_2O) and can be determined by the freezing point depression method with an osmometer or can be calculated by the following formula:

Osmolality (mOsm/kg)

$$= 2\ (\text{serum Na}^+ + \text{K}^+)(\text{mEq/L}) + \frac{\text{blood glucose (mg/dl)}}{18} + \frac{\text{BUN (mg/dl)}}{2.8}$$

The majority of patients are azotemic, which may be renal as well as prerenal in origin. Serum sodium and potassium levels can be high, normal, or low. Normokalemia is associated with depleted total body potassium stores. Therefore if the patient is initially hypokalemic, the clinician should interpret this value as a reflection of a profound total body potassium deficit.

Some patients with NKHDS have a metabolic acidosis despite the absence of detectable blood and urinary ketones. It should be noted that the standard nitroprusside reagent tablets and strips (Acetest reagent tablets and Ketostix reagent strips for the detection of urine ketones; Ames Division, Miles Laboratorics, Inc., Elkart, IN 46514) available for urine ketone determinations detect only acetone and acetoacetate, whereas β-hydroxybutyrate measurements require special laboratory techniques. The cause of the acidosis might be attributed to lactate accumulation, acute renal insufficiency, and unidentified organic acids.[62]

Treatment

The main goals of therapy include reestablishing normal hydration and adequate urine output, using insulin judiciously to avoid a precipitous decline in blood glucose levels, and providing ample amounts of potassium supplementation to make up the total body potassium deficit. The general techniques involving these treatment modalities are described in the section on ketoacidotic diabetes. Only the important exceptions concerning NKHDS are discussed in this section.

A common question regarding fluid therapy is whether the patient should initially receive 0.9% or 0.45% saline. In general, if the patient has a normal blood pressure and an elevated serum sodium level, 0.45% saline can be used initially.[41] If the patient is hypotensive and has normal or decreased serum sodium levels, 0.9% saline is the initial fluid of choice.[16,41] Often 0.9% saline is given during the first 2 hr of intravascular volume resuscitation, and then the fluids are switched to 0.45% saline for the maintenance volume infusion.

The regular insulin requirements for the nonketotic hyperosmolar diabetic are often less than in diabetic ketoacidosis.[41] Therefore close monitoring of the blood glucose levels is essential. Once it declines to approximately 250 mg/dl, the parenteral fluids should be switched to 5% dextrose in 0.45% saline in order to prevent a brisk lowering of the serum osmolality, which might cause cerebral edema.[16,41]

Potassium replacement has already been described in the ketoacidosis section. Insofar as many of these patients have some degree of renal failure, care should be taken to avoid creating hyperkalemia in the oliguric and anuric patient.

The complications of treatment are similar to those mentioned for the ketoacidotic diabetic. These are described in Table 5-2.

HYPOGLYCEMIA

There are numerous derangements in carbohydrate metabolism which may cause the blood glucose concentration to fall to abnormally low levels. Regardless of etiology, severe hypoglycemia is a medical emergency, as neuronal function is dependent on an adequate glucose supply. Irreversible damage to the central nervous system (CNS) or death may result from prolonged and profound hypoglycemia.[26]

Pathophysiology

Normally, glucose is the only energy metabolite used in significant quantities by the brain, yet carbohydrate reserves in nervous tissue are extremely limited.[26] As the blood glucose concentration decreases, the cerebral cortex and other areas of the brain with high metabolic rates are affected initially followed by the more slowly respiring vegetative centers in the diencephalon and hindbrain.[26] Prolonged hypoglycemia results in irreversible neuronal death, the cerebral cortex being damaged first and the lower centers later. Death of the patient is due to damage to the respiratory center.

Hypoglycemia is a potent stimulus for increased secretion of catecholamines, particularly epinephrine. This is a protective reflex as one of the effects of epinephrine is to increase hepatic glycogenolysis. Increased secretion of epinephrine by the adrenal medulla is accompanied by increased adrenocortical secretion, which also tends to compensate for the hypoglycemia by stimulating gluconeogenesis. A decrease in blood glucose also stimulates glucagon secretion and growth hormone secretion, two additional counterregulatory hormones. Glucagon increases both gluconeogenesis and glycogenolysis. Growth hormone, by decreasing utilization in peripheral tissues, tends to make more glucose available to the brain.

Recognition

The blood glucose concentration at which clinical signs of hypoglycemia appear is highly variable. In fact, severity of signs is believed to be related to the rate at which the blood glucose falls rather than to the degree of hypo-

Table 5-3. Clinical Signs of Hypoglycemia[4,22]

Hyperepinephrinemic Phase	Cerebral Phase
Tremors	Episodic incoordination
Nervousness	Posterior paresis
Hyperactivity	Syncope
Polyphagia	Blindness
Weakness	Barking or yelping
Tachycardia	Depression
	Generalized seizures
	Coma
	Death

glycemia.[38] Normal dogs may have fasting glucose levels as low as 40 mg/dl. Signs are usually intermittent and do not always correlate with feeding.[43] The clinical manifestations of hypoglycemia are due to either sympathetic overactivity or neuronal injury and may be classified according to the underlying pathogenetic mechanism (Table 5-3). Signs associated with the hyperepinephrinemic phase usually, but not consistently, precede those of the cerebral phase. Severe, generalized seizures are the most common sign of hypoglycemia in dogs.[22]

Management

The owner of an animal that is suffering from a hypoglycemic reaction may be instructed over the telephone to rub Karo syrup (Best Foods, Englewood, NJ) into the buccal mucosa. Most animals respond to this treatment within 30–60 sec.[22] Owners should never attempt, however, to pour the syrup into the mouth of a convulsing or comatose animal.

A venous blood sample is obtained immediately from any animal with signs suggestive of hypoglycemia as the initial step in management. The blood glucose concentration may be quickly estimated from this sample with Chemstrip reagent strips. The serum is submitted for simultaneous insulin and glucose determinations. If an immediate blood glucose determination is unavailable, dextrose is administered as a therapeutic trial. A solution of 50% dextrose is infused intravenously slowly to effect (usually 1.0 ml/kg). An intravenous infusion of 5–10% dextrose is then started and continued until serial blood glucose determinations reveal normoglycemia.

Inability to alleviate clinical signs with dextrose administration may indicate concomitant cerebral hypoxia and edema or neuronal death, and anticonvulsants, mannitol, dexamethasone, and local hypothermia (ice pack on the head of the dog) may be indicated.[13,22,38]

Blood samples are collected for follow-up glucose determinations at 1- to 2-hr intervals until the animal is stable. The underlying etiology and precipitating factors are then investigated.

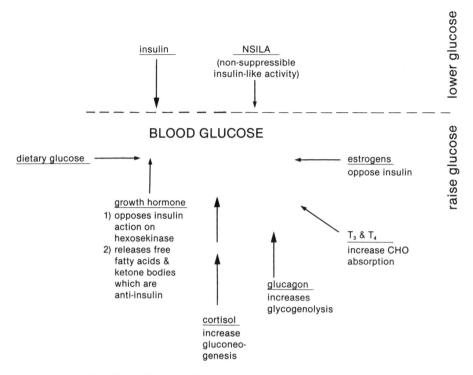

insulin

NSILA
(non-suppressible
insulin-like activity)

lower glucose

BLOOD GLUCOSE

raise glucose

dietary glucose ⟶

⟵ estrogens
oppose insulin

growth hormone
1) opposes insulin
   action on
   hexosekinase
2) releases free
   fatty acids &
   ketone bodies
   which are
   anti-insulin

T₃ & T₄
increase CHO
absorption

glucagon
increases
glycogenolysis

cortisol
increase
gluconeo-
genesis

Fig. 5-1.   Factors affecting blood glucose concentration.

Mechanisms of Hypoglycemia

Several homeostatic mechanisms operate to maintain the blood glucose concentration within a normal range (Figure 5-1). Decreased blood glucose levels may be the result of increased insulin or insulin-like activity, regardless of the source, as insulin enhances movement of glucose into peripheral cells, stimulates phosphorylation of glucose via hexosekinase, enhances oxidation of glucose-6-phosphate via the glycolytic and pentose phosphate pathways, and increases glycogen synthesis.[44] Hypoglycemia may be the result of decreased glycogenolysis, a process dependent on catecholamines and glucagon as well as on adequate tissue stores of glycogen. Decreased gluconeogenesis (e.g., glucocorticoid deficiency) and lack of peripheral insulin antagonism (e.g., growth hormone deficiency) are other mechanisms. Finally, decreased absorption of glucose from the gastrointestinal tract has been described as a mechanism by which hypoglycemia occurs.[4,26]

Differential Diagnosis

There are numerous causes of hypoglycemia, and long-term therapy must be specific for the underlying etiology (Table 5-4). Drug-induced hypoglycemia may occur in diabetic animals receiving exogenous insulin as a result of in-

Table 5-4. Differential Diagnosis of Hypoglycemia

Drug-induced hypoglycemia
Pancreatic islet cell tumors
Extrapancreatic neoplasia
Starvation
Advanced pregnancy
Glycogen storage disease
Adrenocortical hypofunction
Diffuse hepatic disease
Severe sepsis

judicious control of diet, medications, or exercise. Hypoglycemia in some insulin-dependent human diabetic patients has resulted from inadequate counterregulatory mechanisms,[7] but this has not been documented in the dog or cat.

Functional pancreatic islet cell tumors have been reported in both the dog and cat, adenocarcinoma being most common in both species.[63] The diagnosis of an islet cell tumor is strongly suggested by the presence of an elevated insulin level that is inappropriate for the blood glucose level. In a recent study of 25 dogs with insulin-secreting islet cell tumors, the amended insulin/glucose (I/G) ratio

$$\text{Amended I/G} = \frac{\text{serum insulin (microunits/ml)} \times 100}{\text{blood glucose (mg/dl)} - 30}$$

was compared to other recommended diagnostic tests and found to be the most reliable method of diagnosis.[43] (A value > 30 suggests inappropriate hyperinsulinism.) In addition, this method is simple, inexpensive, and of minimal risk to the animal.

Hypoglycemia has also been associated with extrapancreatic neoplasia, particularly mesothelioma, adrenocortical carcinoma, hepatocellular carcinoma, gastrointestinal carcinoma, and lymphosarcoma.[4,18,26,60] It has been shown that hypoglycemia in human patients with nonpancreatic neoplasia may be due to production of a nonsuppressible insulin-like factor by the tumor.[30,34]

Starvation can produce clinical manifestations of hypoglycemia in puppies, especially those which are heavily parasitized. Depleted glycogen stores[13] and immaturity of glucose homeostatic mechanisms have been incriminated.[81] Hypoglycemia in fasted toy breeds has been described and may be the result of limited hepatic glycogen storage[13] or merely an exaggeration of the neonate's inability to tolerate fasting.[81] Seizures believed to be secondary to low blood glucose have been described in fasted hunting dogs.[13] However, the mechanism is unclear, and there are no available clinicopathologic data in the literature to document hypoglycemia as the underlying abnormality in these dogs.

Clinical manifestations of hypoglycemia may be seen during late gestation in some bitches.[35,36] The pathogenetic mechanism causing low blood glucose in these animals is unknown. Hypoglycemia has also been reported in German shepherd dogs with type III glycogen storage disease.[10,64] In humans, hypoglycemia may occur in association with adrenal insufficiency. Although there are some data to suggest that clinically apparent hypoglycemia secondary to adrenal dysfunction also occurs in the dog, this remains controversial.[36]

It is generally believed that severe, diffuse liver disease of any etiology may result in hypoglycemia, as the liver is the major site of glycogenolysis and gluconeogenesis.[39,79] Although this category has been documented in humans, hepatic disease is not a well-established cause of hypoglycemia in dogs and cats.[36]

Finally, hypoglycemia has been described in dogs with both experimentally induced and naturally occurring sepsis.[6,9,32] This is presumably why some dogs with parvoviral enteritis develop hypoglycemia. Several mechanisms have been postulated, including increased glucose utilization and decreased glucose production.

In conclusion, regardless of the underlying etiology, severe hypoglycemia must be recognized and the appropriate emergency care rendered. Determination of the specific cause allows definitive therapy to follow. Failure to recognize and rapidly reverse the clinical manifestations of hypoglycemic crisis may result in death.

THYROTOXICOSIS

In man, thyrotoxicosis can result in "hyperthyroid storm," a serious but rather infrequent medical emergency caused by the sudden and massive release of thyroid hormone. Death in affected individuals occurs from severe hyperpyrexia and from pulmonary edema associated with cardiac arrhythmias, shock, and coma.[4] Although "hyperthyroid storm" is not generally recognized in the dog and cat, thyrotoxicosis due to functional thyroid neoplasms and thyroid adenomatous hyperplasia are seen, and potentially lethal arrhythmias as well as congestive heart failure have been described.[5,33,52,55,65] Hyperthyroidism, particularly in cats, warrants immediate medical intervention to prevent or reverse the serious adverse effects of excessive thyroid hormone on the myocardium.

Pathophysiology

The normal thyroid gland maintains a level of metabolism in the tissues that is optimal for function. Most of the widespread effects of thyroid hormones are secondary to their calorigenic action, although they also affect growth, lipid metabolism, and intestinal absorption of carbohydrate.[26] The constellation of clinical manifestations of thyrotoxicosis has heretofore been considered an exaggeration of hormonal action, but it is recently suggested that there may also be changes in target organ responsiveness, particularly in the myocardium.[4,26,47,84]

The hyperdynamic circulatory effects of excessive thyroid hormone resemble those of β-adrenergic stimulation, and the administration of sympathetic antagonistic agents reduces the heart rate, cardiac output, pulse pressure, and

Table 5-5. Clinical Signs of Hyperthyroidism[5,33,52,55,66]

Signs attributed to enhanced catecholamine effects
  Hyperactivity/nervousness
  Tremors
  Tachycardia
  Arrhythmias
  Heat intolerance (panting)
  Forceful femoral pulse
Signs attributed to hypermetabolism
  Pyrexia
  Polyphagia
  Polyuria/polydipsia[a]
  Weight loss
  Myopathy (weakness)
  Cardiac hypertrophy
Signs attributed to increased autonomic nervous activity
  Diarrhea
  Large, bulky stools

[a] Polyuria may also be due to interference with the action of antidiuretic hormone on the renal tubule.

myocardial oxygen consumption of hyperthyroidism to nearly normal.[15,76,82] Yet there is also evidence to suggest independent action of thyroxine on the myocardium.[24,26] Although excessive thyroid hormone causes cardiac hypertrophy in several species,[77,78] it is not clear if hyperthyroidism causes congestive heart failure independent of other cardiac abnormalities. It is important to note, however, that administration of thyroxine to a group of normal dogs did result in congestive heart failure in one-third of the animals.[61]

Recognition

The actions of the thyroid hormones and the catecholamines are intimately related, and the clinical signs of hyperthyroidism are attributable to the direct action of these hormones on intermediary metabolism, to thyroxine-catecholamine interaction, and to increased autonomic nervous system activity. Table 5-5 summarizes the clinical manifestations of hyperthyroidism in the dog and cat. The cardiac effects of excessive thyroid hormone are potentially life-threatening and merit special consideration. These effects are summarized in Table 5-6. As in human patients, treatment of thyrotoxicosis resolves the ECG abnormalities, cardiac hypertrophy, and hyperdynamic circulatory state in most animals.[33,59,82]

Management

Laboratory confirmation of the diagnosis of thyrotoxicosis requires the finding of elevated serum thyroxine (T_4), triiodothyronine (T_3), or both. Because the cat and dog rarely present in a "hyperthyroid storm," definitive therapy can often await laboratory confirmation. Occasionally, however, a hyperthyroid animal requires initiation of treatment for lethal tachyarrhythmias or congestive heart failure before T_3 and T_4 results are available.

Table 5-6. Effects of Thyrotoxicosis on the Cardiovascular System

Arrhythmias[33,52,59]
    Severe sinus tachycardia[a]
    Ventricular tachycardias
    Ventricular preexcitation
Other ECG abnormalities[59]
    Intraventricular conduction defects
    Increased R wave amplitude in lead II
    Prolonged QRS duration
    Shortened QT interval
Left ventricular hypertrophy[33,59]
Augmented myocardial contractility[15,82]
Increased cardiac output[15,82]
Increased myocardial oxygen consumption[15,82]
Decreased cardiac reserve[24]

[a] Most common abnormality.

As previously discussed, an extremely important aspect of hyperthyroidism, especially its deleterious cardiovascular effects, is the interaction between thyroid hormones and catecholamines. Accordingly, propranolol, a β-adrenergic antagonist, is used to block this interaction. This drug is administered orally or, if needed, by intravenous administration with ECG monitoring. There are data which suggest that thyrotoxic patients require a higher propranolol dosage than euthyroid patients,[21] and the optimal dose must be individualized with a suggested range of 2.5–10 mg PO three times daily in cats and 10–40 mg PO three times daily in dogs. Whereas the use of propranolol is contraindicated in the presence of congestive heart failure of other etiology, it is quite useful in the high output failure of thyrotoxicosis.[4] Signs of congestion, if present, are controlled with diuretics and oxygen in addition to propranolol.

Although the β-adrenergic blocking action of propranolol counters the effects of excessive thyroid hormone on the heart, it has no effect on the elevated thyroid hormone concentrations. A saturated solution of potassium iodide (SSKI) may be used in conjunction with propranolol to retard release of T_3 or T_4 from the thyroid gland.[4,55] The recommended feline dosage is 70–100 mg PO (2–3 drops) daily.[55] A major disadvantage of SSKI is its unpleasant taste, which results in ptyalism and anorexia in some cats.

Surgical removal of functional neoplastic or hyperplastic tissue is the preferred treatment of hyperthyroidism and should be strongly considered, especially in the canine where most functional tumors are malignant.[5,66] All cats are prepared for surgery not only with propranolol and possibly iodides, but also with propylthiouracil (PTU) at a dosage of 50 mg PO three times daily.[56] This agent acts by inhibiting thyroid hormone synthesis, thereby lowering elevated thyroid hormone concentrations within 2–3 weeks. Once the animal has been euthyroid for 2–4 weeks, most of the systemic manifestations of thyrotoxicosis will have resolved and surgical complications, e.g., hyperthermia, disorientation, cardiac dysfunction, and hemorrhage, will be markedly reduced. PTU may be used indefinitely to maintain a euthyroid state in cats who are high surgical risks for other reasons or whose owners refuse surgical intervention. However, surgery is the therapy of choice in most cats.[33] For hyperthyroid dogs, immediate surgical removal of abnormal tissue is indicated unless cardiac abnormalities are apparent.[5,33,66]

REFERENCES

1. Adrogue HJ, Wilson H, Boyd III AE, et al: Plasma acid-base patterns in diabetic ketoacidosis. N Engl J Med 307:1603, 1982
2. Albin J, Rifkin H: Etiologies of diabetes mellitus. Med Clin North Am 66:1209, 1982
3. Arieff AI, Kleeman CR: Studies on mechanisms of cerebral edema in diabetic comas—effects of hyperglycemia and rapid lowering of plasma glucose in normal rabbits. J. Clin Invest 52:571, 1973
4. Bacchus H: Hypoglycemic crisis. In: Metabolic and Endocrine Emergencies—Recognition and Management. p. 87. University Park Press, Baltimore, 1977
5. Belshaw BE: Thyroid diseases. In Ettinger SJ (ed): Textbook of Veterinary Internal Medicine. 2nd Ed. p. 1542. Saunders, Philadelphia, 1983
6. Berk JL, Hagen JF, Beyer WH, et al: Hypoglycemia of shock. Ann Surg 171:400, 1970
7. Boden G, Reichard GA, Hoeldtke RD, et al: Severe insulin-induced hypoglycemia associated with deficiencies in the release of counter-regulatory hormones. N Engl J Med 305:1200, 1981
8. Boyer MH: Hyperosmolar anacidotic coma in association with glucocorticoid therapy. JAMA 202:95, 1967
9. Breitschwerdt EB, Loar AS, Hribernik TN, et al: Hypoglycemia in four dogs with sepsis. J Am Vet Med Assoc 178:1072, 1981
10. Ceh L, Hague JG, Svenkerud R, et al: Glycogenosis type III in the dog. Acta Vet Scand 17:210, 1976
11. Chastain CB: Intensive care of dogs and cats with diabetic ketoacidosis. J Am Vet Med Assoc 179:972, 1981
12. Chastain CB, Nichols CE: Low-dose intramuscular insulin therapy for diabetic ketoacidosis in dogs. J Am Vet Med Assoc 178:561, 1981
13. Chrisman CL: Problems in Small Animal Neurology. Lea & Febiger, Philadelphia, 1982
14. Clements RS Jr, Prockop LD, Winegrad AI: Acute cerebral edema during treatment of hyperglycemia—an experimental model. Lancet 2:384, 1968
15. Cohen MV, Schulman IC, Spenillo A, et al: Effects of thyroid hormone on left ventricular function in patients treated for thyrotoxicosis. Am J Cardiol 48:33, 1981
16. Daniels JS, Fishman N: Diabetes mellitus and hyperlipidemia. In Freitag JJ, Miller LW (eds): Manual of Medical Therapeutics. 23rd Ed. p. 349. Little, Brown, Boston, 1980
17. DeFronzo RA, Cook CR, Andres R, et al: The effect of insulin on renal handling of sodium, potassium, calcium, and phosphate in man. J Clin Invest 55:845, 1975
18. DeSchepper J, Van Der Stock J, DeRick A, et al: Hypercalcemia and hypoglycemia in a case of lymphatic leukemia in the dog. Vet Rec 94:602, 1974
19. Ettinger PO, Regan TJ, Oldewurtel HA: Hyperkalemia, cardiac conduction and the electrocardiogram: a review. Am Heart J 88:360, 1974
20. Fajans SS, Floyd JD: Fasting hypoglycemia in adults. N Engl J Med 294:766, 1976

21. Feely J, Stevenson IH, Crooks J, et al: Increased clearance of propranolol in thyrotoxicosis. Ann Intern Med 94:472, 1981
22. Feldman EC: Hyperinsulinism. In Veterinary Clinical Endocrinology. Program Notes, San Diego's 4th Annual Veterinary Conference, February 1981
23. Feldman EC, Tyrrell JB, Bohannon NV: The synthetic ACTH stimulation test and measurement of endogenous plasma ACTH levels: useful diagnostic indicators for adrenal disease in dogs. J Am Anim Hosp Assoc 14:524, 1978
24. Forfar JC, Muir AL, Sawers SA, et al: Abnormal left ventricular function in hyperthyroidism. N Engl J Med 307:1165, 1982
25. Gabow PA, Kaehny WD, Fennessey PV, et al: Diagnostic importance of an increased serum anion gap. N Engl J Med 303:854, 1980
26. Ganong WF: Review of Medical Physiology, 10th Ed. Lange Medical Publications, Los Altos, CA, 1981
27. Gerich JE, Martin MM, Recant L: Clinical and metabolic characteristics of hyperosmolar nonketotic coma. Diabetes 20:228, 1971
28. Goldberg M: Hyponatremia. Med Clin North Am 65:251, 1981
29. Gonzales RB: Selected emergency endocrinologic problems. In Schwartz GR, Safar P, Stone JH, et al (eds): Principles and Practice of Emergency Medicine. p. 1078. Saunders, Philadelphia, 1978
30. Gordon P, Hendricks CM, Kahn CR, et al: Hypoglycemia associated with non-islet cell tumor and insulin-like growth factors. N Engl J Med 305:1452, 1981
31. Hartsfield SM, Thurmon JC, Benson GJ: Sodium bicarbonate and bicarbonate precursors for treatment of metabolic acidosis. J Am Vet Med Assoc 179:914, 1981
32. Hinshaw LB: Concise review: the role of glucose in endotoxin shock. Circ Shock 3:1, 1976
33. Holzworth J, Theran P, Carpenter JL, et al: Hyperthyroidism in the cat: ten cases. J Am Vet Med Assoc 176:345, 1980
34. Hyodo T, Megyeski K, Kahn CR, et al: Adrenocortical carcinoma and hypoglycemia: evidence for production of nonsuppressible insulin-like activity by the tumor. J Clin Endocrinol Metab 44:1175, 1977
35. Irvine GHG: Hypoglycemia in the bitch. NZ Vet J 169:811, 1964
36. Jackson RF, Bruss ML, Growney PJ, et al: Hypoglycemia-ketonemia in a pregnant bitch. J Am Vet Med Assoc 177:1123, 1980
37. Joffe BI, Krut LH, Goldberg RB, et al: Pathogenesis of nonketotic hyperosmolar diabetic coma. Lancet 1:1069, 1975
38. Johnson RK: Insulinoma in the dog. Vet Clin North Am 7:629, 1977
39. Johnson RK, Atkins CE: Hypoglycemia in the dog. In Kirk RW (ed): Current Veterinary Therapy VI. p. 1010. Saunders, Philadelphia, 1977
40. Kleeman CR, Narins RG: Diabetic acidosis and coma. In Maxwell MH, Kleeman CR (eds): Clinical Disorders of Fluid and Electrolyte Metabolism. 3rd Ed. p. 1339. McGraw-Hill, New York, 1980
41. Kozak GP, Rolla AR: Diabetic comas. In Kozak GP (ed): Clinical Diabetes Mellitus. p. 109. Saunders, Philadelphia, 1982
42. Kreisberg RA: Diabetic ketoacidosis: new concepts and trends in pathogenesis and treatment. Ann Intern Med 88:681, 1978
43. Kruth SA, Feldman EC, Kennedy PC, et al: Insulin-secreting islet cell tumors: establishing a diagnosis and the clinical course for 25 dogs. J Am Vet Med Assoc 181:54, 1982
44. Lehninger AL: Biochemistry. 2nd Ed. p. 820. Worth Publishers, New York, 1975

45. Ling GV, Lowenstine LJ, Pulley LT, et al: Diabetes mellitus in dogs: a review of initial evaluation, immediate and long-term management and outcome. J Am Vet Med Assoc 170:521, 1977
46. Maccario M: Neurological dysfunction associated with nonketotic hyperglycemia. Arch Neurol 19:525, 1968
47. McConnaughey MM, Jones LR, Watanabe AM, et al: Thyroxine and propylthiouracil effects of alpha- and beta-adrenergic receptor number, ATPase activities, and sialic acid content of rat cardiac membrane vesicles. J Cardiovasc Pharm 1:609, 1979
48. McGarry JD, Foster DW: Ketogenesis and its regulation. Am J Med 61:9, 1976
49. Miller RH: Textbook of Basic Emergency Medicine. 2nd Ed. p. 117. Mosby, St. Louis, 1980
50. Morgan RV: Endocrine and metabolic emergencies. Part I. Compend Contin Educ Pract Vet 4:755, 1982
51. Morris LR, McGee JA, Kitabchi AE: Correlation between plasma and urine glucose in diabetes. Ann Intern Med 94:469, 1981
52. Mulnix JA, Stokof AA, van Nes JJ, et al: Hyperthyroidism and cardiac changes in a dog. Can Pract 3:38, 1976
53. Narins RG, Gardner LB: Simple acid-base disturbances. Med Clin North Am 65:321, 1981
54. Nelson DH: The adrenal cortex: physiological function and disease. In Smith LH Jr (ed): Major Problems in Internal Medicine. Vol. 18. p. 113. Saunders, Philadelphia, 1980
55. Peterson ME: Feline hyperthyroidism. In: Veterinary Clinical Endocrinology. Program notes, San Diego's 4th Annual Veterinary Conference, February 1981
56. Peterson ME: Propylthiouracil in the treatment of feline hyperthyroidism. J Am Vet Med Assoc 179:485, 1981
57. Peterson ME, Feinman JM: Hypercalcemia associated with hypoadrenocorticism in sixteen dogs. J Am Vet Med Assoc 181:802, 1982
58. Peterson ME, Javanovic L, Peterson CM: Insulin resistant diabetes mellitus associated with elevated growth hormone concentrations following megestrol acetate treatment in a cat. In: ACVIM Scientific Proceedings. p. 63. July 1981
59. Peterson ME, Keene B, Ferguson DC, et al: Electrocardiographic findings in 45 cats with hyperthyroidism. J Am Vet Med Assoc 180:934, 1982
60. Peterson ME, Nesbitt GH, Schaer M: Diagnosis and management of concurrent diabetes mellitus and hyperadrenocorticism in thirty dogs. J Am Vet Med Assoc 178:66, 1981
61. Piatnek-Leunissen D, Olson RE: Cardiac failure in the dog as a consequence of exogenous hyperthyroidism. Circ Res 20:242, 1967
62. Podolsky S: Hyperosmolar nonketotic coma in the elderly diabetic. Med Clin North Am 62:815, 1978
63. Priester WA: Pancreatic islet cell tumors in domestic animals: data from 11 colleges of veterinary medicine in the United States and Canada. J Natl Cancer Inst 53:227, 1974
64. Rafiquzzman M, Svenkerud R, Strande A, et al: Glycogenosis in the dog. Acta Vet Scand 17:196, 1976
65. Reid CF, Persinger RR, Ferrigon W, et al: Functioning adenocarcinoma of the thyroid gland in a dog with mitral insufficiency. Am J Vet Radiol 4:36, 1963
66. Rijnberk A: Canine hyperthyroidism. In Veterinary Clinical Endocrinology. Program notes, San Diego's 4th Annual Veterinary Conference, February 1981.

67. Schaer M: Clinical survey of thirty cats with diabetes mellitus. J Am Anim Hosp Assoc 13:23, 1977
68. Schaer M: Diabetic hyperosmolar nonketotic syndrome in a cat. J Am Anim Hosp Assoc 11:42, 1975
69. Schaer M: Disorders of potassium metabolism. Vet Clin North Am 12:399, 1982
70. Schaer M: Feline diabetes mellitus. Vet Clin North Am 6:453, 1976
71. Schaer M: Hypoadrenocorticism. In Kirk RW (ed): Current Veterinary Therapy— Small Animal Practice VII. p. 983. Saunders, Philadelphia, 1980
72. Schaer M: Medical treatment of diabetes mellitus in the cat. AAHA's 50th Annual Meeting Proceedings. p. 167. 1983
73. Schaer M, Scott R, Wilkens R, et al: Hyperosmolar syndrome in the non-ketoacidotic diabetic dog. J Am Anim Hosp Assoc 10:357, 1974
74. Schall WD, Cornelius LM: Diabetic ketoacidosis. In Kirk RW (ed): Current Veterinary Therapy VII—Small Animal Practice, p. 1016. Saunders, Philadelphia, 1980
75. Shapiro AP, Benedek TG, Small JL: Effect of thiazides on carbohydrate metabolism in patients with hypertension. N Engl J Med 265:1028, 1961
76. Skelton CL: The heart and hyperthyroidism. N Engl J Med 307:1206, 1982
77. Skelton CL, Sonnenblick EH: Heterogeneity of contractile function in cardiac hypertrophy. Circ Res 34/35(Suppl 2):83, 1974
78. Sterling K: Thyroid hormone action at the cell level. N Engl J Med 300:173, 1979
79. Strombeck DR: Small Animal Gastroenterology. p. 365. Stonegate Publishing, Davis, CA, 1979
30. Strombeck DR, Krum S, Meyer DJ, et al: Hypoglycemia and hypoinsulinemia associated with hepatoma in a dog. J Am Vet Med Assoc 169:811, 1976
81. Strombeck DR, Rogers Q, Freedland R, et al: Fasting hypoglycemia in a pup, J Am Vet Med Assoc 173:299, 1978
82. Taylor RR, Covell JW, Ross J, et al: Influence of the thyroid state on left ventricular tension-velocity relations in the intact, sedated dog. J Clin Invest 48:775, 1969
83. Tilley LP: Essentials of Canine and Feline Electrocardiography. p. 158. Mosby, St. Louis, 1979
84. Tse J, Wrenn RW, Kuo JF, et al: Thyroxine-induced changes in characteristics and activities of β-adrenergic receptors and adenosine 3',5'-monophosphate and guanosine 3',5'-monophosphate systems in the heart may be related to reputed catecholamine sensitivity in hyperthyroidism. Endocrinology 107:6, 1980
85. Willard MD, Schall WD, McCaw DE, Nachreiner RF: Canine hypoadrenocorticism: report of 37 cases and review of 39 previously reported cases. J Am Vet Med Assoc 180:59, 1982

6 | Urogenital Emergencies

Dennis J. Chew

Emergencies of the urogenital system are common in small animal practice. The major categories include renal failure, urinary tract trauma, obstructive uropathy, and genital medical emergencies.

RENAL FAILURE (AZOTEMIA)

Renal failure is defined as a level of renal dysfunction that results in retention of nitrogenous wastes. By definition, the serum creatinine and serum urea nitrogen (SUN, BUN) are elevated (azotemia). The detection of elevated serum creatinine or BUN should trigger a methodical search for the cause(s). There is a sense of urgency in identifying the cause(s) of azotemia, as permanent renal failure may result when correctable conditions are overlooked.

It must be emphasized that the magnitude of the azotemia does not determine its origin (prerenal, postrenal, or intrarenal), nor does it indicate whether a condition is acute or chronic, reversible or irreversible.[16] The BUN and serum creatinine must be integrated with history, physical examination, radiographs, and other laboratory findings (particularly a complete urinalysis). Laboratory data should be collected before drug or fluid therapy is given as they can alter results. Serial measurements of BUN and serum creatinine are frequently necessary to assess adequacy of therapy.

Prerenal Azotemia

Patients with newly recognized azotemia obligate consideration that prerenal, primary intrarenal, or postrenal factors are creating the disorder. Prerenal azotemia, the most frequent type, is associated with conditions that result in decreased delivery of blood to the kidney, e.g., shock, dehydration, or heart failure. Healthy kidneys are capable of excreting the nitrogenous load if adequate blood flow is presented to them. Thus prerenal azotemia characteristically declines rapidly as the kidney receives improved perfusion through fluid therapy (extracellular fluid volume expansion) or improved cardiodynamics.

The importance of determining that azotemia is prerenal is that it directs attention away from the kidney as the cause for the azotemia and focuses attention on dysfunction or illness in other organ systems that may cause reduced effective extracellular fluid volume (ECFV). Another consideration is that severe and/or protracted prerenal azotemia may eventually lead to primary renal azotemia (see later discussion on ischemic nephrosis). Consequently, rapid restoration of circulating fluid volume in patients with prerenal azotemia is essential (Ch. 4) and may be accomplished through administration of isotonic electrolyte solutions. Prerenal azotemic patients usually have urine concentrated to > 1.030 specific gravity.

Physical examination may disclose dehydration (estimated from skin turgor), cardiac murmurs or arrhythmias, and weak pulses. The clinician should look for a source for fluid loss, including sequestration detected by thoracic percussion or abdominal palpation. Abdominal radiographs should reveal normal kidney size and shape. Severely dehydrated or hypovolemic animals may show microcardia on thoracic radiography, or cardiac enlargement and pulmonary edema if severe cardiac disease with congestive failure exists. Although prerenal azotemia may be the sole origin of azotemia, it commonly coexists with primary intrarenal and postrenal causes of azotemia.

Postrenal Azotemia

Postrenal azotemia is usually readily diagnosed by physical examination and abdominal radiographs. It arises when there is obstruction to flow of urine formed by both kidneys, or when there is a tear in the excretory pathway resulting in urine leakage into the peritoneal cavity (uroabdomen). These causes of postrenal azotemia are further discussed under "Urinary Tract Trauma" and "Obstructive Uropathy." Initially, the kidneys are normal and capable of excreting waste products if the obstruction is relieved or the leak repaired. Longstanding obstruction can result in permanent loss of kidney function, ECFV depletion, and ischemic renal injury.

Primary Intrarenal Azotemia

Primary intrarenal azotemia can be caused by a wide variety of disorders that all have in common structural or functional lesions within the kidney. Three-fourths or more of the functional nephron mass must be nonfunctioning before azotemia occurs. Acute renal failure (ARF) is a syndrome characterized by an abrupt deterioration in renal function, recent onset of azotemia, and a failure of the kidney to adequately regulate solute and water balance. A concept of great clinical importance is that this functional state is potentially reversible.[27] Recently recognized azotemia due to intrarenal causes can fall into one of two categories: ARF or chronic renal failure that was not detected earlier.

Table 6-1. Etiology of Nephritis Causing Acute Renal Failure

Leptospirosis
Pyelonephritis
Glomerulonephritis
Viral
Drug-induced (allergic)

ARF superimposed on previously existing chronic renal failure or chronic renal disease must also be considered.

Nephritis. Nephritis and nephrosis are the two major divisions of primary intrarenal ARF. Nephritis capable of creating ARF must have inflammatory lesions involving more than three-fourths of the functional nephron mass. The potential causes are listed in Table 6-1.

Leptospirosis is occasionally encountered as a cause of ARF due to nephritis. The diagnosis may be suggested by concomitant liver disease, as well as renal/muscle pain, fever, casts in the urine, and oliguria. Serology demonstrating a rising leptospirosis titer helps secure the diagnosis. Definitive culture is difficult, and demonstration of leptospiruria is unreliable. Leptospirosis is treated with penicillin and streptomycin to rid tissues of the organism. Parenteral fluid therapy is also important.

Overwhelming bacterial infection of the kidney from an ascending route (pyelonephritis) or from hematogenous embolic seeding of bacteria can also result in primary ARF. Renal pain, fever, excessive casts in the urine (notably white blood cell casts), pyuria, and bacteriuria are all suggestive of bacterial nephritis. Quantitative urine culture usually reveals one type of bacteria growing in abundance. Kidneys are usually normal or slightly enlarged on palpation and radiography. Intravenous pyelography can support a diagnosis of pyelonephritis if dilated proximal ureters, diverticular blunting, or renal pelvic dilatation are found, but these abnormalities can be transient and are not found in every case.[2] Neutrophilic leukocytosis with left shift can also be seen.[18] Urine concentration is disrupted early in the development of pyelonephritis. Depending on the stage, urine volume may initially be increased but is decreased later as dehydration and renal inflammation become more severe.

Early recognition and treatment of symptomatic bacterial infection in the kidney that has caused ARF is important to prevent not only irreversible loss of nephron mass but also the consequences of bacteremia. Because most of these patients are seriously ill, the intravenous route of administration of replacement and maintenance fluid is required. Initial antimicrobial treatment is given intravenously while awaiting the results of susceptibility tests and organism identification. An agent should be chosen that achieves high tissue and urine concentration and is not nephrotoxic. The cephalosporins (Keflex) are often chosen because of their wide spectrum of activity, relative nontoxicity to the kidney, and the high urine and tissue concentrations they achieve. Dosage is employed at 11–18 mg/kg IV t.i.d. Ampicillin at 22 mg/kg IV t.i.d. can also be used, particularly when gram-positive organisms are identified. Chloramphenicol is an alternative drug at 33 mg/kg IV t.i.d. Changing from one drug

Table 6-2. Etiology of Nephrosis

Hypoperfusion (ischemia)[a]
Nephrotoxins[a]
Thrombosis/embolization
Pigments (myoglobinuria/hemoglobinuria)

[a] Most important.

to another may be advised if no symptomatic improvement is seen within 24 hr of treatment or if a superior drug is indicated by identification of the organism (e.g., *Klebsiella* and cephalosporin[30] or *Pseudomonas* and gentamicin[31]) or by susceptibility tests. It should be noted that Kirby-Bauer susceptibility disk testing may report back drugs as ineffective that actually are effective in urine due to the high concentration of agent there when excreted. Reculture of urine while on the agent is advised after 48 hr of therapy. If organisms are still growing, another agent should then be substituted. Treatment with nephrotoxic antibiotics may be unavoidable if resistant organisms are encountered. When this is necessary, it is wise to ensure adequate hydration prior to starting agents such as aminoglycosides.

Nephrosis. Nephrosis classically exists when there are degenerative or necrotic lesions within the renal tubules without primary inflammatory lesions. Intrarenal ARF can result from obvious lesions of the tubules, but sometimes minimal or no light microscopic lesions can be found, even though severe functional derangement exists. The etiologies of nephrosis are listed in Table 6-2.

Renal hypoperfusion (Table 6-3) is a common predisposition to nephrosis in veterinary patients. It is frequently not possible to predict which patients will progress to intrarenal ARF, but those with the longest duration and most severe degree of ischemia are most likely to develop primary ARF. Many of the conditions listed in Table 6-3 produce catecholamine-induced vasoconstriction which reduces the glomerular filtration rate (GFR) and renal blood flow (RBF), resulting in renal ischemia. The renal tubule cell has high-energy production and consumption requirements which make it especially susceptible to the effects of ischemia.

Nephrotoxin exposure is another common cause of nephrosis (Tables 6-4 and 6-5). Increased numbers of patients with ARF due to nephrotoxins may be anticipated with more widespread use of potent nephrotoxic antibiotics. Ethylene glycol poisoning and exposure to the potent aminoglycoside antibiotics pose the greatest risks for nephrotoxic ARF.

Table 6-3. Renal Hypoperfusion (Ischemia)

Dehydration	Surgery
Hypovolemic shock	Sepsis
Hemorrhage	Burns
Trauma	Body temperature extremes
Anesthesia	Pigments

Table 6-4. Nephrotoxins

Antibiotics
Heavy metals
Organic compounds (ethylene
    glycol)[a]
Anesthetics
Hypercalcemia
Radiographic contrast agents
Snake venom

[a] Most important.

The lesions in nephrotoxic ARF are most obvious in the proximal tubule but may affect all levels of the nephron, depending on the severity of the insult. Nephrotoxins in general exert their effect after attaching to tubular cell membranes and altering cell permeability, which then affects nutrient transport, energy production, and cell volume, causing cell death.[38]

The patient who survives ischemic or nephrotoxic ARF goes through three phases: latent, maintenance, and recovery. The latent phase is the period from the toxic or ischemic insult until there is a detectable increase in BUN or serum creatinine or a detectable change in urine volume. Initially, urine specific gravity becomes progressively more dilute, but no other abnormality in the urinalysis is detected. Because clinical signs are minimal at this stage, it is unlikely for animals to be presented for evaluation at this time. It is possible that patients who develop ARF while in a veterinary hospital may be detected during this stage if carefully observed. Reversibility is most feasible during this stage.

The maintenance phase (Table 6-6) implies that a predictable course of renal dysfunction has been entered and that removal of the inciting insult at this point will not result in the immediate return of normal renal function. The duration of renal failure during this stage typically lasts 7–14 days regardless of urine volume. During this stage the serum creatinine and BUN increase progressively until a plateau of azotemia is reached. Regardless of urine volume, urine concentration is low (low specific gravity). Urine sediment may be active, showing casts and/or renal epithelia. In addition, proteinuria can be anticipated, and occasionally glucosuria occurs due to tubular injury.

Improving GFR and decreasing BUN and serum creatinine characterize the recovery phase. Previously oliguric cases enter a diuretic phase before or during the decline of BUN and creatinine. Polyuric ARF cases gradually return

Table 6-5. Nephrotoxic Antibiotics

Aminoglycosides[a]
Amphotericin B[a]
Cephaloridine
Sulfonamides
Polymixin B
Vancomycin
Bacitracin
Tetracycline

[a] Most important.

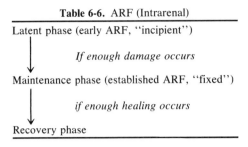

Table 6-6. ARF (Intrarenal)

Latent phase (early ARF, "incipient")

    If enough damage occurs

Maintenance phase (established ARF, "fixed")

    if enough healing occurs

Recovery phase

to normal urine production. Subclinical defects in maximal urine concentration and acidification do remain, though BUN and creatinine return to normal.[27]

The pathophysiology of oliguria and retention of nitrogenous wastes encountered in primary ARF include failure of glomerular filtration to occur, passive back-leak of filtrate along damaged tubules, and obstruction to flow along the nephron.[23,27] Conversion to nonoliguria and a decreasing level of nitrogenous waste accumulation can be explained by the correction of the factors just discussed. Additionally, defective solute resorption by the proximal tubule, excretion of solutes retained during the maintenance phase, excretion of iatrogenic volume overload during the maintenance phase, and medullary washout may contribute to diuresis.[27]

Table 6-7 lists criteria for differentiating chronic renal failure, acute renal failure, and prerenal failure. No single criterion is capable of pinpointing intrarenal ARF; thus careful integration of findings from the history, physical examination, and selected laboratory or radiographic studies is necessary to establish a diagnosis. In some cases it may also be necessary to obtain a renal biopsy before an appropriate diagnosis can be made.

Table 6-8 notes the various factors which predispose a patient to developing intrarenal ARF.

Treatment of Intrarenal ARF

Because the existing renal lesions of intrarenal ARF cannot be directly changed, the goal of therapy is to keep the patient alive long enough to allow "natural healing" of the kidney to occur. The earlier the therapeutic intervention, the more likely is a successful outcome. Supportive measures consisting of fluids, electrolytes, alkali, blood transfusion, and various drugs are aimed at minimizing disturbances of internal homeostasis. Treatment and patient monitoring for ARF are summarized in Tables 6-9 and 6-10

Parenteral fluid therapy is necessary to support the intrarenal ARF patient throughout much of the maintenance phase (see "Fluid Therapy" in Ch. 4). Though fluid therapy is essential, the potential for overhydration poses a serious problem, as the excretory capacity of the ARF kidney is severely reduced. Volumes of infused fluid must be carefully calculated and adjusted according to urine output and adequacy of hydration. Rehydration can be accomplished with 0.9% NaCl or lactated Ringer's solution as commonly available isotonic

Table 6-7. Clinical Findings in CRF, Intrarenal ARF, and Prerenal Failure

Clinical Finding	CRF	Intrarenal ARF	Prerenal Failure
Serum urea nitrogen*	↑	↑	↑
Serum creatinine*	↑	↑	↑
Urine specific gravity* (urine osmolality)	↓	↓	↑
Urine sediment*	Inactive	Active	Inactive
Kidney size* (palpation, x-ray)	N or ↓	N or ↑	N
Anemia* (nonregenerative)	+	– (Early)	–
Response to fluid therapy* (decline in serum urea nitrogen or serum creatinine)	Minimal	Minimal	Dramatic
Longstanding polyuria/polydipsia (historical)	+	–	–
Toxin, drug exposure	–	+	–, +
Ischemic episode	–	+	+, –
Renal pain (history, physical)	–	+	–
Oliguria	– (Unless near terminus)	+, –	+
Polyuria	+	–, +	–
Hypothermia	–	+	–
Fractional clearance of Na	↑	↑↑	↓
U/S creatinine ratio	↓	↓	↑
U/S osmolality ratio	↓	↓	↑
Serum phosphorus	N or ↑	↑	N or ↑
Serum calcium	N or ↓	N or ↓	N
Serum potassium	N or ↓	↑ or N	N
Metabolic acidosis	Mild	Moderate to severe	N or mild

(CRF) chronic renal failure. (ARF) acute renal failure. (N) normal. (↑) increased or elevated. (↓) decreased. (U) urine. (S) serum. (*) most important considerations.

solutions. Once rehydration has been accomplished, maintenance needs can best be met with 0.45% NaCl in 2.5% dextrose (or in water) to prevent sodium overload. The maintenance infusion should be chosen and modified after evaluation of serum electrolytes. The patient is weighed twice daily as an accurate monitor of developing overhydration or dehydration. The initial fluid electrolyte composition should also be relatively free of potassium, particularly during any oliguric periods. On the other hand, during phases of diuresis and anorexia, potassium supplementation of fluids will likely be necessary (the technique of potassium supplementation is described in Chapter 4). Fluid therapy is fre-

Table 6-8. Predisposing Factors for Intrarenal ARF

Use of nephrotoxic drugs
Trauma/hypovolemia
Dehydration
Anesthesia—prolonged and deep
Surgery—prolonged
Preexisting renal disease
Old age
Combinations of the above

Table 6-9. Checklist for Initial Treatment of Intrarenal ARF

1. Rule out obstructive uropathy and uroperitoneum
2. Rule out pyelonephritis, leptospirosis
3. Rule out hypercalcemic nephropathy
4. Correct all prerenal factors (ensure adequate hydration)
5. Monitor urine output for initial 24 hr to determine oliguria vs. nonoliguria
6. Correct all serious acid-base/electrolyte abnormalities
7. Create mild fluid volume expansion
8. Pay meticulous attention to fluid/electrolyte regimen
9. Administer diuretics (mannitol/furosemide/dopamine)
10. Control hyperphosphatemia (aluminum hydroxide)
11. Control gastric hyperacidity (H_2-receptor antagonist)
12. Institute early dialysis during established ARF
13. Consider nutritional therapy (hyperalimentation)
14. Stop all nephrotoxic drugs
15. Avoid prescribing nephrotoxic drugs
16. Prescribe specific antidotes for nephrotoxins if available
17. Avoid episodes of hypotension/anesthesia/surgery

quently required for 7–14 days to support the animal until adequate renal function can be restored, if recovery is to happen at all.

Though intrarenal ARF patients do not show anemia initially, they often develop it during the course of hospitalization for a variety of reasons. This anemia is occasionally severe enough to require blood transfusion.

Recent evidence seems to indicate that control of hyperphosphatemia in intrarenal ARF may be important in preventing further deterioration of renal function and progression of renal lesions.[45] The use of aluminum hydroxide antacids that "bind" phosphorus in the intestine (e.g., Amphojel) is advocated as one means to help prevent hyperphosphatemia. Dietary restriction of phosphorus intake is also recommended (as in k/d or u/d), although many patients during the maintenance phase of ARF are anorexic.[34,37]

Severe metabolic acidosis can occur in intrarenal ARF and requires alkali therapy, as described in Chapter 4. Aggressive alkali replacement is not routinely recommended, however, as tetany may be precipitated in patients with low-normal calcium or hypocalcemia. Also, sodium overload can occur as sodium is infused along with bicarbonate. Patients with symptomatic hyperka-

Table 6-10. Monitoring During Therapy of Intrarenal ARF

1. Avoid overhydration/dehydration
   a. Weigh two to three times daily initially
   b. PCV/TPP twice daily
2. Monitor urine output
3. ECG frequently, particularly if oliguric
4. Daily electrolytes—Na, K, Cl
5. Blood gases initially
6. BUN, serum creatinine daily at first
7. Consider renal biopsy if diagnosis in doubt or if renal failure persists

lemia induced by ARF [altered electrocardiogram (ECG)] require more aggressive alkali therapy as an emergency measure to decrease serum potassium.

Therapy may also be aimed at reducing the severity of vomiting that is often encountered in ARF patients. The antacids used to control hyperphosphatemia may also help to coat uremic ulcers in the gastrointestinal tract and reduce gastric hyperacidity. Cimetidine has recently come into common clinical use in veterinary uremic patients to help reduce gastric acidity through its H_2-receptor blocking properties. The initial dosage is 10 mg/kg IV for the first dose, then 5 mg/kg IV b.i.d. until oral medication can be tolerated.[42] Clinical effectiveness for this regimen remains to be proved; however, the author believes that it is beneficial. Centrally acting antiemetics (Compazine) can also be helpful in controlling severe vomiting.

What role do diuretics play in the treatment of intrarenal ARF patients? Diuretics may lessen the severity of an ongoing insult or may change the course of intrarenal ARF such that earlier return of renal function can occur. Experimental studies indicate that diuretics can lessen injury when given before or shortly after the insult, but the beneficial effects on renal function are much less when given later during the maintenance phase of intrarenal ARF. Diuretics can result in increased formation of urine, but this increase in volume is often due to decreased resorption of filtrate, rather than increased GFR.[28] Consequently, the response of urine volume to diuretics cannot be directly equated with improvement in renal function. The author advocates the use of diuretics in intrarenal ARF (particularly oliguric cases) on the basis that GFR and RBF may be improved and that conversion from oliguria to nonoliguria facilitates successful fluid therapy with less tendency for overhydration and hyperkalemia.

Mannitol may be the diuretic of choice in intrarenal ARF cases that are not overhydrated. A dosage of 0.25–0.50 g/kg is given intravenously in a 20–25% solution of mannitol. Diuresis should occur within the hour. If diuresis fails, it is acceptable to repeat the dose or to combine a repeat dose with furosemide. Furosemide is given at a dose of 2–4 mg/kg IV. If diuresis fails, the dose may be doubled and repeated within the hour. Some patients respond better to one diuretic than the other. Combination mannitol and furosemide may result in diuresis in some instances where either agent alone was not successful.

Dopamine (Intropin) is also a diuretic that can be prescribed as an infusion at 2–10 µg/kg/min but may be effective at 1–3 µg/kg/min with fewer side effects.[1,20] If dopamine is infused too rapidly, serious cardiac arrhythmias can be created and renal vasoconstriction rather than renal vasodilatation occurs. If this diuretic is chosen, the volume infused must be precisely monitored and the drugs adjusted carefully to achieve the desired rate. There is experimental evidence in dogs with intrarenal ARF that dopamine (3 µg/kg/min) acts synergistically with furosemide (1 mg/kg bolus, then 1 mg/kg/hr) in creating diuresis.[29] The author has successfully used this regimen in a limited number of cases.

Table 6-11. Factors Favoring Survival in Intrarenal ARF

Reversible nonrenal disease, if present
No underlying chronic renal disease
Mild degree of toxic or ischemic insult
Young age
Nonoliguria, rather than oliguria
Few serum biochemical abnormalities
    (acid-base, K, Na, Ca, PO_4)
Short time interval for recognition/treatment

Regardless of which diuretic is used, it is important to prevent dehydration by matching excessive fluid lost from increased urinations with parenteral fluid replacement. Diuretics are discontinued if no beneficial response is gained after adjusting or repeating the initial doses.

Dialysis may be necessary for patient survival if fluid and diuretic therapy fail to restore adequate renal function.[35] Severe symptomatic uremia, persistent metabolic acidosis, persistent hyperkalemia, and overhydration can all be indications to start dialysis Dialysis should be considered during the maintenance phase of intrarenal ARF before patients become moribund from advancing uremia. Peritoneal dialysis with the recently developed column disk catheter can be successfully performed in private practice or at referral centers.[41] In cases that cannot be adequately controlled with peritoneal dialysis, referral for hemodialysis may be of benefit.[10]

Nutritional support with parenteral hyperalimentation may improve the prognosis in selected cases of intrarenal ARF.[14,43] The special techniques involved and complications encountered with hyperalimentation make it difficult to adequately perform even at referral centers. Further discussion of hyperalimentation is beyond the scope of this book.

The prognosis for intrarenal ARF cases in dogs and cats is poor, even with the best of care. Table 6-11 list a variety of factors that may affect prognosis. Though the renal lesions of intrarenal ARF are potentially reversible, animals often die from uremia before adequate renal healing has had time to occur. The complexities of biochemical and metabolic abnormalities encountered in the uremia of intrarenal ARF patients make successful clinical management difficult. Patients may require hospitalization for 2–3 weeks before adequate renal function can be reclaimed. In most instances, these patients can best be managed at referral centers after initial stabilization by the local practitioner. The enormous expense involved in these cases is chosen by few clients. Euthanasia of a patient whose owner cannot afford dialysis is justifiable after medical treatments with fluids and diuretics have failed to improve renal function or if accompanied by progressive clinical deterioration of the animal because of uremia.

Acute Decompensation of Chronic Renal Disease

Patients with chronic renal disease (CRD) or chronic compensated renal failure (CRF) are at risk for developing transient episodes of ARF due to prerenal factors. Obligatory loss of electrolytes and water in the urine of CRD patients predisposes them to rapid development of dehydration if water intake cannot be maintained. The principles discussed above for ARF also apply here. Rapid correction of dehydration is important to restore prior levels of GFR and RBF. This helps to prevent an episode of intrarenal ARF superimposed on CRD and prerenal azotemia. Rehydration and maintenance fluid infusion often allows return of enough glomerular filtration such that the level of azotemia and clinical signs subside. Diuretic therapy has been recommended in CRF patients on the basis that waste products are turned over and excreted more rapidly.[17] However, the benefit of diuretic therapy over fluid volume expansion alone is questionable.

Anemia is common in CRF and may be severe enough to require blood transfusion. In such instances, severe anemia may be one of the factors responsible for decompensating the patient.

Fluid replacement is accomplished with an isotonic polyionic solution, e.g., lactated Ringer's solution.[4,9,11] Anorexia, polyuria, and perhaps gastrointestinal loss often lead to hypokalemia, which should be treated with potassium supplementation of administered fluids. Continued urine output in the absence of food intake can result in hyponatremia, which may benefit from 0.9% NaCl. Metabolic acidosis during decompensation can be severe enough to require alkali ($NaHCO_3$) supplementation; however, vigorous alkali therapy is not recommended because of the possible tetany that can result, as discussed earlier. The volume of fluid should initially be infused intravenously so as to replace hydration needs, provide maintenance needs, and keep up with losses in vomiting or diarrhea. The volume of urine output is usually large during therapy; consequently, calculations of daily fluid maintenance needs should take this extra loss into consideration (normal maintenance volume requirement is 44–66 cc/kg/day, but CRF patients require more than this). Many CRF patients survive an occasional bout of decompensation merely through correction of the prerenal factors. The BUN and serum creatinine in these instances may decline substantially as hydration is reestablished, but the values do not return completely to the normal range.

Therapeutic endeavors must be undertaken simultaneously to minimize losses of fluid and electrolytes through uremia-induced vomiting and diarrhea. The use of promazine-derivative tranquilizers (Compazine), cimetidine, and antacids may be helpful as discussed previously.

When rehydration has been accomplished, the BUN and serum creatinine have fallen, and the patient seems stable, fluid therapy is then gradually tapered. During this taper, renal function and hydration are carefully monitored. Success is judged by the animal who maintains hydration and a stable (although elevated) BUN and serum creatinine. If no improvement occurs after standard medical therapy, it is possible that so few nephrons are able to function that the degree of associated azotemia may not be compatible with life. In such cases euthanasia is warranted. Peritoneal dialysis for a short duration may benefit some CRF patients by altering the uremic environment temporarily such that clinical signs decline, allowing standard medical therapy to take over. This is rarely recommended. Once the predisposing cause(s) of dehydration (gastritis, enteritis, pancreatitis, accidental water deprivation, "stress," e.g., in surgery or boarding) has resolved and the patient is feeling better, further attention is directed toward minimizing uremic signs by restricting dietary protein and phosphorus intake. Standard texts should be consulted for detailed information about protein restriction and diets in renal failure.

URINARY TRACT TRAUMA

Major abdominal trauma can create emergencies from damage to the urinary tract.[24] Fortunately, the kidneys are relatively well protected by the ribs, skeleton, and epaxial musculature. All abdominal trauma victims must be routinely evaluated for potential injury to the urinary tract, particularly those with fractures of the pelvis, extensive damage to soft tissue overlying the abdomen, or penetrating abdominal wounds. Radiographs of the abdomen are essential to evaluate renal shadows, retroperitoneal density, distention of the bladder, and accumulation of fluid in the peritoneal cavity.[36,39] Abdominocentesis is of value in identifying any peritoneal fluid. Although the following discussion pertains to urinary tract injury, all injuries sustained by the traumatized patient must be considered and prioritized during diagnosis and treatment.

Bladder

Blunt abdominal trauma from vehicular accidents, falls from height, or other forceful blows to the abdomen often result in transient self-limiting hematuria. Ruptured bladder is the most common injury to the urinary tract that constitutes an emergency.[24] Urine leakage into the peritoneal cavity (uroabdomen) results in resorption of nitrogenous waste products across the peritoneum as a form of acute postrenal failure (azotemia). Shifts of water from the body into the peritoneal cavity may also occur during uroabdomen, tending to accelerate dehydration.[7]

The diagnosis of ruptured bladder may not be initially apparent in the multiinjured animal with complex major abdominal trauma undergoing shock therapy. The initial clue may be when the patient's bladder fails to fill properly after adequate fluid therapy. Abdominal distention and ballotable fluid may become apparent only after aggressive intravenous fluid therapy has been given. Serum urea nitrogen and creatinine remain normal for several hours after the rupture. As more time elapses, progressive elevations of BUN and serum creatinine become detectable. Inability to palpate the bladder or pain in that region alerts the clinician to consider rupture as a possibility from the start, and pelvic fractures increase the level of suspicion.

Radiographic evaluation can confirm the presence of abdominal fluid, inability to visualize the bladder, and pelvic fractures. An animal with a small tear radiographed shortly after trauma may not always reveal peritoneal fluid. A positive-contrast cystogram is performed to evaluate the integrity of the bladder. Pneumocystography can be used to detect leaks, but it is more difficult to confirm the leak with this method than with positive contrast.[7]

Abdominocentesis may reveal the presence of urine-like fluid. A negative fluid aspirate, however, does not exclude the possibility that uroabdomen exists, particularly early when the quantity of peritoneal fluid may be small. The physical appearance alone of fluid withdrawn from the abdomen should not be relied on to diagnose uroabdomen. Aspirated fluid is chemically and cytologically analyzed to confirm it as urine or urine modified with peritoneal effusion. The test of choice is to determine the creatinine content of the suspect fluid and then compare it simultaneously with the patient's serum creatinine level. If the suspect fluid is urine, a substantial gradient will exist such that creatinine in the fluid exceeds that in serum. The same ratio can be measured using urea nitrogen, but the gradient may not be as obvious, as urea more readily diffuses across the peritoneal membranes back into the body than does creatinine.[7]

History may yield some clues as to the likelihood of a ruptured bladder. An animal who urinated shortly before the traumatic event has less chance for rupture to occur. Voiding of a large volume of urine after the trauma also lessens the likelihood of rupture, although some volume of urinations can and do occur from patients with known ruptured bladder. Some animals with a ruptured bladder show signs of acute dysuria or stranguria.

Urinary catheterization and the retrieval of fluid should not be relied on to indicate whether a ruptured bladder does or does not exist. Depending on the location of the tear in the bladder wall, urine may spill into the peritoneal cavity while some still flows into the bladder. Also, the catheter sometimes passes into the abdominal cavity through the tear, allowing fluid retrieval. Air injected through the catheter may fail to distend the bladder or to keep it distended as air leaks out. Occasionally hissing sounds are heard as air is injected through the catheter and rapidly leaks through the tear.

Iatrogenic rupture of the bladder occurs uncommonly as the result of poor technique during urinary catheterization. Friable neoplastic tissue or devitalized inflammatory tissue may be perforated more readily during catheterization. The bladder may also rupture during attempts at expressing urine by manual compression if intravesical pressure is increased too rapidly or is too high. Occasionally, animals with complete obstruction of the urethra end up with bladder rupture from overdistention; these animals were already uremic before the rupture, and consequently their metabolic status is much worse from uremia than with other types of bladder rupture.

Surgical repair of the rent in the bladder is undertaken as soon as the patient is adequately stabilized. Hyperkalemia and severe metabolic acidosis can occur late in the course of experimental ruptured bladder (days later)[7] but may occur earlier in the clinical setting of severe tissue trauma and shock. Hyperkalemia and metabolic acidosis are treated prior to anesthesia and surgery with infusions of sodium bicarbonate according to the guidelines in Chapter 4. Use of antibiotics in the perioperative arena is also recommended. It is not necessary for the BUN and serum creatinine to be normal before the repair is performed. In critically ill cases where fluid therapy alone does not improve the patient's status, surgery may be safely delayed if drainage of urine from the peritoneal cavity can be accomplished by passing a catheter through the bladder tear into the peritoneal cavity. An alternative is to place drains surgically under local anesthesia across the abdominal wall. This can be quickly and easily accomplished with Penrose drains or Brunswick feeding tubes secured in the peritoneal cavity, wrapped with sterile gauze, and bandaged to prevent contamination. Conducting urine outside the body in this manner may dramatically lessen the degree of azotemia and improve patient survival when surgery can be performed later. A few exchanges with peritoneal dialysis fluids, when drains are in place, may be used to more rapidly reduce azotemia prior to surgery.

Urethra

Postrenal azotemia as discussed above can also result when urine accumulation in the abdomen occurs from a tear in the proximal urethra. Azotemia may also be present if urine leaks into the tissues surrounding a more distal urethral tear. Concomitant obstruction at the site of the tear frequently occurs from inflammation and contraction of tissue.

The frequency of urethral tears in trauma patients is much greater when pelvic fractures are present.[39] Iatrogenic perforations can occur with poor technique during urethral catheterization or during attempts to dislodge urethral calculi. Most tears of the urethra are partial, and only rarely does the tear result in avulsion.

Suspicion for ruptured urethra must be entertained when uroabdomen occurs and when the bladder cannot be well visualized. Confirmation depends on demonstrating leakage of dye with positive-contrast urethrography. Distal urethral rupture results in urine accumulation within the tissues of the perineum and thighs, causing cellulitis and possible sloughing of skin in those areas. Catheterization of the bladder may be difficult as tissue reaction, compression, and contraction at the site of the tear occur.

Emergency medical treatment with fluid therapy, alkali, antibiotics, and sometimes drains is similar to that described previously. A urethral catheter is passed into the bladder and then secured in place for 5–7 days to allow small tears to heal as urine is diverted away from the damaged area. Diverting urine away from larger tears helps lessen any uremia and reduces tissue reaction at the site of the tear, but surgical closure of the tear is usually necessary. If a catheter cannot be advanced, surgery will be necessary as soon as emergency stabilization has been accomplished. The same applies for complete avulsion of the urethra. Surgical details are described in the next book of this series, *Surgical Emergencies*.

Kidney/Ureter

Violent trauma to the sublumbar area occasionally causes clinically significant injury of the kidney or ureter. The most serious emergency, major blood loss from trauma to the kidney, can be rapidly fatal. Trauma to the excretory pathway of the renal pelvis or ureters can result in uroperitoneum or urine accumulation retroperitoneally. Abdominal radiographs may reveal fluid free within the peritoneal cavity or fluid density expanding the retroperitoneal space, causing loss of ability to visualize the renal shadows.[36] Often pain is present upon palpation near the costovertebral angle and sublumbar areas. Increasing abdominal girth may also be noticeable. Abdominocentesis is necessary to characterize the peritoneal fluid as either blood or urine. It is not possible by radiography alone to tell whether an increased retroperitoneal density is due to hemorrhage or urine accumulation.

Renal trauma with major blood loss is usually diagnosed after emergency shock therapy fails to stabilize the patient and blood loss is found to be ongoing within the abdomen. Emergency abdominal celiotomy identifies the site of hemorrhage, and usually nephrectomy is necessary. Nephrectomy is performed if renal artery avulsion is found or if extensive laceration, fracture, or pulpefaction of the traumatized kidney is discovered.[8] Partial nephrectomy can be performed if only one pole of the kidney is damaged.

Not all patients with blood loss from an injured kidney continue to actively bleed. In such instances, intravenous pyelography (IVP) is valuable for identification of the site and severity of renal injury, though surgery may still not be necessary.

The patient with renal/ureteral trauma may present with only increased fluid density of the retroperitoneal space. IVP is essential to assess the integrity of the excretory pathway. If the IVP reveals normal renal pelvis and ureters, the fluid accumulation is due to hemorrhage. Careful attention to the nephrogram phase of the IVP may reveal irregularities of kidney shape and contour induced by the renal trauma that may indicate the site of the initial hemorrhage. Hemorrhage in this area, however, more often comes from damaged small vessels of soft tissue in the sublumbar region. The patient with retroperitoneal hemorrhage alone usually does not require surgical repair.

Surgical intervention is necessary to correct retroperitoneal leakage of urine. Tears in the renal pelvis or avulsion of the proximal ureter from the renal pelvis are not reparable due to constraints of size and hence require nephrectomy. More distal tears of the ureter may be repaired by primary anastomosis and ureteral stenting, or by transposition of the ureter into the bladder.[4,8] Further discussion of surgical treatment is beyond the scope of this book.

Often uroabdomen rather than retroperitoneal accumulation results when urine leaks from a damaged kidney or ureter, even though they are retroperitoneal structures, because the peritoneum is also traumatized and perforated. Repair is the same as described above. Stabilization of the patient with uroabdomen should be achieved, as discussed before, regardless of the source of the urine leak. The earlier the surgical repair the less tissue reaction there will be secondary to urine extravasation and the greater is the chance for surgical success.

Sharp trauma to the kidney/ureters may result from knife or bullet wounds. Renal biopsy, particularly blind keyhole punch procedures, can also cause serious renal injury. Hemorrhage and/or extravasation of urine can result, depending on the depth of the injury and whether the lumen of the renal pelvis or ureter was entered.

Blood loss from major renal trauma or avulsion of the renal artery requires transfusion of whole blood before and probably during surgery. Because blood loss can be massive, autotransfusion of blood from the patient's own abdominal cavity should be considered during the initial treatment to stabilize the animal before surgery. Blood is aspirated into routine blood collection bottles or bags, anticoagulated, and immediately reinfused intravenously through a filter.[12] Additional blood from storage or fresh from donors may be required.

In some cases, blood loss from a damaged kidney can be reduced by the use of an abdominal compression bandage to increase the pressure against the kidney. An Ace bandage can be wrapped around a cotton roll placed under the abdomen and pressure applied. This wrap is released every 20–30 min and then reapplied if necessary. This is not a substitute for surgical repair but may allow some time to improve the patient's condition prior to anesthesia and surgery. In some cases bleeding from the kidney may cease, and surgery can be avoided. In other cases severe ongoing hemorrhage necessitates immediate surgery.

OBSTRUCTIVE UROPATHY

Complete obstruction to outflow of urine from the body results in death within a time period that varies from 3 to 5 days.[3,6,15] Signs directly attributable to uremia (acute postrenal failure/azotemia) do not occur until after 24 hr of complete obstruction but may develop rapidly thereafter. Signs related directly to the cause of the obstruction may be observed earlier, e.g., stranguria, dysuria, pollakiuria, abdominal pain from increased pressure, hematuria, narrowing of urine stream diameter, and eventual cessation of any urine voiding. Death from urine outflow obstruction can be attributed to hyperkalemia, severe metabolic acidosis, dehydration, and retention of uremic toxins.

Etiology

Complete obstruction to urine outflow most commonly is caused by a lesion in the urethra. The most frequent cause of urethral obstruction in dogs is urinary calculi that have lodged within the urethra, usually in males. In cats the most common lesion is a struvite plug within the urethral lumen, a manifestation of the so-called feline urologic syndrome (FUS), which occurs almost exclusively in males. Other lesions capable of causing severe urethral obstruction and uremia are much less common; they include urethral foreign bodies; clots from hemorrhaging lesions in the urethra or bladder that become lodged; urethral or periurethral neoplasia; strictures of the urethra after trauma or infection; iatrogenic misplacement of a ligature around the urethra; acute periurethral trauma with edema, hemorrhage, and inflammation (e.g., vehicular trauma with pelvic fractures); severe urethritis (granulomatous urethritis); and possibly detrussor-urethral dyssynergia from a neurologic lesion.

Bilateral obstructive lesions of the kidneys or ureters would be necessary to create renal failure, assuming both kidneys were normal prior to the obstruction. It is an extraordinarily remote possibility that both renal pelves or both ureters would become entirely obstructed at the same time from any of the processes mentioned under urethral obstruction. Obstruction of one kidney or ureter could result in renal failure if the nonobstructed kidney was already significantly diseased.

Diagnosis

Diagnosis of urethral obstruction is usually obvious on physical examination. A large, turgid, painful bladder is usually palpable, and there is inability to express urine during mild pressure. Visualization of the urethral orifice in male cats may reveal protrusion of the offending plug material. Urethral calculi in male dogs may be palpable caudal to the os penis, within the perineal urethra, and occasionally per rectum within the pelvic urethra. A rectal examination in all dogs with suspected obstruction is performed to evaluate the urethra for intraluminal calculi, neoplasia, or severe inflammation. Neurologic examination with emphasis on evaluation of long spinal tracts and segmental reflexes of the lumbar and sacral regions is performed when no obvious structural cause of obstruction is found yet urine cannot be expelled, which suggests detrussor-urethral dyssynergia. In those patients with ureteral or renal pelvic obstruction, pain at or near the area of obstruction may be elicited during palpation. Physical examination in longstanding complete obstruction reveals a depressed patient who may be hypothermic and severely dehydrated. Bradycardia, arrhythmia, and systemic hypotension may be detected if hyperkalemia is severe. The patient may also present in a state of acute collapse.

Passage of a urinary catheter may be difficult or impossible. Sometimes the catheter slips around an intraluminal obstruction and the clinician erroneously concludes that obstruction does not really exist. Similarly, passage of a catheter through the lumen of the urethra may not be difficult in some instances where the obstruction is caused by extraluminal compression.

Radiography provides further indication of the location and cause of the obstruction. Plain abdominal radiographs reveal most urethral calculi. Positive-contrast urethrography is needed in some instances to identify the site of urethral obstruction. IVP identifies the rare case with bilateral renal pelvic or ureteral obstruction.

Biochemical evaluation of the severely obstructed patient often reveals marked elevation in BUN and serum creatinine, serum phosphorus, and an elevation in serum potassium, whereas serum calcium is usually decreased. It is not unusual for a cat with severe urethral obstruction to present with a serum creatinine level that exceeds 10–20 mg/dl, a BUN greater than 200 mg/dl, and a serum phosphorus in excess of 10 mg/dl. We have occasionally observed a serum calcium as low as 3–4 mg/dl, possibly due to the acute mass law effect of extremely elevated phosphorus. Hyperkalemia of 6.0–11.0 mEq/L can be observed in cats with severe urethral obstruction.

Treatment

The aggressiveness of medical treatment depends on how long the obstruction has been present and the particular patient's clinical status. Patients with early obstruction are not true emergencies but can rapidly progress to emergency status if the obstruction is not relieved. Only a small percentage of obstructed patients are presented in the severe, advanced stage of obstruction, manifesting hyperkalemia, metabolic acidosis, arrhythmias, and collapse.[6,13] Further discussion below centers on these critically ill animals.

Initial treatment is directed at establishing an intravenous line and infusing isotonic fluids that do not contain potassium (0.9% NaCl or 0.45% NaCl in 2.5% dextrose) to combat hypovolemia and circulatory collapse. An ECG is monitored initially. Even though arrhythmias or bradycardia may not be auscultable or palpable when feeling the pulse, the ECG may reveal striking abnormalities in electrical conduction. If the ECG is normal, the clinician proceeds with urethral unblocking procedures. When the ECG is abnormal in the setting of urinary obstruction, it is likely due to the effects of hyperkalemia and metabolic acidosis, possibly with contributions from hypocalcemia and other electrolyte derangement. The most typical ECG abnormalities and arrhythmias of hyperkalemia include bradycardia, tall tent-shaped T waves, flattened P waves, increasing P-R interval, atrial standstill, sinoventricular rhythm, ventricular fibrillation, and finally asystole. When these rhythm and conduction disturbances are present, they are treated as life-threatening cardiac emergencies prior to urethral unblocking procedures.

The initial treatment of choice for conduction disturbances and arrhythmias created by hyperkalemia is the infusion of sodium bicarbonate at 1.1–2.2 mEq/kg as a slow bolus infusion followed by another infusion at the same dosage if the ECG fails to show any response. Often the ECG normalizes within minutes after the alkali infusion. The presumed mechanism for this beneficial effect is that as acidosis is corrected there is a shift of potassium ions from the extracellular space to the intracellular space, thereby reducing the level of hyperkalemia. Some animals whose ECGs do not respond to alkali infusion benefit from a slow infusion of calcium gluconate (1–10 cc 10% solution) either because they are hypocalcemic or because the calcium infusion provides direct cardioprotection against still-existing hyperkalemia. Management of hyperkalemia is further discussed in Chapter 4.

Relief of obstruction is the next priority. If the obstruction is intraluminal, hydropulsion techniques are performed using a urethral catheter to dislodge the obstruction. After the catheter is introduced into the urethra, a bolus injection of sterile physiological solution is made so as to dilate the urethra and propel the obstructing material into the bladder where it can later be removed surgically if necessary. Sometimes a small-diameter catheter can be maneuvered around the obstruction, allowing drainage of the bladder; then hydropulsion techniques are tried again. If the obstruction is extraluminal, urethral catheterization with a small-diameter catheter is necessary to accomplish bladder drainage.

The urinary catheter, once successfully placed, is left there to ensure adequate outflow of urine until the patient's condition improves and uremia resolves. Urine is collected into a sterile container, and the urine volume produced is measured to facilitate calculation of the volume of fluid to be infused intravenously.

In some patients it is not possible to relieve urethral obstruction via urinary catheterization. In these instances emergency urethrostomy in conjunction with cystotomy may be necessary. Patients who are moribund or those who have severely traumatized urethral and/or periurethral tissues may benefit from temporary tube cystostomy drainage under local anesthesia. This allows better patient and tissue condition prior to more permanent corrective surgery. Cystocentesis with a 25-gauge needle can decompress the bladder, but rupture of the bladder can occur as a complication. Consequently, this procedure is recommended only when other options are not available.

In the unlikely event that bilateral ureteral or renal pelvic obstruction exists, surgical intervention is advisable as soon as medical treatment has stabilized the patient. Tube nephrostomy under local anesthesia is potentially available as a technique to relieve pressure from the kidney and to allow urine drainage to outside the body. As the patient's clinical condition improves, a more definitive surgery can then be performed. So long as the kidney is relieved of the obstruction temporarily by the tube nephrostomy, the uremia should subside if the kidney itself was healthy before the onset of the obstruction. Renal function can recover even after 2 weeks of total obstruction to one kidney.[44]

Following relief of obstruction via catheterization or surgery, a phenomenon referred to as postobstructive diuresis may occur.[6,13] A variety of reasons for this diuresis have been proposed, including retention of osmotically active solute accumulated during anuria, ADH insensitivity, and decreased ability for tubular resorption of sodium. Diuresis is usually immediate following the release of obstruction, and it may be voluminous. Usually the magnitude of diuresis tends to become self-limiting as azotemia resolves. If careful attention is not paid to urine volume during this phase, dangerous dehydration and even shock may develop. At the same time, there is accelerated loss of both sodium and potassium. Consequently, the parenteral fluid chosen during this phase is usually 0.9% NaCl or lactated Ringer's supplemented with potassium chloride, as described in Chapter 4. In the absence of potassium supplementation during this diuretic phase, hypokalemia may develop and prolong the hospital recovery period.

GENITAL MEDICAL EMERGENCIES[33]

Tables 6-12 and 6-13 provide an overview of medical and surgical genital emergencies in both sexes, but only medical situations are discussed in the text.

Table 6-12. Genital Emergencies in the Male

Penis
  Paraphimosis—edema/necrosis
  Trauma—Laceration/hemorrhage
          Contusion
          Bite wound
          Fracture of os penis
Testes
  Orchitis—acute[a]
    Traumatic
    Infectious—*Brucella*, other bacteria
  Torsion—Traumatic
          Spontaneous intraabdominal
Scrotum
  Trauma
Prostate
  Prostatitis, acute bacterial[a]
  Prostatic abscess
  Ruptured prostatic abscess
  Trauma

[a] Topics considered medical emergencies that are discussed in the text; all other listed topics are covered in the companion book *Surgical Emergencies*.

Acute Orchitis

The testes and epididymides may both become inflamed due to either trauma or infectious agents, and frequently are affected simultaneously. *Brucella canis* is the most common cause of epididymitis/orchitis in the dog but is usually insidious. Bacterial organisms from an infected prostate or urinary tract infection can enter the vas deferens as a retrograde portal of entry.[25]

Dogs with acute orchitis may be reluctant to move or may assume an unusual posture and gait to avoid placing pressure on the painfully enlarged testes and/or epididymides. Excessive licking of the scrotum may be observed, sometimes creating scrotal abrasion and dermatitis. Severely affected dogs may appear depressed and anorexic.

Physical examination may reveal fever from infection or inflammation. Swollen testes and/or epididymides may be palpated, usually with pain. The testes may be pulled up higher than normal within the scrotum, and scrotal dermatitis may be seen.

Table 6-13. Genital Emergencies in the Female

Vaginal hyperplasia/prolapse
Uterine prolapse
Pyometra
Acute metritis[a]
Abnormalities of gestation/parturition dystocia—maternal/fetal

[a] Topic considered medical emergency to be discussed in text; all other listed topics are covered in the companion book *Surgical Emergencies*.

Acute orchitis is not considered a threat to life, but it is extremely painful and a threat to reproductive capacity. Thermal injury to the testes, resulting from increased blood flow and inflammation, can cause testicular degeneration and subsequent atrophy.

With orchitis due to trauma, application of cold compresses can be beneficial if treatment is started shortly after the injury. Glucocorticosteroids are given in high doses initially to help reduce the inflammatory response. Antibiotics are administered if severe tissue trauma and devitalization has occurred and in all cases caused by penetrating wounds (e.g., bite wounds). Castration may be necessary in cases with trauma-induced pulpefaction.

If orchitis is due to bacteria other than *Brucella*, vigorous antibiotic therapy is started immediately. The most common isolates are gram-negative bacteria, *Staphylococcus* sp., and *Streptococcus* sp. Culture and sensitivity tests of urine or an ejaculate are obtained before initiating antibacterial therapy. Concomitant glucocorticosteroids can be used to reduce the damage and scarring if the infection seems to be confined to the testes/epididymides; however, caution must be employed if infection also resides within the urinary tract or prostate. Suppurative inflammation and formation of multiple abscesses may not respond to medical treatment, thus requiring castration.

If the inflammatory response is due to infection with *Brucella canis*, medical treatment may not be warranted. Even after orchitis/epididymitis subside, the *B. canis* organism can be shed in semen for a long time intermittently and is difficult to eliminate. Due to potential human health hazards, euthanasia of the dog should be offered as an option. If the owner understands the risks and the difficulties in treatment, castration is performed to remove a major site of sequestration of the infection and to help prevent spread of the disease from venereal contact with other dogs. Protracted treatment with tetracycline-streptomycin or minocycline-streptomycin may be required for months to attempt a cure, but frequently antibiotics only temporarily interrupt the *B. canis* bacteremia characteristic of the disease.[19]

Work-up of the orchitis patient routinely includes a serum titer for *B. canis*. Initially a screening plate test (Pittman Moore) is performed, and if it is positive for *B. canis* confirmatory testing is performed using either a tube agglutination titer for *B. canis* or blood culture. These two additional tests confirm *B. canis* infection. If the screening plate test is negative, it is unlikely that *B. canis* is playing a role in the infection. In these dogs, bacterial culture of catheterized urine or ejaculated semen should be submitted for isolation of other bacteria that may be causing orchitis. When orchitis is associated with severe trauma, catheterization of the urethra ensures that the urethra is intact. Antibacterial medication is adjusted when results of bacterial susceptibility testing are available.

Acute Prostatitis

Acute prostatitis can be a medical emergency in some affected dogs who develop systemic signs. *Escherichia coli* is the most frequently isolated cause of bacterial prostatitis, although other gram-negative organisms, e.g., *Proteus* and *Pseudomonas* spp., can also be found, and occasionally gram-positive *Staphylococcus* and *Streptococcus* are isolated.[3,22]

Clinical Features. Depression, anorexia, vomiting, rectal tenesmus, reluctance to walk, postural/gait changes due to pain, shivering, and hemorrhagic or purulent urethral discharge unassociated with urination may be observed by the owner. Signs referrable to concomitant urinary tract infection with cystitis and urethritis may also be seen (pollakiuria, stranguria, hematuria).

Physical examination often reveals fever, depression, and painful rectal palpation of the prostate. Enlargement of the prostate, loss of symmetry, or change in texture per rectal examination is quite variable. Benign prostatic hypertrophy is common in older dogs, predisposing them to develop bacterial prostatitis, and can contribute to any enlargement that is palpated. Sometimes the external urethral orifice appears inflamed, and a hemorrhagic or purulent urethral discharge may be observed during the examination. The presence of bacteremia and urinary tract infection contributes to increased severity of the illness at initial presentation. Dehydration and shock may be present in these instances.

Diagnosis. Urine collected by cystocentesis is submitted for urinalysis, culture, and susceptibility studies. Urinalysis may reveal hematuria, pyuria, and bacteriuria, but these findings do not localize the process to the prostate. Neutrophilic leukocytosis with a left shift can also be found in severe prostatitis. The infected prostate may reflux organisms into bladder urine, or concomitant urinary tract infection may be documented. Culture of any urethral discharge after cleansing the tip of the penis gently with a sterile gauze sponge and saline may be helpful in isolating the infecting organism. In the absence of urethral discharge, urethral catheterization, prostatic massage, and flushing with sterile solutions to remove prostatic fluid can be used to obtain culture specimens for analysis.

Collection of semen for cytologic studies and culture can be helpful, but dogs with acute prostatitis often have too much pain to ejaculate. If the prostate is palpable per abdomen, fine needle aspiration may be successful in obtaining material for culture. Blood culture is considered in patients who are suspected of having bacteremia associated with the prostatitis. Culture of prostatic tissue sampled by wedge or punch biopsy can also be considered.

Treatment. In acute prostatitis, the normal blood-prostate barrier has broken down. Consequently, many antimicrobial drugs enter the prostate that would not otherwise be able to do so in the normal animal or in those with chronic prostatitis. Because *E. coli* is the most common pathogen, initial drug therapy is chosen for a high likelihood of activity against this organism and an ability to achieve high tissue and urinary levels. The cephalosporins, ampicillin, trimethoprim-sulfa, and chloramphenicol have all been used successfully in the management of acute prostatitis. Systemically ill patients may require intravenous fluid support. Antimicrobials can be given intravenously until the dog is stable enough to be taken off fluids, then continued orally for at least 14 days.

Diethylstilbestrol at low doses (1.0–5.0 mg/day initially followed by 1.0 mg daily for less than a week) may be beneficial for initial reduction of prostatic size (atrophy). Reduced prostatic size may relieve rectal tenesmus when present and may aid elimination of bacteria from the prostate (but this is not proved). Stool softeners may also help to relieve constipation and tenesmus from an enlarged prostate.

Acute prostatitis occasionally compromises the prostatic urethra, causing obstruction and urine retention. Therefore the bladder is frequently palpated to assess its size and a urinary catheter is passed if needed to relieve bladder distention.

Acute Metritis

Acute metritis is a severe bacterial infection of the uterus that usually occurs shortly after parturition. *E. coli* is the most common bacterial cause, although some cases are due to *Streptococcus* or *Staphylococcus*.[21,26,32] Retained fetuses or placenta may be predisposing factors, as may infection after obstetric manipulation during dystocia. The diseased uterus, after abortions and subinvolution of the placental sites, may also facilitate uterine infection. Postestral infection occurs rarely after natural breeding or from contamination during artificial insemination.

Clinical Features and Diagnosis.   Acute bacterial metritis is considered a medical emergency because the condition can progress rapidly, leading to toxemia and bacteremia. Most often the bitch presents 7–14 days after parturition with the owner's complaint of a foul-smelling purulent or sanguino-purulent vaginal discharge. Anorexia, depression, and vomiting are commonly reported and sometimes polydipsia as well. She may display decreasing interest in her pups, or the pups may not be able to get enough milk. In some cases the bitch presents with a history of acute collapse if septic shock has intervened.

Physical examination usually reveals fever, typically 104°F and higher. The vagina is hyperemic and swollen, and contains a purulent or sanguino-purulent exudate. Dehydration may be detectable after evaluating skin turgor and dryness of mucous membranes. Abdominal palpation discloses a turgid and enlarged uterus. Palpation for possible retained fetuses is always performed. Those dogs in septic shock will be in a state of collapse with weak pulses and slow capillary refill time.

Culture of the uterine exudate is taken from a swab of the cranial vagina or cervical region before starting treatment. Hematology studies reveal a neutrophilic leukocytosis, usually with a left shift; dehydration may produce an elevated packed cell volume and total protein concentration. Cytologic study of the vaginal discharge shows purulent inflammation with bacteria. Abdominal radiography confirms uterine enlargement as well as the presence of any retained fetus.

Treatment.   The treatment of choice following patient stabilization is ovariohysterectomy if the bitch is of no breeding value. An intravenous line for fluid support or shock therapy is necessary in advanced cases. Broad-spectrum systemic antibiotics are given intravenously after samples for vaginal culture have been taken. Ampicillin, cephalosporins, chloramphenicol, and amino-glycosides, e.g., gentamicin, are appropriate.

If the bitch is a valuable breeding animal, medical therapy alone can be attempted. One method of evacuating the exudate from the uterus has included ergonovine 0.1–0.2 mg twice daily for 2–3 days or oxytocin 5–10 units every 3 hr for three injections. Surgical insertion of a Foley catheter through the cervix and into the uterine lumen has been used for drainage and irrigation of the uterus. These older methods have more recently been replaced by the use of prostaglandin $F_{2\alpha}$ at 250 µg/kg/day SC as a highly effective method to evacuate uterine exudate and increase uterine blood flow; side effects at this dosage include staggering, salivation, diarrhea, and a dazed look that is transient and of little consequence. It may be necessary to continue these injections for 2–10 days in conjunction with antibiotic therapy until expulsion of uterine exudate ceases.[5,40]

REFERENCES

1. Adams HR, Parker JL: Pharmacological management of circulatory shock: cardiovascular drugs and corticosteroids. J Am Vet Med Assoc 175:86, 1979
2. Barber DL, Finco DR: Radiographic findings in induced bacterial pyelonephritis in dogs. J Am Vet Med Assoc 175:1183, 1979
3. Barsanti JA, Finco DR: Treatment of bacterial prostatitis. In Kirk RW (ed): Current Veterinary Therapy VIII—Small Animal Practice. p. 1101. Saunders, Philadelphia, 1983
4. Brace JJ, Chew DJ: Urinary system emergencies. In Kirk RW (ed): Current Veterinary Therapy VII—Small Animal Practice. p. 1042. Saunders, Philadelphia, 1980
5. Burke TJ: Prostaglandin $F_{2\alpha}$ in the treatment of pyometra-metritis, Vet Clin North Am :107, 1982
6. Burrows CF, Bovee KC: Characterization and treatment of acid-base and renal defects due to urethral obstruction in cats. J Am Vet Med Assoc, 172:801, 1978
7. Burrows CF, Bovee KC: Metabolic changes due to experimentally induced rupture of the canine urinary bladder. Am J Vet Res 35:1083, 1974
8. Carlton CR Jr: Injuries of the kidney and ureter. In Harrison JH, Gittes RF, Perlmutter AD, et al (eds): Campbell's Urology. p. 881. Saunders, Philadelphia, 1978
9. Cornelius LM: Fluid therapy in the uremic patient. In Kirk RW (ed): Current Veterinary Therapy VIII—Small Animal Practice. p. 989. Saunders, Philadelphia, 1983
10. Cowgill LD: Current status of veterinary hemodialysis. In Kirk RW (Ed) Current Veterinary Therapy VII—Small Animal Practice. p. 1111. Saunders, Philadelphia, 1980
11. Cowgill LD, Low DG: Emergency management of the acute uremic crisis. In Kirk RW (Ed): Current Veterinary Therapy VIII—Small Animal Practice. p. 981. Saunders, Philadelphia, 1983
12. Crowe DT: Autotransfution in the trauma patient, Vet Clin North Am 10:581, 1980
13. Finco DR: Induced feline urethral obstruction: response of hyperkalemia to relief of obstruction and administration of parenteral electrolyte solution. JAAHA 12:198, 1976

14. Finco DR, Barsanti J: Parenteral nutrition during a uremic crisis. In Kirk RW (Ed): Current Veterinary Therapy VIII—Small Animal Practice. p. 994. Saunders, Philadelphia, 1983

15. Finco DR, Cornelius LM: Characterization and treatment of water, electrolyte, and acid-base imbalances of induced urethral obstruction in the cat. Am J Vet Res 38:823, 1977

16. Finco DR, Duncan JR: Evaluation of blood urea nitrogen and serum creatinine concentrations as indicators of renal dysfunction: a study of 111 cases and a review of related literature. J Am Vet Med Assoc 168:593, 1976

17. Finco DR, Low DG: Intensive diuresis in polyuric renal failure. In Kirk RW (Ed): Current Veterinary Therapy VII—Small Animal Practice. p. 1091. Saunders, Philadelphia, 1980

18. Finco DR, Shotts EB, Crowell WA: Evaluation of methods for localization of urinary tract infection in the female dog. Am J Vet Res 40:707, 1979

19. Flores-Castro R, Carmichael LE: Canine brucellosis. In Kirk RW (Ed): Current Veterinary Therapy VII—Small Animal Practice. p. 1303. Saunders, Philadelphia, 1980

20. Henderson IS, Beattie TJ, Kennedy AC: Dopamine hydrochloride in oliguric states. Lancet 18:827, 1980

21. Herron MA, Stein B: Prognosis and management of feline infertility. In Kirk RW (Ed): Current Veterinary Therapy VII—Small Animal Practice. p. 1234. Saunders, Philadelphia, 1980

22. Hornbuckle WE, Kleine LJ: Medical management of prostatic disease. In Kirk RW (Ed): Current Veterinary Therapy VII—Small Animal Practice. p. 1146. Saunders, Philadelphia, 1980

23. Hostetter RH, Wilkes BM, Brenner BM: Mechanisms of impaired glomerular filtration in acute renal failure. In Brenner BM, Stein JG (Eds): Acute Renal Failure. p. 52. Churchill Livingstone, New York, 1980

24. Kolata RJ, Johnston DE: Motor vehicle accidents in urban dogs: a study of 600 cases. J Am Vet Med Assoc 167:938, 1975

25. Lein DH: Canine orchitis. In Kirk RW (Ed): Current Veterinary Therapy VI—Small Animal Practice. p. 1255. Saunders, Philadelphia, 1977

26. Lein DH: Pyometritis in the bitch and queen. In Kirk RW (Ed): Current Veterinary Therapy VIII—Small Animal Practice. p. 942. Saunders, Philadelphia, 1983

27. Levinsky NG, Alexander EA, Venkatachalam MA: Acute renal failure. In Brenner BM, Rector FC (Eds): The Kidney. 2nd Ed. p. 1181. Saunders, Philadelphia, 1981

28. Levinsky NG, Bernard DB, Johnston PA; Enhancement of recovery of acute renal failure: effects of mannitol and diuretics. In Brenner BM, Stein JH (Eds): Acute Renal Failure. p. 163. Churchill Livingstone, New York, 1980

29. Linder A, Cutler RE, Goodman WG: Synergism of dopamine plus furosemide in preventing acute renal failure in the dog. Kidney Int 16:158, 1979

30. Ling GV, Ruby AL: Cephalexin for oral treatment of canine urinary tract infection caused by Klebsiella pneumoniae. J Am Vet Med Assoc 182:1346, 1983

31. Ling GV, Ruby AL: Gentamicin for treatment of resistant urinary tract infections in dogs J Am Vet Med Assoc 175:480, 1979

32. Lipowitz AJ, Larsen RE: Acute metritis. In Kirk RW (Ed): Current Veterinary Therapy VII—Small Animal Practice. p. 1214. Saunders, Philadelphia, 1980

33. Morgan RV: Urogenital emergencies. Part II. Compend Contin Educ 5:43, 1983

34. Osborne CA, Polzin DJ: Conservative medical management of feline chronic polyuric renal failure. In Kirk RW (Ed): Current Veterinary Therapy VIII—Small Animal Practice. p. 1008. Saunders, Philadelphia, 1983

35. Parker HR: Current status of peritoneal dialysis. In Kirk RW (Ed): Current Veterinary Therapy VII—Small Animal Practice. p. 1106. Saunders, Philadelphia, 1980
36. Pechman RD: Urinary trauma in dogs and cats: a review. JAAHA 18:33, 1982
37. Polzin DJ, Osborne CA: Conservative medical management of canine chronic polyuric renal failure. p. 997. In Kirk RW (Ed): Current Veterinary Therapy VIII—Small Animal Practice. Saunders, Philadelphia 1983
38. Porter GA, Bennett WM: Nephrotoxin-induced acute renal failure. In Brenner BM, Stein JH (Eds): Acute Renal Failure. p. 123. Churchill Livingstone, New York, 1980
39. Selcer BA: Urinary tract trauma associated with pelvic trauma. JAAHA 18:785, 1982
40. Sokolowski JR: Prostaglandin $F_{2\alpha}$-THAM for medical treatment of endometritis, metritis, and pyometritis in the bitch. JAAHA 16:119, 1982
41. Thornhill JA: Continuous ambulatory peritoneal dialysis. In Kirk RW (Ed): Current Veterinary Therapy VIII—Small Animal Practice. p. 1028. Saunders, Philadelphia, 1983
42. Thornhill JA: Control of vomiting in the uremic patient. In Kirk RW (Ed): Current Veterinary Therapy VIII—Small Animal Practice. p. 1022. Saunders, Philadelphia, 1983
43. Toback FG: Amino acid treatment of acute renal failure. In Brenner BM, Stein JH (Ed): Acute Renal Failure. p. 202. Churchill Livingstone, New York, 1980
44. Wright FS, Howards SS: Obstructive injury. In Brenner BM, Rector FC (Eds): The Kidney. 2nd Ed. p. 2008. Saunders, Philadelphia, 1981
45. Zager RA: Hyperphosphatemia: a factor that provokes severe experimental acute renal failure. J Lab Clin Med 100:230, 1982

7 | Medical Emergencies of the Digestive Tract and Abdomen

Susan Johnson

Medical emergencies of the digestive tract and abdomen are categorized for discussion into hepatic failure, acute pancreatitis, peritonitis, abdominal trauma, gastrointestinal emergencies, and splenic emergencies.

HEPATIC FAILURE

Liver failure in the dog and cat may be classified as acute or chronic (Tables 7-1 and 7-2). Hepatotoxins, infectious agents, vascular malformations, and certain metabolic diseases can induce either acute or chronic liver failure; however, in many clinical cases the inciting etiology is not identified.[14] Liver biopsy is usually required to evaluate causes of liver failure. When histopathologic evaluation is not diagnostic for a specific etiology, descriptive morphologic characteristics, i.e., acute necrosis, steatosis, chronic active hepatitis, fibrosis, and cirrhosis, aid in classification of hepatic disease. The histologic description provides information concerning the chronicity and reversibility of the disease and may suggest potential etiologies. Furthermore, the clinical course of certain disorders, e.g., cirrhosis and feline lipidosis, can be predicted even though the underlying mechanisms are poorly understood.

Clinical signs and laboratory data reflect the functional aspects of hepatic failure but fail to distinguish acute from chronic disease. Accordingly, emergency management of hepatic failure is directed toward symptomatic and supportive treatment of the metabolic derangements, allowing time to pursue a definitive diagnosis and to determine if specific treatment is available.

213

Table 7-1. Etiology of Acute Liver Failure

Hepatotoxins
  Exogenous
    Drugs
      Acetaminophen (feline)
      Arsenicals
      Halothane
      Ketoconazole
      Mebendazole
      Methoxyflurane
      Phenytoin
      Phenazopyridine (feline)
      Sulfonamides (sulfadiazine/trimethoprim)
      Tetracycline
    Environmental toxins
      Aflatoxin
      Carbon tetrachloride
      Dimethylnitrosamine
      Heavy metals
      Herbicides
      Pesticides
      Phosphorus
      Pyrrolizidine alkaloids
      Selenium
  Endogenous
    Bacterial endotoxins
Infectious agents
  Infectious canine hepatitis virus
  Leptospira spp.
  Salmonella spp.
  Feline infectious peritonitis virus (feline)
  Toxoplasma gondii
  Bacillus piliformis (Tyzzer's disease)
Others
  Pancreatitis
  Septicemia
  Inflammatory bowel disease
  Acute hemolytic anemia

Etiology and Principles of Diagnosis

The presence of hepatic disease may be initially suspected from historical information, physical examination findings, and laboratory tests. Because a routine data base is necessary to detect liver disease, appropriate patient evaluation as described in Table 7-3 is the first step to proper management. Initial diagnostic efforts in the animal in hepatic failure are directed toward differentiation of acute and chronic hepatic disease. This classification in turn suggests specific etiologies of each category. Moreover, the long-term prognosis of chronic diseases, e.g., cirrhosis, is poor and may not warrant the intense symptomatic and supportive care that would be well justified in acute, reversible disorders, e.g., leptospirosis. As mentioned previously, liver biopsy is the test of choice to determine the etiology and reversibility of hepatic disease; however, certain features of the history, physical examination, laboratory evaluation, and radiographic examination may suggest the etiology and chron-

Table 7-2. Chronic Liver Diseases Resulting in Liver Failure

Chronic active hepatitis
    Idiopathic
    Copper-associated liver disease of Bedlington terriers
    Leptospira interrogans serovar *grippotyphosa*
    Chronic active hepatitis of Doberman pinschers
Cirrhosis
    Idiopathic
    Anticonvulsant-associated
    Subsequent to chronic active hepatitis
Hepatic fibrosis
Chronic drug therapy
    Anticonvulsants
    Methotrexate
    Tolbutamide
    Corticosteroids
Fungal hepatitis
    Histoplasmosis
    Coccidioidomycosis
    Others
Metabolic
    Diabetes mellitus
    Amyloidosis
Hepatic neoplasia
Vascular malformations
    Congenital portosystemic shunt
    Hepatic AV fistula
Feline lipidosis
Feline cholangiohepatitis

icity of a disorder. Clinical features that indicate chronicity include protracted clinical signs, ascites, emaciation, hypoalbuminemia, decreased blood urea nitrogen (BUN), and microhepatia.[40]

Acute Liver Failure. The most frequently recognized causes of acute liver failure are hepatotoxins and infectious agents that result in hepatic necrosis or steatosis.[33] Hepatotoxins may be exogenous or endogenous in origin (Table 7-1). Categories of exogenous hepatotoxins include drugs and environmental toxins. Although numerous substances have the potential to induce hepatic damage, confirmation of these toxin-induced diseases is difficult to obtain in the clinical setting. The potential for drugs such as thiacetarsamide sodium to induce hepatic disease is readily apparent. However, most hepatic drug reactions are idiosyncratic in nature, making cause-and-effect relationships difficult to establish. Clinical diagnosis of hepatotoxicity is often based on circumstantial evidence that incriminates a particular drug or toxin. Frequently a potential hepatotoxin cannot be identified, and the clinical diagnosis is based on suggestive histologic lesions, e.g., acute hepatic necrosis or steatosis, in an animal who had previously been healthy. Bacterial endotoxins are endogenous causes of hepatic necrosis and steatosis.[14] Although primarily originating from the gut, infection in any body system may be associated with endotoxin production and subsequent hepatic dysfunction. The clinical diagnosis is difficult to establish but may be suspected when the use of intestinal

Table 7-3. Clinical Evaluation of Patients with Suspected Liver Failure

Clinical Findings	Comments
History: problems that suggest liver disease Emesis Diarrhea Anorexia Weight loss Stunted growth Drug intolerances Polydipsia, polyuria Abnormal behavior Seizures	Clinical signs are not specific for liver disease. Signs may be acute or chronic. If chronic, they are often intermittent. CNS signs may be precipitated by a high protein meal. Patients may be intolerant of tranquilizers, sedatives, anesthetics, etc. Inquire about previous drug therapy and vaccination status (ICH, leptospirosis).
Physical examination: findings suggestive of liver disease Hepatomegaly Pain elicited by liver palpation Jaundice Ascites Emaciation Acholic stools Pigmented urine (orange) Diffuse cerebral encephalopathy	Only hepatomegaly, hepatic pain, and acholic stools are specific for liver disease. Causes of hepatomegaly include infiltrative disease (fat, neoplasia), inflammation, congestion, biliary obstruction, and nodular hyperplasia. Signs of encephalopathy frequently wax and wane.
Laboratory: tests potentially abnormal with liver disease Enzymes: SGPT (ALT), SGOT (AST), alkaline phosphatase Liver function tests: BSP retention, blood NH_3, bilirubin, albumin, glucose, cholesterol, BUN, bile acids Urine analysis: dilute urine, bilirubinuria, urobilinogen, bilirubin and NH_4 biurate crystals, darkfield microscopy for spirochetes (leptospirosis) RBC characteristics: target cells, acanthocytes, microcytes Hemostatic parameters: OSPT, APTT, ACT, FDPs, platelets Serology: histoplasmosis, coccidioidomycosis, leptospirosis, toxoplasmosis, FIP Others: serum protein electrophoresis, amylase, lipase, abdominal fluid analysis and cytology, fecal occult blood	Liver enzymes may be normal in congenital portal vein anomalies, cirrhosis, and neoplasia. The presence of steroid-induced alkaline phosphatase isoenzyme suggests steroid hepatopathy. Blood NH_3 concentration before and after oral NH_4Cl administration is the best test to identify hepatic encephalopathy. Hyperbilirubinemia caused by hepatic and posthepatic disease must be differentiated from that caused by hemolytic disorders. Hypoalbuminemia suggests chronicity. Hypoglycemia caused by hepatic failure is a poor prognostic sign and must be differentiated from endotoxemia-induced hypoglycemia. Urinary NH_4 biurate crystals are most frequently observed with congenital portosystemic shunts.
Radiographic findings Hepatomegaly—focal or generalized Microhepatia Mineralization of hepatic parenchyma or biliary tree Gas density in liver or gallbladder Ascites Renomegaly	*See* causes of hepatomegaly under "Physical Examination." Microhepatia may indicate cirrhosis or a portosystemic shunt. Confirmation of portosystemic shunting of blood requires splenoportography or cranial mesenteric angiography. Renomegaly may be observed with congenital portal vein anomalies. Sophisticated testing with ultrasonography may provide additional information in hepatic disorders, e.g., biliary obstruction or hepatic neoplasia.

(ICH) infectious canine hepatitis. (SGPT) serum glutamic pyruvic transaminase. (ALT) alanine aminotransferase. (SGOT) serum glutamic oxalacetic transaminase. (AST) aspartate aminotransferase. (BUN) blood urea nitrogen. (OSPT) one-stage prothrombin time. (APTT) activated partial thromboplastin time. (ACT) activated clotting time. (FDP) fibrin degradation products. (FIP) feline infectious peritonitis. (CAH) chronic active hepatitis.

Table 7-3. (*continued*)

Clinical Findings	Comments
Hepatic biopsy	Special stains to detect the presence of fungal
Histopathology	organisms, fibrosis, copper, and amyloid are
Cytology	indicated in certain cases. Fungal or
Cultures of parenchyma and bile	bacterial cultures may be submitted. Hepatic
Copper analysis	copper concentrations are increased, >350
Toxin analysis	μg/g dry weight, in Bedlington liver disease
Electron microscopy	and CAH in Doberman pinschers. Chemical
	analysis of the liver may be indicated to
	detect toxins, i.e., lead, arsenic.

antibiotics or toxin adsorbers, e.g., cholestyramine, result in improved hepatic function.

Infectious agents that are important causes of hepatic necrosis include *Leptospira* spp., *Bacillus piliformis* (Tyzzer's disease), infectious canine hepatitis (ICH) virus, feline infectious peritonitis (FIP) virus, and *Toxoplasma gondii*.[14,33] Because of the generalized nature of such infections, liver failure may be but one of several concurrent clinical manifestations. These associated extrahepatic manifestations may provide important diagnostic clues to the cause of liver disease. For example, sudden onset of concurrent hepatic and renal failure in a dog might suggest leptospirosis, and concurrent uveitis and liver disease in a cat may indicate FIP, toxoplasmosis, or a feline leukemia virus-related disease.

Other causes of acute liver failure are pancreatitis, septicemia, inflammatory bowel disease, and acute hemolytic anemia.[39] These diseases cause secondary hepatic necrosis; however, the clinical signs are primarily attributable to disease in other organs. In acute pancreatitis, jaundice and marked liver enzyme elevations that are occasionally seen have been attributed to pancreatic enzyme-induced hepatic injury or to pancreatic swelling and extrahepatic biliary obstruction. Differentiation from primary hepatobiliary disease is substantiated by detection of increased serum amylase and lipase activity. The cause of acute hepatic necrosis associated with inflammatory bowel disease is unknown. Endotoxemia, septicemia, and immune-mediated inflammatory disease have been suggested as possible mechanisms. Hemolytic anemia causes acute hypoxia and results in centrolobular hepatic necrosis.

Chronic Liver Disease. Chronic liver diseases frequently progress to hepatic failure (Table 7-2). The final phase of hepatic decompensation in such chronic diseases may represent a state of acute metabolic emergency. Despite the association of certain etiologies, e.g., copper-associated hepatitis in Bedlington terriers and *Leptospira*-induced chronic active hepatitis (CAH), with the histopathologic lesions of CAH, the inciting event in most clinical cases is not apparent.[14] An increased incidence of CAH in Doberman pinschers suggests a hereditary predisposition, and female dogs of all breeds also seem to be at increased risk.[14,16] The initiation and perpetuation of CAH by immunologic mechanisms, although generally accepted in humans, has yet to be

Table 7-4. General Therapy for Liver Failure

Goals of Therapy	Product and Dose	Comments
Correct dehydration and maintain fluid and acid-base balance	NaCl 0.45% or 0.9% IV; give NaHCO₃ if metabolic acidosis present	Avoid alkalosis. Use 0.45% NaCl in chronic liver disease to prevent excessive sodium and water retention.
Prevent hypoglycemia	Add 2.5–5% dextrose to IV fluids	
Avoid hypokalemia	Add 14 mEq KCl to each 500 cc of maintenance fluids	Monitor serum potassium daily and adjust potassium supplementation accordingly.
Control hepatic encephalopathy		
Avoid use of anticonvulsants, sedatives, tranquilizers, organophosphates, and diuretics		If oral anticonvulsant therapy is unavoidable, use phenobarbital at reduced doses.
Prevent production and absorption of enteric toxins	Cleansing enemas q 6 h Retention enemas q 6 h with: Neomycin 15 mg/kg *or* Lactulose 50% solution + water in a 1:2 ratio: 50–200 cc total *OR* Neomycin 10–20 mg/kg PO q.i.d. Lactulose 15–30 cc PO q.i.d.	For retention enema, place Foley catheter in colon and inflate balloon. Keep in place for 1 hr. If comatose, use retention enema, otherwise oral therapy is preferable.

Control GI hemorrhage	Correct coagulopathy (see below) Diagnose and treat concurrent GI parasites Cimetidine 20–40 mg/kg PO, IV divided t.i.d.	Use cimetidine if a gastric ulcer is suspected.
Dietary manipulations	Low protein, low fat, high carbohydrate, e.g., k/d, u/d, cottage cheese, boiled rice, spaghetti	NPO[a] in initial stages of HE[b]. For chronic therapy, give as much protein as clinical signs will tolerate. Vegetable protein may be superior to animal protein.
Control coagulopathy	Vit K_1, 5–20 mg IM q 12 h Fresh plasma transfusion If DIC: heparin therapy 5–10 units/kg SC b.i.d.–t.i.d.	Cautious use of heparin is advised. May incubate heparin with plasma before infusion.
Control ascites	Low sodium diet Abdominocentesis if dyspneic Spironolactone 1–2 mg/kg PO b.i.d. Furosemide 0.25–0.5 mg/kg PO, IV, IM divided b.i.d.	Use diuretics cautiously. May worsen encephalopathy by causing hypokalemia, alkalosis, dehydration, and azotemia.
Control infection and endotoxemia	Penicillin, ampicillin, cephalosporins, gentamicin, kanamycin	Reduce dosage of drugs that are dependent on hepatic metabolism, i.e., chloramphenicol.

[a] (NPO) nothing per os.
[b] (HE) hepatic encephalopathy.

proved in dogs. In any event, CAH as a histologic diagnosis can be established only by liver biopsy.

Cirrhosis, or end-stage liver disease, is characterized histologically by fibrosis, nodule formation, and disruption of the lobular architecture. Numerous insults to the liver, including CAH, may progress to cirrhosis; however, in most animals the inciting cause is unidentified.[14] A noteworthy association between long-term anticonvulsant therapy and cirrhosis has been suggested in dogs, although a cause-and-effect relationship has not yet been established.[5]

A history of chronic drug administration may suggest drug-induced liver disease. However, as with acute drug-induced hepatic disease, the clinical diagnosis is usually based on circumstantial evidence.

A diagnosis of congenital portosystemic shunt should be suspected in any young dog with a history of stunted growth, gastrointestinal disturbances, or neurologic abnormalities (hepatic encephalopathy). Routine biochemical and hematologic data are often unremarkable except for hypoproteinemia, low BUN, target cells, and microcytosis; consequently, the diagnosis must be suspected from clinical signs.[14] Although abnormal BSP (Bromsulphalein) retention and ammonia intolerance support the diagnosis, confirmation requires demonstration of the vascular anomaly by contrast radiography. In older animals, acquired portosystemic communications evolve as a physiological response to portal hypertension, which is frequently caused by cirrhosis. In such cases, a liver biopsy in conjunction with contrast radiography is required for diagnosis. Other chronic hepatic disorders listed in Table 7-2 are primarily diagnosed by liver biopsy, although serologic studies and contrast radiography may provide a definitive diagnosis in certain diseases.

Pathophysiology and Basis for Therapy

The metabolic derangements that are a consequence of hepatic failure merely reflect disruption of normal hepatic function. The liver plays a central role in such diverse activities as carbohydrate, fat, and protein metabolism; detoxification and excretion of drugs and other substances; and formation and elimination of bile. An understanding of the pathophysiological mechanisms of hepatic failure is essential to accurately formulate appropriate therapy. General and specific recommendations for treatment are listed in Tables 7-4 and 7-5.

Hepatic Encephalopathy.   Hepatic encephalopathy (HE) is a syndrome of altered central nervous system (CNS) function resulting from hepatic insufficiency. Clinical signs include depression, behavioral changes, ataxia, staggering, head pushing, circling, pacing, blindness, seizures, and coma. Despite considerable research, the precise cellular mechanisms responsible for HE are unknown. Several recent reviews have summarized current pathophysiological mechanisms and are recommended to the reader.[14,34,36] Postulated mechanisms of HE include interference with brain energy metabolism, disturbances of neuronal membrane function, and impaired synaptic transmission caused by a derangement in the balance of neurotransmitters. Of clinical importance is the concept that the principal "lesion" of HE is a biochemical, not a structural,

Table 7-5. Specific Therapy for Liver Failure

Disorder	Product and Dose	Comments
Drug-induced liver disease	Recognition and avoidance of suspected drug	
Bacterial hepatitis/cholangitis		
Leptospirosis	Procaine penicillin G 20,000 units/kg IM, SC s.i.d.–b.i.d.	
Others	Dihydrostreptomycin 10 mg/kg IM, SC t.i.d. Penicillin, ampicillin, cephalosporins	
Mycotic hepatitis	Amphotericin B 0.25–0.5 mg/kg IV q 2/days Ketoconazole 10 mg/kg PO t.i.d.	
Chronic active hepatitis	Prednisolone 0.5–1.0 mg/kg/day PO Decrease gradually to ADT[a] Continue for at least 6 wk Azathioprine 2 mg/kg PO s.i.d. in conjunction with prednisolone.	Monitor serum enzyme activity and liver biopsy to determine response to therapy.
	D-Penicillamine 125–250 mg/day in adult dogs 30 min prior to eating	D-Penicillamine may be useful to chelate hepatic copper in Bedlington liver disease and CAH of Doberman pinschers.
	Ascorbic acid (vit C) 500–1,000 mg/day	Vitamin C may augment urinary copper excretion.
Feline cholangiohepatitis	Ampicillin Prednisolone 2 mg/kg/day PO	Use antibiotics first if bacterial cholangitis is suspected.
Congenital portosystemic shunts	Surgical ligation of shunt	
Hepatic neoplasia	Chemotherapy or surgical resection	

[a] ADT = alternate day therapy.

alteration in the CNS. Consequently, the clinical signs of HE are potentially reversible if hepatic function can be improved or if the metabolic imbalances or accumulation of toxins can be reversed. Whereas the brain is morphologically normal in acute HE, a lesion of astrocytosis has been observed in chronically encephalopathic dogs.[36] In humans, cerebral edema infrequently complicates fulminant hepatic failure and encephalopathy.[34]

Interactions between a variety of toxins and the metabolic imbalances of liver failure are probably responsible for the clinical manifestations of HE. Inadequate hepatic clearance of enteric toxins has long been suspected to cause HE. The clinical improvement seen in patients treated with intestinal antibiotics suggests that bacteria do play a role in this syndrome. Potential toxins thought to originate from the gut include ammonia, mercaptans, short-chain fatty acids (SCFA), indoles, skatols, biogenic amines, and γ-aminobutyric acid.[14,34,36]

The toxin most frequently incriminated in HE is ammonia, which is generated by urease-producing colonic bacteria.[14,34,36] The primary substrate is intestinal urea, although dietary amino acids also contribute to ammonia production. Normally, ammonia is absorbed into the portal blood and converted to urea in the liver by the Krebs-Henseleit urea cycle. Most newly formed urea is excreted in the urine, although as much as 25% may undergo enterohepatic circulation and ultimately be hydrolyzed to ammonia in the gut. Portosystemic shunting of blood or hepatic disorders severe enough to interrupt hepatic extraction or metabolism of ammonia result in excessive accumulation of ammonia in the blood, brain, and cerebrospinal fluid (CSF). Rarely, signs of hyperammonemia may be attributed to a deficiency of hepatic urea cycle enzyme activity. Elevated venous blood ammonia concentrations are detected most frequently in dogs with portosystemic shunting of blood; however, plasma ammonia levels do not correlate well with the degree of encephalopathy, which may indicate that other factors influence intracerebral ammonia concentrations, e.g., alkalosis and hypokalemia. Other toxins, e.g., SCFA and mercaptans, have been shown to potentiate the effects of hyperammonemia.

Mercaptans are produced by bacterial degradation of dietary methionine and have been implicated as a toxin of encephalopathy.[34,36] As with ammonia, inadequate hepatic clearance leads to excess plasma accumulation. Mercaptans can induce a reversible coma in dogs. Furthermore, the administration of methionine-containing lipotropic drugs has been associated with worsening of encephalopathy in dogs. Thus methionine should not be empirically administered to dogs with severe liver disease, as this amino acid may potentiate the development of HE.

SCFAs are also suspected to be important in HE.[34,36] These substances are derived from ingested fat and can be shown experimentally to induce coma. Both SCFA and mercaptans interrupt ammonia detoxification and enhance the toxicity of hyperammonemia. The free fatty acids that accumulate secondary to hepatic dysfunction may also increase plasma and CSF tryptophan, which in turn has been implicated in the pathogenesis of HE.

In addition to toxins of gut origin, imbalances of CNS neurotransmitters and their precursor amino acids have also been suspected to contribute to encephalopathy.[34,36] Dogs with acute hepatic failure have increases of most plasma amino acids. This has been attributed to excessive hepatocellular release and impaired hepatic clearance. With chronic hepatic disorders, plasma aromatic amino acids (AAAs) (phenylalanine, tyrosine, and tryptophan) and methionine are increased, and branched-chain amino acids (BCAAs) (leucine, isoleucine, and valine) are decreased. The BCAA/AAA ratio in normal dogs is 3:1–4:1, whereas ratios of 1.0–1.5 or less are detected in dogs with portosystemic vascular shunting and acquired hepatic insufficiency. Elevations of AAA are attributed to delayed hepatic clearance, and BCAA concentrations are decreased owing to their increased utilization for energy. The hormonal derangement resulting from hepatic failure, specifically increases in insulin and glucagon, may also contribute to the amino acid imbalance. Alterations in amino acid ratios generally correlate with the degree of encephalopathy in dogs.[14,36] Moreover, normalization of the amino acid ratio by administration of BCAA is associated with improvement of clinical signs in dogs with experimentally induced hepatic insufficiency. These derangements probably alter intracerebral amino acid metabolism and synthesis of neurotransmitters.[34,36]

Metabolic imbalances frequently precipitate signs of hepatic encephalopathy in dogs with hepatic insufficiency.[14,36] Most cases can be attributed to potentiation of one of the previously discussed pathophysiological mechanisms for hepatic coma. Many factors, for example, can increase ammonia production in the gut, including high-protein diets, gastrointestinal hemorrhage, and constipation. Prevention and control of HE necessitates detection and treatment of these precipitating events (Table 7-4).

The use of antibiotics, e.g., neomycin, metronidazole, or ampicillin, is recommended to reduce the numbers of urea-splitting bacteria and thus inhibit ammonia production. The nonabsorbable, nonmetabolizable synthetic disaccharide lactulose is used to lower blood ammonia concentrations in HE. The means by which this is accomplished include: (1) acidification of the colon with trapping of NH_4^+; (2) catharsis; (3) alteration of colonic bacterial flora; and (4) increasing stool nitrogen content. Lactulose may also exert a beneficial antiendotoxin effect. Although objective data are lacking, orally administered lactulose, alone or in combination with neomycin, seems to be effective in dogs with HE.[36]

The administration of stored blood to dogs with liver disease can be deleterious as it contains 170 μg NH_3/100 ml after 1 day and increases progressively with further storage.[34,36] Hypovolemia can cause azotemia and retention of nitrogenous wastes, which precipitate hepatic decompensation. Moreover, the direct depressive effects of uremia on the cerebrum may potentiate signs of HE. Consequently, correction of volume deficits and maintenance of normal hydration improve signs of HE. Bacterial infections are treated with appropriate antibiotic therapy as infection has a catabolic effect and increases endogenous nitrogen load.

The inability of dogs with chronic liver disease to tolerate recommended doses of CNS depressant drugs, i.e., tranquilizers, anticonvulsants, and anesthetics, may be partly attributed to impaired hepatic metabolism but also to increased "cerebral sensitivity" to such drugs.[14,36] The potential for impaired hepatic metabolism and subsequent accumulation of drugs should be considered before administering any substance. Although specific drug and dose modifications are unavailable, the veterinarian should attempt to determine whether the liver is important for metabolism of that particular drug and decrease the dose accordingly.

Hypoglycemia may complicate HE and may be caused by impaired gluconeogenesis or endotoxemia.[14] Intravenous dextrose therapy is recommended to prevent hypoglycemia and possibly increase the uptake of ammonia by glutamate.

Acid-Base and Electrolyte Disturbances.   Acute and chronic hepatic failure in dogs may be accompanied by disorders in acid-base balance. Any acid-base disorder may occur secondary to extrahepatic complications, but respiratory alkalosis is most common and has been attributed to direct stimulation of the respiratory center by toxins.[44] Ammonia has been suspected, as the intravenous administration of ammonium acetate induces hyperammonemia and respiratory alkalosis in dogs.[31] In addition, metabolic alkalosis may be precipitated by excessive loss of hydrogen ion from the gastrointestinal tract (vomiting) or urinary tract (hyperaldosteronism) and by intracellular shifting of hydrogen ion as a result of hypokalemia. Alkalosis is particularly deleterious as it can potentiate signs of hepatic encephalopathy by converting ammonium ion to ammonia, which freely diffuses into cells.[36] On the other hand, metabolic acidosis may develop when circulatory collapse and lactic acidosis complicate hepatic failure.[44]

Although the potential for total body potassium depletion exists with chronic hepatic disorders, evaluation of serum potassium may not be a reliable indicator of this problem.[44] Hypokalemia usually results from anorexia, emesis, diarrhea, and loss of potassium in the urine. The latter may be augmented by secondary hyperaldosteronism or by diuretic therapy, which causes hypokalemia and contraction alkalosis. Metabolic alkalosis causes hypokalemia by shifting potassium intracellularly, increasing the potassium available for sodium exchange in the distal convoluted tubule.

Ascites.   Ascites, the accumulation of extracellular fluid in the peritoneal cavity, is a frequent complication of chronic hepatic disorders, especially cirrhosis. Factors implicated in the formation of ascites include portal hypertension, hypoalbuminemia, and renal retention of sodium and water.[14] Concurrent portal hypertension and hypoalbuminemia are usually present in dogs with liver disease and ascites. The traditional theory of ascites formation invokes portal hypertension and hypoalbuminemia as the primary events. The subsequent accumulation of peritoneal fluid results in a loss of fluid and electrolytes from intravascular spaces and a decreased "effective" plasma volume. The renal response to this volume depletion is activation of the renin-angiotensin-aldosterone system. Despite the renal sodium and water retention that ensues, this fails to restore an "effective" plasma volume because of continuous fluid losses into the abdominal cavity, creating a vicious cycle. More recently, it has been suggested that there is a primary inability of the kidneys to excrete sodium and water. Retention of salt and water results in an expanded plasma volume. In the presence of portal hypertension and hypoalbuminemia, ascites develops.

In any event, sodium retention is a key perpetuating factor in ascites toward which medical therapy can be directed. Reducing sodium intake is essential when treating ascites. Diuretic therapy augments urinary loss of sodium and water; however, the potential for worsening of HE must be considered. Diuretics that work by antagonizing aldosterone, i.e., spironolactone, may have additional benefits in this situation (Table 7-4).

Abnormalities of Hemostasis. The liver is the major site for production of most coagulation factors, including factors I, II, V, VII, VIII, IX, X, XI, and XII.[40] The liver also synthesizes activators and inhibitors of the fibrinolytic system and catabolizes activated procoagulant factors and fibrin degradation products. Consequently, it is not surprising that hepatic disease often disrupts the normal hemostatic mechanisms, although clinical evidence of excessive bleeding is infrequent. Fifteen percent of dogs with various hepatic disorders in one study had abnormal values for the one-stage prothrombin time (OSPT) or activated partial thromboplastin time (APTT) without evidence of bleeding.[3] When the OSPT and APTT were performed on serial dilutions of platelet-poor plasma, 66% had at least one abnormal test. These results suggest that subclinical coagulation disorders may be frequent in dogs with liver disease.

Hemostatic defects associated with hepatobiliary disease may be attributed to disseminated intravascular coagulation (DIC), primary failure of the liver to synthesize clotting factors, or the vitamin K deficiency caused by biliary obstruction.[14,40] The first two mechanisms are probably most frequent. DIC has been described as a complication of infectious canine hepatitis, acute hepatic necrosis, aflatoxicosis, leptospirosis, and chronic active hepatitis and is discussed further in Chapter 8. Primary failure of hepatocytes to synthesize clotting factors must be differentiated from biliary obstruction causing impaired production of the vitamin K-dependent factors II, VII, IX, and X. Administration of vitamin K_1 intramuscularly should correct the coagulopathy caused by biliary obstruction within 24–48 hr. An attempt has been made to identify abnormalities in activity of selected clotting factors in dogs with various liver diseases.[2] Results suggest that specific patterns may be characteristic of certain disorders, including cirrhosis and hepatic neoplasia; however, further evaluation is needed before the diagnostic significance of factor quantitation is known. A fresh blood or plasma transfusion may temporarily improve coagulopathies due to hepatic failure; however, the long-term prognosis is poor.

Thrombocytopenia associated with liver disease most frequently results from DIC, although splenic sequestration as a consequence of portal hypertension is possible.[14] Platelet function defects occur in humans with hepatic failure, but similar studies in dogs are lacking.

Gastrointestinal Bleeding. In the presence of a mild bleeding tendency, gastric ulcers or venous congestion caused by portal hypertension may induce significant gastrointestinal blood loss.[40] The pathogenesis of gastric ulcers in liver disease is unknown. Failure of the liver to inactivate a secretagogue, possibly gastrin, has been proposed. Blood lost into the gastrointestinal tract is a substrate for ammonia production; thus there is potential for precipitation of encephalopathy in animals with hepatic failure. If gastrointestinal ulceration is suspected, cimetidine therapy may be useful to decrease gastric acid secretion and promote mucosal healing (Table 7-4).

Endotoxemia. Impaired hepatic reticuloendothelial cell function may predispose the patient with liver disease to developing endotoxemia.[14] Removal of bacteria and endotoxins from the portal blood is a necessary hepatic function. Endotoxemia may in turn cause extrahepatic signs of liver disease, e.g., hypergammaglobulinemia, renal vasoconstriction, acute tubular necrosis, DIC, fever, and myocardial depression. Furthermore, these toxins have been incriminated in the pathogenesis of hepatocellular injury. Oral antibiotics or toxin-adsorbing drugs, e.g., cholestyramine, have been recommended to decrease endotoxin production.

ACUTE PANCREATITIS

Acute pancreatitis is a common clinical diagnosis in dogs but is infrequently recognized in cats.[15,32] The clinical signs of acute pancreatitis are determined by the extent and severity of pancreatic and peripancreatic inflammation and the presence of extrapancreatic complications. Edematous pancreatitis, for example, can be mild and self-limiting, whereas hemorrhagic necrotizing pancreatitis can progress to hypovolemic shock and death despite appropriate therapy. Because the etiology of acute pancreatitis is infrequently identified in the clinical setting, therapy is focused on early recognition and treatment of fluid and electrolyte imbalances, suppression of pancreatic secretory stimuli, and control of complications including peritonitis, sepsis, cardiac arrhythmias, DIC, and hypovolemic or endotoxemic shock.

Etiology

The cause of acute pancreatitis is not identified in most clinical cases.[15,27,32] However, experimental models of pancreatitis suggest a number of mechanisms capable of initiating pancreatic injury. These include obesity, hyperlipemia, biliary tract disease, bile reflux, duodenal reflux, pancreatic duct obstruction, infectious agents, uremia, hypercalcemia, immunologic injury, trauma, and drugs, particularly corticosteroids.[15,29,33] As one or more of these mechanisms could contribute to the development of pancreatitis in the individual patient, successful treatment and prevention of recurrences could hinge on a knowledge of the predisposing cause. However, of these factors, only obesity and hyperlipemia are observed with any frequency in clinically diagnosed cases of acute pancreatitis. Obesity seems to be the most significant predisposing factor, as acute pancreatitis occurs most frequently in overweight dogs and is uncommon in animals on a balanced diet and in good physical condition.[15,32] Although lipemic serum is frequently detected in patients with acute pancreatitis, this may be the result rather than the cause of pancreatic inflammation. Hyperlipemia is thought to cause pancreatitis in humans due to fatty-acid-induced pancreatic ischemia.[32] It is conceivable that dogs with diseases causing abnormal lipid metabolism, i.e., hypothyroidism, diabetes mellitus, or idiopathic hyperlipoproteinemia, could be predisposed to developing pancreatitis.[32] Furthermore, the frequent observation that a high-fat meal was consumed prior to the onset of pancreatitis may incriminate hyperlipemia as a cause of pancreatitis.

Corticosteroid administration and hyperadrenocorticism in dogs is occasionally associated with clinical and laboratory findings suggestive of pancreatitis.[15,29,32] The mechanism is unknown, although ductal obstruction caused by increased viscosity of pancreatic secretions and ductal epithelial hyperplasia has been proposed.[15] In one study, dexamethasone therapy in normal dogs resulted in increased serum lipase activity but decreased serum amylase activity and no histologic evidence of pancreatitis.[29] These results suggest that detection of increased serum lipase activity is unreliable in confirming pancreatitis in dexamethasone-treated dogs, whereas an increase in serum amylase activity may be more significant.

Isolated cases of canine pancreatitis have been attributed to hypercalcemia, bile duct occlusion, trauma, and L-asparaginase therapy.[13,15,32] In cats, pancreatic fluke infestation, toxoplasmosis, feline infectious peritonitis, and cholangitis have been associated with pancreatitis.[33]

Pathophysiology

Regardless of the inciting cause, the pathophysiological mechanisms of pancreatitis involve pancreatic acinar cell damage, increased cell membrane and lysosomal permeability, and subsequent pancreatic autodigestion.[15,27,32] Activation of pancreatic enzymes leads to a complex series of events resulting in pancreatic and extrapancreatic disease. For example, trypsin activates phospholipase A, elastase, kallikrein, and bradykinin. Phospholipase A is a potent cytotoxin which causes hemolysis, acinar cell necrosis, and pulmonary dysfunction. Elastase dissolves elastic fibers in pancreatic blood vessels, thereby contributing to the development of hemorrhagic pancreatitis. Kallikrein and bradykinin produce local and systemic vasodilation, increased vascular permeability, leukocyte infiltration, and pain. When pancreatic blood flow is compromised, edematous pancreatitis progresses to the more serious necrotizing form. Factors contributing to impaired pancreatic blood flow include increased sympathetic tone, shock, pancreatic edema, vascular damage, fat embolization, and DIC.

Systemic complications are more likely with hemorrhagic necrotizing pancreatitis and are evidenced by cardiovascular, renal, hepatic, and pulmonary dysfunction.[27,32] Hypotension and hypovolemia are caused by fluid loss (vomiting, diarrhea, ascites), release of vasoactive polypeptides, and decreased cardiac output due to myocardial depressant factor released from ischemic pancreatic tissue. Cardiac arrhythmias may further compromise cardiovascular stability. Dehydration causes prerenal azotemia possibly complicated by toxin-induced nephrosis. Hepatic complications include congestion and focal necrosis. Occasionally, pancreatic inflammation causes extrahepatic biliary obstruction and jaundice. Although respiratory insufficiency is a well-recognized complication of hemorrhagic pancreatitis in humans, it is infrequently encountered in veterinary medicine.

Peripancreatic inflammation due to leakage of activated enzymes causes localized or generalized chemical peritonitis. Septic peritonitis may ensue if translocation of enteric bacteria occurs or if anaerobic conditions allow proliferation of *Clostridium perfringens*, a normal inhabitant of the pancreas.[27]

Diagnosis

The clinical diagnosis of acute pancreatitis in dogs is based on information obtained from the history, physical examination, abdominal radiographs, and laboratory tests.

Pancreatitis occurs most frequently in middle-aged, obese, female dogs.[15,32] A history of recent dietary indiscretion may be obtained from the owner. The most consistent clinical signs are vomiting, anorexia, and depression. Nausea can be present and is suggested by restlessness, constant pacing, ptyalism, or repeated swallowing. Findings of diarrhea, abdominal pain, abdominal distention, and fever are inconsistent. The absence of abdominal pain or, for that matter, vomiting does not eliminate the possibility of acute pancreatitis. Dogs with acute pancreatitis may assume the "position of relief" or seek a cool surface to lie on. In general, signs of acute hemorrhagic pancreatitis are similar to those of edematous pancreatitis but tend to be more severe and accompanied by hypotension, hypovolemia, and shock.

Results of abdominal radiography may suggest that pancreatitis is present but do not confirm the diagnosis. Radiographic signs of pancreatitis include an increased density in the right cranial quadrant, displacement of the duodenum to the right, and a static duodenal or colonic gas pattern in the area of the pancreas.[32] Abdominal radiographs can also be normal. Radiographs are obtained to evaluate other causes of vomiting that must be differentiated from pancreatitis, including gastrointestinal, hepatic, and renal disorders.

Evaluation of serum amylase and lipase activity is the most definitive means of confirming pancreatitis short of exploratory surgery and pancreatic biopsy. However, considerable controversy surrounds the interpretation of these tests. This is likely due to inadequate knowledge of the extrapancreatic sources of serum enzyme activity, the stimuli for enzyme release other than pancreatitis, and the mechanisms of enzyme degradation and clearance. Variation in testing methods also contributes to the confusion. Serum lipase evaluation has been recommended as a more specific test for pancreatitis, as the pancreas is the major tissue source of lipase.[42] Serum amylase, on the other hand, is thought to originate from many organs, including the pancreas. Hyperamylasemia has been detected in nonpancreatic disorders affecting the intestine and kidney.[32] Impaired renal function is thought to result in decreased filtration or tubular degradation of amylase, thereby causing increases in serum amylase activity up to 2.5 times normal.[30] Unfortunately, recent studies also indicate as much as a four-fold increase in serum lipase activity when renal function is impaired.[30] Neither amylase nor lipase values correlate with parameters of renal dysfunction, e.g., BUN or creatinine, thus hyperamylasemia and hyperlipasemia are not reliable indices of concurrent pancreatitis in dogs with primary renal failure.[30]

The following guidelines have been proposed for interpretation of increased serum amylase and lipase activity.[15] When the BUN and creatinine are normal, hyperamylasemia and hyperlipasemia are most likely due to pancreatitis. When azotemia and increased serum enzyme activity are detected, a low urine specific gravity (1.008–1.012) suggests primary renal failure with lack of enzyme degradation, whereas the finding of concentrated urine (>1.020) is more compatible with prerenal azotemia, possibly caused by pancreatitis. Concurrent pancreatitis and primary renal failure are also possible. In general, simultaneous determination and interpretation of both serum amylase and lipase activities is recommended.[32]

Other biochemical abnormalities detected in patients with acute pancreatitis include increased serum alanine aminotransferase (formerly SGPT) and alkaline phosphatase, hyperbilirubinemia, lipemia, transient hyperglycemia, hypoproteinemia, and hypocalcemia.[15,32] Hypocalcemia has been attributed to peripancreatic calcium soap formation, hypoalbuminemia, and blunted parathyroid hormone response. Clinical signs of hypocalcemia usually do not occur. Acid-base and electrolyte disturbances vary with the severity of the disease and its extrapancreatic complications; therefore laboratory analysis is helpful in tailoring fluid therapy to the individual patient's needs, according to the guidelines in Chapter 4.

Hematologic changes in acute pancreatitis include a stress leukogram and possible increased numbers of immature neutrophils.[15,32] The presence of a left shift suggests severe pancreatic inflammation and may indicate septic peritonitis or abscess formation. Detection of fibrin degradation products, thrombocytopenia, and prolonged OSPT, APTT, and activated clotting time (ACT) indicate probable DIC.

Fluid obtained by abdominocentesis may be evaluated for amylase or lipase activity, cytologic evidence of inflammation and sepsis, and bacterial culture.[15]

Treatment

Treatment of acute pancreatitis consists of maintaining adequate hydration, preventing pancreatic secretion, and controlling secondary sepsis and other complications.[15,27,32,44]

Fluid therapy is the single most important aspect of patient management and must provide for fluid deficits, ongoing losses (vomiting, diarrhea, peritonitis), maintenance requirements, and in some instances shock therapy. Parenteral routes of fluid administration are used in all patients with pancreatitis. Intravenous fluid therapy is preferable; however, when clinical signs are mild, the subcutaneous route suffices. A balanced electrolyte solution combined with lactate (lactated Ringer's) is a reasonable choice, as metabolic acidosis is the most common acid-base imbalance. Although additional fluid supplementation with calcium, potassium chloride, bicarbonate, and glucose (septic shock) may be required, these deficits are unpredictable and require prior laboratory confirmation. Low-molecular-weight dextrans (10% dextran at 5 ml/kg/hr IV) have been recommended for treatment of pancreatitis.[27] They are thought to be beneficial in that they decrease blood viscosity, thereby maintaining pancreatic blood flow. However, the expense of these solutions may preclude their use. The reader is referred to Chapter 2 for a discussion of the therapy for shock and to Chapter 4 for discussion of fluid therapy.

Prevention of pancreatic secretion is best accomplished by total restriction of oral intake (food, water, medications). Gastric distention, fat, amino acids, and duodenal acidity are thus prevented from further stimulating the pancreas. Anticholinergic drugs, e.g., atropine (0.04–0.08 mg/kg IV, IM, SQ) and glycopyrrolate (0.01 mg/kg IM, SQ), have traditionally been used in the treatment of acute pancreatitis to inhibit neurogenic pancreatic secretion.[32] However, their efficacy in pancreatitis is unproved. When anticholinergic drugs are administered, the clinician must be aware of their potential for causing delayed gastric emptying and intestinal ileus.

The patient is offered small volumes of water when emesis has not occurred for at least 48 hr. Normalization of serum enzyme activity may not be necessary for the patient to begin tolerating oral intake.[27] If vomiting of water does not occur after 1–2 days, small amounts of a low-fat diet (prescription diet i/d or r/d) are offered. The animal is gradually returned to a regular diet over the next few days. If vomiting occurs at any time, parenteral fluid therapy is resumed, and the animal's oral intake is restricted for at least two more days.

Septic peritonitis, septicemia, or endotoxemia can complicate the course of acute pancreatitis.[15,27,32] However, the efficacy of prophylactic antibiotics has not been proved. Nonetheless, broad-spectrum antibiotics effective against anaerobes and gram-negative organisms, e.g., ampicillin and chloramphenicol, are often routinely administered.[32] When infection is present, bacterial culture and sensitivity tests are performed on blood, infected peritoneal fluid, or abscess contents to determine the most appropriate antibiotic. Peritoneal lavage has also been advocated for treatment of refractory pancreatitis. This procedure is most likely to be beneficial when septic peritonitis is present.[32]

Heparin therapy may be useful to treat acute pancreatitis.[32] Potential beneficial mechanisms include preservation of pancreatic blood flow by preventing local DIC and clearing of lipemia. The dose recommended for the latter effect is 150 IU/kg IV. Guidelines for heparin therapy of DIC are discussed further in Chapter 8.

Glucocorticoids are sometimes used in the treatment of pancreatitis to decrease the inflammatory response.[27,32] Inasmuch as these drugs are also suspected of causing pancreatitis, their use is restricted to treatment of shock.

Analgesic drugs are occasionally used in the treatment of acute pancreatitis to control severe abdominal pain. Meperidine HC1 (10 mg/kg IM BID or TID) is frequently recommended; however, the short plasma half-life of meperidine

Table 7-6. Causes of Peritonitis

Chemical
  Uroperitoneum—rupture of urethra, bladder, and ureter secondary to trauma, catheterization, or urolithiasis
  Bile peritonitis—biliary rupture secondary to trauma, cholangitis, cholelithiasis, neoplasia
  Pancreatitis
  Rupture of the stomach—secondary to penetrating ulcers, neoplasia, trauma, gastric dilatation-volvulus syndrome
Septic
  Ruptured bowel—secondary to trauma, foreign body, ischemic necrosis (volvulus, thrombosis, intussusception), neoplasia
  Penetrating wounds of the abdominal wall
  Urogenital infections—pyometra, prostatic abscess
  Liver abscess
  Surgical contamination
  Complication of peritoneal dialysis
Combination
  Trauma
  Chemical peritonitis with secondary infection

HCl in the dog may decrease its usefulness.[32] Morphine, a potent analgesic in the dog, may be contraindicated as it increases the tone of pancreatic sphincters, thus potentially augmenting stasis of pancreatic secretions.[32]

Early recognition and appropriate treatment of acute pancreatitis are helpful in preventing complications such as septic peritonitis, pancreatic abscesses, endotoxic or hypovolemic shock, and DIC. Measures such as weight reduction and dietary management are useful for preventing further recurrences of pancreatitis and the long-term complications of diabetes mellitus and exocrine pancreatic insufficiency.

PERITONITIS

Etiology

Peritonitis can be classified as primary or secondary and as local or diffuse.[17,21] Feline infectious peritonitis is the only important example of primary peritonitis in animals; however, it is a chronic disease that is unlikely to present as an emergency and thus is not considered here. Secondary peritonitis due to bacterial infection or chemical irritation is an important cause of life-threatening emergency in clinical practice. The causes of chemical and bacterial peritonitis are listed in Table 7-6.[17,21] Chemical peritonitis is often sterile and is frequently secondary to intraabdominal leakage of urine or bile, inflammation of the pancreas, or rupture of the stomach. An accurate diagnosis of chemical peritonitis can usually be made by abdominocentesis, radiography, and clinical laboratory tests. Septic peritonitis, which is always considered a surgical emergency, may be a consequence of ruptured bowel, extension of urogenital infection, or penetrating injury to the abdomen. In septic peritonitis the source of contamination is often not determined until an exploratory operation has been performed. Combinations of chemical and septic peritonitis may result from extensive abdominal trauma or from chemical injury to the bowel, which permits translocation of enteric organisms into the peritoneal cavity.

Pathogenesis

The cause and extent of peritonitis influence both therapy and outcome. Whereas the initial pathophysiological alterations are similar for both chemical and septic peritonitis, infection leads to more profound systemic effects and to septic shock.[21]

The focal nature of some cases of peritonitis favors successful walling off via the inflammatory process.[17,21] Such situations may be manifested clinically by vague abdominal pain, mild splinting, local ileus, and a systemic response, e.g., mild fever and neutrophilia. These are simply the host responses to peritoneal injury and can be accounted for by inflammation. When local inflammation cannot be contained, diffuse peritonitis may result. Regardless of the etiology, diffuse peritonitis causes a significant flux of fluid, protein, and electrolytes into the abdominal space and may result in volume contraction, splanchnic pooling of blood, and ileus. Additional features of septic peritonitis are endotoxic shock, hypoglycemia, bacteremia, and release of myocardial depressant factors.[21] Offending organisms are most likely to be coliforms, nonhemolytic *Streptococcus, Staphylococcus, Clostridium*, and other anaerobes.[17]

Diagnosis

The clinical diagnosis of diffuse peritonitis is often suspected initially from the signs: depression, lethargy, vomiting, ascites, abdominal pain, fever, and ileus. However, these findings are not observed in all patients inasmuch as focal or chemical peritonitis may not lead to fever or detectable ascites. The history can be revealing, particularly when abdominal trauma has been observed or when abdominal surgery has recently been performed. Other clinical and laboratory findings depend on the cause of the peritonitis (Table 7-6). For example, leukocytosis is compatible with inflammation; hyperamylasemia may indicate pancreatitis; and azotemia, hyperkalemia, and hyponatremia may be associated with rupture of the urinary bladder. Radiographs may demonstrate focal or generalized increases in abdominal fluid density, loss of visceral detail, ileus, free abdominal gas, or other organ-associated abnormalities.[17] Contrast radiography may be necessary to identify leakage from the gastrointestinal or urinary tracts; however, cholangiography is unreliable in diagnosing biliary rupture.[43] When rupture is suspected, iodides are used instead of barium sulfate for contrast studies of the gastrointestinal (GI) tract.

Once the diagnosis of peritonitis is suggested by the history, physical examination, and survey abdominal radiographs, confirmation depends on analysis of abdominal fluid obtained by abdominocentesis.[17] The fluid is evaluated by gross inspection, cell count, cytology, biochemical analysis, and bacterial culture. When infection is present, the effusion is cloudy and characterized cytologically by an increased number of degenerate neutrophils and both extra-

and intracellular bacteria. Bile peritonitis is characterized grossly by a dark green fluid that has a higher total bilirubin level than serum, with microscopic evidence of phagocytized bile and acute inflammation.[4] Rarely, bile leakage from a ruptured intestine can be confused with a biliary tear with secondary infection. When fluid concentration of creatinine exceeds that of the serum, urinary rupture is indicated. Similarly, a disproportionately high fluid concentration of amylase suggests pancreatitis.

Treatment

Effective clinical management of peritonitis is predicated on an accurate diagnosis of the inciting cause. In many instances, definitive treatment requires surgical correction of a leaking organ or lavage and drainage of the abdominal cavity. However, immediate surgery is not always necessary or advisable. For example, when bile peritonitis or uroperitoneum is diagnosed, correction of the metabolic consequences of these disorders should be initiated prior to surgical exploration. Conversely, acute leakage of intestinal contents or rupture of a pyometra are surgical emergencies in which medical therapy is initiated simultaneously with preparations for immediate abdominal surgery. It is beyond the scope of this chapter to discuss surgical techniques for organ repair or intermittent peritoneal lavage. The reader is referred to standard surgical texts for this information.

Medical treatment of peritonitis is aimed at control of sepsis and correction of metabolic imbalances before, during, and after surgery. In certain instances, medical therapy alone may be adequate, as with focal peritonitis, pancreatitis, or peritonitis secondary to peritoneal dialysis. Control of sepsis is essential as bacterial peritonitis can lead to endotoxic shock and rapid deterioration. Therefore intravenous antibiotic therapy, e.g., sodium penicillin, sodium ampicillin, or cephalothin, is initiated before obtaining the results of culture and sensitivity testing.[17] Effectiveness against anaerobic bacteria is an important consideration. Under severe life-threatening circumstances, gentamicin is used in combination with these antibiotics to enhance the broad-spectrum activity against gram-negative organisms. The initial selection of an appropriate antibiotic may be assisted by information obtained from a gram stain of bacteria present in abdominal fluid; however, the regimen is adjusted according to the results of culture and sensitivity tests as well as the patient's response to treatment.

The metabolic consequences of peritonitis include hypovolemia, acidosis, electrolyte imbalances, and endotoxic shock.[17,21] The greatest potential for these imbalances to occur is when peritonitis is diffuse and accompanied by bacterial infection. Intravenous fluid therapy is initiated using a balanced electrolyte solution, e.g., lactated Ringer's solution. Hypoglycemia, a complication of endotoxemia, is prevented by adding dextrose to the fluids as needed in a concentration of 2.5–5%. If hypoproteinemia is present, a plasma transfusion may be useful. Principles of fluid therapy and treatment of acid-base abnormalities are discussed in Chapter 4 and should be consulted for details. When uroperitoneum is the cause of peritonitis, complications of renal failure require additional therapeutic considerations (Ch. 6). The treatment of pancreatitis has been discussed previously in this chapter.

Complications

Complications of peritonitis include endotoxic shock, ileus, chronic peritonitis, and abscess and adhesion formation.[17] The clinical signs, diagnosis, and treatment of endotoxic shock are discussed in detail in Chapter 13.

The pathogenesis of the adynamic ileus that develops as a consequence of peritonitis is poorly understood. However, the end result may be functional bowel obstruction and luminal sequestration of water and electrolytes. Specific therapy for ileus is unavailable. Consequently, clinical management is directed at treating the underlying cause of peritonitis and correcting fluid and electrolyte imbalances.

Chronic peritonitis and adhesion formation can result in intestinal obstruction and is manifested clinically by weight loss, vomiting, and anorexia.[17] Treatment of chronic peritonitis and abdominal abscesses frequently requires surgical débridement, abdominal lavage, and antibiotic therapy. Adhesion formation is difficult to prevent. However, corticosteroid therapy has been recommended to minimize primary adhesion formation.[17] It is generally agreed that breakdown of abdominal adhesions at surgery is frequently complicated by further adhesion formation; thus the prognosis is poor when widespread abdominal adhesions are present.

ABDOMINAL TRAUMA

Abdominal trauma is a frequently encountered problem in small animal practice.[8,19] Although results of physical examination, abdominal radiography, and laboratory testing may suggest severe intraabdominal injury, definitive diagnosis and treatment usually require surgical intervention. Nonetheless, appropriate and timely medical management during the preoperative period is vital to a successful outcome. Surgical aspects of the diagnosis and treatment of abdominal trauma will be detailed in an upcoming volume of this series. The present discussion focuses on the diagnosis and medical therapy of traumatized abdominal organs excluding the urogenital system, which is covered in detail in Chapter 6.

Etiology

Blunt trauma to the abdominal cavity is caused by motor vehicles, kicks, and falls from heights.[8,19] These types of injury can cause contusions, lacerations, avulsions, or rupture of abdominal structures. External evidence of abdominal injury may be minimal or absent, thus permitting those potentially life-threatening injuries to be initially overshadowed by more obvious cardiovascular, respiratory, neurologic, and musculoskeletal injuries.

Penetrating injuries are caused by weapons, bite wounds, and occasionally procedures such as percutaneous needle liver biopsy. Potential injury of the abdominal cavity is usually detected by a thorough physical examination; however, the external appearance of the penetration site does not necessarily reflect the extent of the internal injuries. Low-velocity penetrating injuries caused by sticks, knives, shotgun pellets, pistols, and airguns may produce minimal damage to nearby tissues, whereas rifle bullets fired at high velocity often result in extensive, widespread tissue damage.[8] Severe crushing injuries of the abdomen may accompany puncture wounds in cases of dog bite trauma.

Pathophysiology

The clinical sequelae to abdominal trauma can be attributed to: (1) acute hemorrhage; (2) peritonitis; and (3) organ dysfunction.[19] Severe, profuse intraabdominal bleeding can be accompanied by abdominal pain, acute hypovolemia, and shock. The most frequent source of massive intraabdominal hemorrhage is stellate or multiple fissure fractures of the liver.[19] However, injury to the spleen, kidneys, or large intraabdominal vessels can also produce extensive bleeding. When a history of trauma cannot be elicited from the owner and hemoperitoneum is diagnosed, other considerations for bleeding include coagulopathies, ruptured neoplasms (especially splenic hemangiosarcoma), ruptured omental cysts, vascular thrombosis, gastric dilatation-volvulus, splenic torsion, and erosion of the caudal vena cava by a pheochromocytoma. Rupture of gastric and duodenal ulcers can also cause hemoperitoneum and shock.

Peritonitis is a more insidious manifestation of abdominal trauma than hemorrhage, but it is devastating nonetheless.[8,19] Leakage of organ contents caused by lacerations, ruptures, or ischemic necrosis can lead to a chemical or bacterial peritonitis. Rupture of the small intestine and colon are associated with gross bacterial contamination of peritoneal surfaces, whereas urinary, biliary, gastric, and pancreatic secretions are chemical irritants that may predispose to secondary bacterial peritonitis. When bacteria cause peritonitis, clinical signs are fulminant and patients exhibit depression, anorexia, vomiting, fever or hypothermia, abdominal tenderness, splinting, fluid accumulation, and septic shock. On the other hand, extrahepatic biliary rupture may be inapparent for several days after the traumatic injury.[4,43] It is not uncommon to observe gradual progressive accumulation of abdominal fluid for weeks following a biliary tear. Inasmuch as bile is irritating to membranes, a sterile chemical peritonitis results. Secondary bacterial infection is possible, however, and should be considered in patients showing evidence of septic shock. Uroperitoneum due to urinary tract rupture is a relatively common cause of posttraumatic abdominal fluid accumulation (Ch. 6). Occasionally, dogs with ischemic necrosis or rupture of the small intestine appear normal during the first few days after trauma, with signs of peritonitis being delayed for as long as 1 week.[43]

Diagnosis

Trauma may or may not be observed by the owner. A thorough description of a traumatic event is of obvious importance in the initial assessment of the patient. In addition, the owner is questioned regarding blood in the stool or urine, micturition following injury, or rapid deterioration of clinical status. However, an extensive history is postponed until emergency measures to control life-threatening shock, hemorrhage, and thoracic injury have been instituted, as discussed elsewhere in this volume.

Abdominal wounds, entrance and exit lesions, abrasions, umbilical hemorrhage, and tire marks on the skin are suggestive of intraabdominal injury. Ballottement is employed to detect fluid, auscultation is used to assess the presence or absence of intestinal sounds, and systematic but gentle palpation is performed to assess the position, size, and integrity of each major abdominal organ. When initial examination findings are equivocal, serial evaluations are performed to detect developing signs of intraabdominal injury.

Abdominal radiographs may substantiate the presence of intraabdominal injuries by demonstrating free fluid, free gas, or alteration in the position and size of a major abdominal organ. Generalized loss of abdominal contrast indicates accumulation of peritoneal fluid. Hemorrhage cannot be differentiated radiographically from uroperitoneum or from peritonitis; this distinction requires further evaluation by abdominocentesis. Free abdominal air may be caused by rupture of the gastrointestinal tract, contamination with gas-producing organisms, or penetration of the abdominal wall. Contrast radiography can be useful to confirm leakage from the urinary or gastrointestinal tract.

Abdominocentesis may be used to detect intraabdominal trauma.[4,8,19] Use of a peritoneal dialysis catheter is preferable to a needle because of the larger diameter and number of side holes. In cases where peritonitis is suspected and no fluid is obtained, peritoneal lavage with saline 20 ml/kg may provide diagnostic information. Techniques for peritoneal lavage have been described elsewhere.[8,18] Results of abdominal paracentesis may distinguish different types of abdominal injury. For example, hemorrhage as occurs with hepatic or splenic rupture, is typically a bloody fluid with a packed cell volume (PCV) and white blood cell (WBC) count similar to that in peripheral blood. Characteristics of abdominal fluid in peritonitis are discussed in the previous section.

During the early posttraumatic period, laboratory testing may contribute very little to the diagnosis of abdominal trauma. With severe hemorrhage, a drop in the PCV and total protein occurs, especially after fluid therapy. However, the lowest values may not be detected until 12–24 hr later. With the development of peritonitis, a neutrophilia and left shift may be detected in the peripheral blood. In bacterial peritonitis with septic shock, neutropenia can be seen when sequestration of leukocytes in the abdominal cavity surpasses the bone marrow capacity for cell production.[17]

Biliary rupture causes conjugated hyperbilirubinemia and mild to moderate increases in serum alkaline phosphatase and glutamic pyruvic transaminase (SGPT) activity.[4,19,43] Bilirubinuria is also common and merely reflects the presence of conjugated hyperbilirubinemia. Acholic feces and absence of urine urobilinogen suggest a failure of bile pigments to enter the gut but also may be seen with biliary obstruction. The key to distinguishing complete common bile duct rupture from biliary obstruction is to identify the extravasation of bile into the peritoneal cavity that results from a biliary tear. However, diseases causing biliary obstruction, e.g., cholelithiasis, cholangitis, and biliary neoplasia, occasionally lead to secondary rupture of the extrahepatic biliary system.[4] In any event, surgical exploration is required for definitive diagnosis and treatment.

Other biochemical abnormalities are dependent on the individual organs sustaining damage from trauma. For example, increased serum amylase and lipase activity indicate pancreatic damage and leakage of enzymes, whereas detection of increased serum alkaline phosphatase and SGPT activity suggest hepatobiliary injury. The hematologic and biochemical sequelae of a ruptured urinary tract have important diagnostic and therapeutic relevance and are summarized in Chapter 6.

Treatment

The medical management of acute abdominal hemorrhage induced by trauma is directed toward treatment of the life-threatening complications of acute blood loss: hypovolemia and shock. Thus the primary goal is to establish an effective circulating blood volume by administering a whole blood transfusion or intravenous crystalloid fluids, e.g., lactated Ringer's solution. Additional measures to combat hypovolemic shock include the administration of glucocorticoids, sodium bicarbonate, and antibiotics. Specific recommendations for shock therapy are detailed in Chapter 2. Central venous pressure, capillary refill time, oral mucous membrane color, heart rate, femoral pulse quality, and urine output can be monitored to determine patient response to therapy. Even patients with continuous abdominal hemorrhage usually show initial improvement when given shock doses of intravenous fluids. However, when fluid therapy is decreased to maintenance rates, these patients relapse with deterioration of clinical parameters. A blood transfusion should be considered when the PCV is less than 25% and the plasma protein less than 3.5 mg/dl. If the patient cannot be stabilized by these means or there is continued loss of blood, immediate abdominal surgery is indicated to locate and arrest the source of bleeding. Abdominal pressure wraps may be helpful, but they must not be relied on for serious abdominal hemorrhage.[8] In certain situations where abdominal hemorrhage is acute and massive, survival of the animal may be accomplished only with immediate abdominal exploration.

When physical examination, abdominocentesis, and abdominal radiographs suggest the presence of septic peritonitis, abdominal surgery must not be delayed. The medical management of septic and chemical peritonitis has been discussed previously.

Complications

Complications of trauma-induced septic peritonitis include endotoxic shock, ileus, chronic peritonitis, and adhesions.[8,17,43] Occasionally, trauma causes disruption of the blood supply to an organ (i.e., intestine) or severe maceration and devitalization of tissue (i.e., liver), and the full extent of the damage is not evident for several days. In time, necrosis and abscessation develop, producing peritonitis. As mentioned previously, biliary rupture may be overlooked for days or weeks. Thus the veterinarian must be aware that even close observation of a traumatized animal for 24 hr does not eliminate the possibility of a delayed complication. Effective education of and communication with the owner are of obvious importance.

GASTROINTESTINAL EMERGENCIES

Vomiting

Dogs and cats are frequently presented to the emergency service for treatment of vomiting. Because vomiting is a clinical sign rather than a diagnosis, the historical, physical, laboratory, and radiographic findings must be correlated to determine the underlying etiology. Causes of vomiting range from nonspecific self-limiting gastroenteritis to severe life-threatening acute intestinal obstruction. Thus appropriate management of the vomiting patient necessitates identification and treatment of the underlying problem. Moreover, as severe, profuse emesis can lead to serious metabolic disturbances, timely symptomatic and supportive medical therapy is also crucial.

Etiology and Pathophysiology. Vomiting is associated with numerous metabolic, infectious, inflammatory, mechanical, and toxin-induced disorders (Table 7-7).[9,41] It is beyond the scope of this chapter to discuss in detail the pertinent clinical data associated with each disease; however, many of these disorders are covered in other sections of this book.

Vomiting is a reflex that results in expulsion of gastric contents through the oral cavity.[9,41] Neural integration of this reflex occurs in the vomiting center of the medulla oblongata. Afferent stimuli to the vomiting center originate from three different sources: (1) the cerebral cortex; (2) the chemoreceptor trigger zone (CRTZ); and (3) the peritoneum and abdominal viscera. Knowledge of the mechanisms of vomiting has clinical application, inasmuch as antiemetic drugs act in different ways on the vomiting reflex and are effective under different circumstances. The properties of antiemetic drugs are discussed further in the "Treatment" section.

Whereas infrequent vomiting causes few metabolic consequences, profuse emesis is associated with electrolyte depletion, acid-base imbalance, and dehydration. Protracted vomiting most often produces hyponatremia, hypokalemia, and hypochloremic metabolic alkalosis.[9] Although loss of water, electrolytes, and hydrogen in the vomitus contributes to these imbalances, compensatory renal mechanisms potentiate loss of potassium in the urine and

Table 7-7. Etiology of Vomiting and Basis for Diagnosis

Disorder	Diagnosis
Infectious diseases	
Feline panleukopenia	History, CBC
Canine parvovirus	CBC, fecal HA
Canine distemper	History, PE, conjunctival scrapings, CBC
Leptospirosis	BUN, UA, SGPT, SAP, lepto titer, darkfield microscopy of urine
Salmonellosis	Fecal culture
Infectious canine hepatitis	SGPT, SAP, liver biopsy
Inflammatory diseases	
Pyometra	PE, rads, CBC
Prostatitis	PE, rads, CBC
Peritonitis	PE, rads, abdominocentesis
Gastric ulcers	History, rads, endoscopy
Pancreatitis	Amylase, lipase, rads, CBC
Gastroenteritis	CBC, rads, fecal assimilation tests, fecal flotation, biopsy
Mechanical obstruction	
Intestinal FB, volvulus, intussusception, neoplasia	Rads
GDV	Rads
Pyloric stenosis	Rads
Metabolic diseases	
Renal failure	BUN, creatinine, K^+, UA, rads
Hypoadrenocorticism	Na^+, K^+, cortisol levels
Liver disease	SGPT, SAP, bilirubin, BSP, UA, rads, biopsy
Diabetic ketoacidosis	Glucose, UA
Toxins and drugs	
Heavy metals, pesticides, solvents	History
Digitalis, salicylates, mebendazole, D-penicillamine, chloramphenicol, erythromycin, antineoplastic drugs	
Others	
Miscellaneous	
CNS disease	History, neurologic examination
HGE	History, PE, CBC
Hairballs	

(CBC) complete blood count. (HA) hemagglutination. (PE) physical examination. (BUN) blood urea nitrogen. (UA) urinalysis. (SGPT) serum glutamic pyruvic transaminase. (SAP) serum alkaline phosphatase. (rads) radiographs. (GDV) gastric dilatation-volvulus. (BSP) 30 min sulfobromophthalein retention. (HGE) hemorrhagic gastroenteritis.

perpetuate metabolic alkalosis (for further details see Ch. 4). Occasionally metabolic acidosis, rather than alkalosis, is a consequence of vomiting, particularly when the vomitus contains large volumes of bicarbonate-rich fluid from the proximal small intestine.[44] Also, the primary cause of emesis may contribute to metabolic acidosis, i.e., ketoacidotic diabetes and renal failure. Thus serum electrolyte determination and blood gas analysis are performed, when possible, before initiating therapy.

Diagnosis. When vomiting is the primary presenting sign, a complete history and physical examination are first performed to assess the potential causes and evaluate the gravity of the situation. The history elicits the frequency and duration of vomiting, a description of the vomitus, diet modifi-

Table 7-8. Antiemetic Drug Therapy

Product	Dose	
	Dog	Cat
Phenothiazine derivatives		
Chlorpromazine (Thorazine)	3.3 mg/kg PO s.i.d.–q.i.d.	Same
	0.55–1.1 mg/kg IV, IM s.i.d.–q.i.d.	Same
Prochlorperazine (Compazine)	1.0 mg/kg IM, IV	Same
Promethazine (Phenergan)	0.2–1.0 mg/kg PO, SC b.i.d.–t.i.d.	None
Antihistamines		
Diphenhydramine (Benadryl)	2–4 mg/kg PO t.i.d.	Same
	5–50 mg IM, IV b.i.d.	
Dimenhydrinate (Dramamine)	25–50 mg PO t.i.d.	12.5 mg PO t.i.d.
Anticholingergics		
Atropine	0.05 mg/kg IV, IM, SC q.i.d.	Same
Glycopyrrolate	0.01 mg/kg IM, SC	None
Others		
Prochlorperazine,	0.14–0.22 ml/kg SC b.i.d.	Same
isopropamide (Darbazine)	2–7 kg: 1 #1 capsule PO b.i.d.	None
	7–14 kg: 1–2 #1 capsules PO b.i.d.	
	Over 14 kg: 1 #3 capsule PO b.i.d.	
Metoclopramide (Reglan)	0.2–0.5 mg/kg PO, SC, IV t.i.d.– q.i.d.	Same

cations, previous illnesses, vaccination and deworming status, presence of systemic signs, and exposure to drugs, toxins, or potential foreign bodies. Vomiting must be clinically differentiated from regurgitation. A thorough physical examination is performed, emphasizing gentle but meticulous abdominal palpation. Clinical findings that are suggestive of potentially serious underlying disease include profuse vomiting, hematemesis, weakness, severe depression, anorexia, palpation of an abdominal mass, fever, abdominal pain, abdominal distention, dehydration, and shock. When these abnormalities are detected, it is particularly important to evaluate the animal further with laboratory tests and radiographs (as specified in Table 7-7) in order to identify specific disorders and their metabolic complications. It is imperative that diseases requiring immediate medical or surgical therapy, e.g., severe gastroenteritis or intestinal obstruction, are recognized and treated without delay. Determination of serum electrolyte concentrations and blood gas parameters are useful to detect and monitor metabolic imbalances incurred by frequent or persistent emesis.

When the history and physical examination of an acutely vomiting patient are unremarkable, further diagnostic evaluation may be postponed, pending response to symptomatic and supportive therapy.

Treatment. Symptomatic and supportive treatment of the patient with profuse vomiting is directed toward pharmacologic control of emesis and correction of metabolic imbalances and hypovolemia.

Vomiting can be controlled by administering drugs with antiemetic properties (Table 7-8).[6,9,41] Phenothiazine derivatives are most effective because they inhibit the vomiting center, which is the final common pathway of the vomiting reflex.[41] However, these drugs are also peripheral α-adrenergic agents, and hence hypotension can be a complication of their usage. Phenothiazine derivatives are effective antiemetics at a lower dose than that required for tranquilization. Examples include chlorpromazine, prochlorperazine, and promethazine. Antihistamines can block vomiting that is stimulated through the CRTZ, as occurs with vestibular disease, uremic toxins, and digitalis administration. Anticholinergic drugs, e.g., atropine and isopropamide, are peripheral antiemetics and effective only when vomiting is stimulated by cholinergic-induced enteric smooth muscle spasms. As this is infrequently the primary stimulus for vomiting, the antiemetic action of the combination drug Darbazine (isopropamide and prochlorperazine) is primarily attributed to the phenothiazine component. Metoclopramide, a recently marketed gastrointestinal promotility agent, also possesses central (CRTZ) and peripheral antiemetic properties.[6] Inasmuch as vomiting frequently precludes oral administration of antiemetic drugs, parenteral therapy is recommended.

When frequent emesis occurs, food is withheld for at least 24 hr. If the patient is to be treated on an outpatient basis, the owners are instructed to offer small amounts of water or ice cubes frequently throughout the day. If emesis resolves, a bland low-fat diet (e.g., i/d, r/d, or lean meat and cooked rice) is offered in small amounts. After 1–2 days, the regular diet is gradually substituted for the bland food. When adequate hydration cannot be maintained by the oral route or if dehydration is detected on the initial physical examination, fluid therapy is indicated.

Mild dehydration, in the absence of other systemic signs, is best treated with hypodermoclysis. Intravenous fluid therapy is preferred for moderate to severe dehydration or for hypovolemia. Daily fluid requirements are dependent on the degree of dehydration, ongoing fluid losses, and maintenance needs, and are discussed in detail in Chapter 4. The fluid of choice for the patient with profuse vomiting is 0.9% NaCl; however, when electrolyte and acid-base status are unknown, a balanced electrolyte solution, e.g., Ringer's solution, is satisfactory. Hypokalemia, a frequent complication of persistent vomiting, must be anticipated. Thus the serum potassium is monitored daily, and fluids are supplemented with potassium chloride according to guidelines in Chapter 4. When hypovolemia and hypokalemia are effectively treated, metabolic alkalosis usually resolves spontaneously. Metabolic acidosis is treated with fluids containing lactate or sodium bicarbonate, as described in Chapter 4.

Protectorants and adsorbents, e.g., kaolin and pectin (Kaopectate) 1–2 ml/kg PO QID and bismuth subsalicylate (Pepto-Bismol) 10–30 ml QID, are administered to patients when vomiting is attributed to gastroenteritis. However, the efficacy of these products is questionable, and they may provoke further emesis.

Vomiting that persists longer than 48–72 hr despite appropriate symptomatic therapy indicates a need for further diagnostic studies to identify the underlying problem (Table 7-7).

Acute Diarrhea

Diarrhea is an increased frequency, fluidity, or volume of feces. Acute diarrhea, a common clinical problem, can be caused by both intestinal and systemic disorders. Enteric diseases that cause acute diarrhea can be mild and self-limiting (as with dietary indiscretion) or severe and life-threatening (as with parvoviral enteritis, hemorrhagic gastroenteritis, ancylostomiasis in neonates, and intestinal obstruction). Patients with extraintestinal disease, e.g., hypoadrenocorticism, renal failure, and liver disease, frequently exhibit diarrhea in addition to other systemic signs. Therefore appropriate clinical management of patients with acute diarrhea entails identification and correction of the underlying etiologies and symptomatic and supportive treatment to control fluid and electrolyte loss and septicemia.

Etiology and Pathophysiology.   The causes of acute diarrhea are varied and include infectious and parasitic diseases, toxicosis, metabolic derangements, and mechanical disorders (Table 7-9).[35]

Despite the large number of diagnostic considerations, some general principles of diagnosis are important to review. Puppies are likely to be affected by nematodes, sudden changes in diet, lactose (milk) intolerance, viral enteritis, ingestion of spoiled foods and foreign bodies, intestinal intussusception, and bacterial enteritis. Neoplasia, metabolic disease, and inflammatory bowel diseases are additional considerations in mature animals. The following discussion centers on severe diarrhea of acute onset; however, the clinician must be aware that many chronic bowel disorders are also characterized by intermittent exacerbations of profuse diarrhea.

There are four important mechanisms invoked to explain the pathogenesis of diarrhea: osmotic diarrhea, intestinal hypersecretion, exudation, and hypermotility.[35] All result in increases in intestinal water content. Of these, hypermotility is least likely to be a primary cause of diarrhea; however, it may occur secondary to increased volume within the intestinal lumen. Bacterial enterotoxins may induce hypersecretion, and microorganisms may directly invade the intestine causing an exudative process. Osmotic diarrhea is common, as evidenced by the problems of lactose intolerance and malabsorption secondary to parvovirus infection. These abnormalities are described in detail elsewhere.[35]

The clinician must be cognizant of serious systemic and metabolic consequences of acute diarrhea and intestinal injury. Endotoxic shock may lead to hypoglycemia, leukopenia, and vascular collapse. Significant hypoproteinemia can also occur owing to inflammation and exudation in the intestine. Moreover, these hematologic changes are often accompanied by electrolyte disorders and hemoconcentration resulting from isotonic fluid loss in the gut. Acute diarrhea represents a loss of fluid into the intestinal lumen accompanied by relatively large amounts of bicarbonate, sodium, chloride, and potassium.[44] Volume contraction and metabolic acidosis are anticipated derangements, although the acid-base picture may be altered by concurrent emesis. Thus serum biochemical determinations are valuable in guiding the therapy of such patients, and fluids such as lactated Ringer's, possibly supplemented with dextrose, potassium chloride, and infusions of sodium bicarbonate, are usually required.

Diagnosis.   The diagnostic work-up is guided by the history, results of physical and rectal examinations, and the severity of clinical signs. Whereas elaborate function tests of digestion and absorption are not usually indicated

Table 7-9. Etiology of Acute Diarrhea

Disease	Basis for Diagnosis
Metazoan parasites	
Hookworms, ascarids, *Strongyloides* spp., whipworms	Fecal flotation
Protozoan parasites	
Giardia spp., *Trichomonas* spp., coccidia, *Balantidium coli, Entamoeba histolytica*	Fecal saline smears
Dietary indiscretion or intolerance	History, response to diet modification
Drug- or Toxin-induced	
Corticosteroids, aspirin, nonsteroidal antiinflammatory drugs, dithiazanine, Mg antacids, antiparasitic drugs, antineoplastic drugs	History
Heavy metals, insecticides, herbicides, fungicides	History
Viral	
Coronavirus	History, PE
Parvovirus	CBC, fecal HA
Canine distemper	History, PE, conjunctival scrapings, CBC
Infectious canine hepatitis	SGPT, SAP, liver biopsy
Bacterial	
Salmonella spp.	
Campylobacter jejuni	Fecal cultures
Yersinia enterocolitica	
Leptospira spp.	BUN, SGPT, SAP, lepto titer, darkfield microscopy of urine
Bacillus piliformis (Tyzzer's disease)	Intestinal biopsy
Clostridium spp.	
Enteropathogenic *E. coli*	Serotyping, inoculation studies
Rickettsia	
Neorickettsia helminthoeca (salmon poisoning)	Fecal sedimentation, cytology of lymph node aspirate
Metabolic diseases	
Renal failure	BUN, creatinine, UA, rads
Hypoadrenocorticism	Na^+, K^+, cortisol levels
Liver disease	SGPT, SAP, bilirubin, BSP, liver biopsy
Others	
HGE	History, PE, CBC
Intestinal obstruction	Rads

(PE) physical examination. (CBC) complete blood count. (HA) hemagglutination. (SGPT) serum glutamic pyruvic transaminase. (SAP) serum alkaline phosphatase. (BUN) blood urea nitrogen. (UA) urinalysis. (rads) radiographs. (BSP) 30 min sulfobromophthalein retention. (HGE) hemorrhagic gastroenteritis.

in acute diarrhea, a careful history is necessary to elicit the possibility of infectious disease or dietary indiscretion. If the physical examination fails to demonstrate hypothermia, fever, dehydration, marked abdominal pain, palpable intestinal mass lesion, or clinical signs of systemic involvement, simple tests (e.g., fecal flotation and saline smears) to rule out parasitism should suffice. Abdominal radiographs are indicated if a foreign body, intussusception, or peritonitis is suspected. A complete blood count, fecal hemagglutination (HA), and possibly stool cultures are appropriate in dogs exhibiting signs of infectious enteritis. Dogs with pallor may be shocky or simply anemic from hookworm infestation. Fetid, bloody, or jam-like stools are often found on rectal examination of dogs with parvovirus or hemorrhagic gastroenteritis (HGE). Severe depression, dehydration, or evidence of systemic infection warrant a data base including complete blood count (CBC), chemistry profile, fecal flotation, fecal cultures, and examination for leukocytes in feces. Other tests, e.g., a barium series for gastrointestinal obstruction or intussusception, are appropriate in selected cases (Table 7-9).

Treatment.   Most acute cases of diarrhea are self-limiting and resolve regardless of therapy. Often simply removing the inciting cause, as with a dietary, parasitic, or drug-induced diarrhea, is all that is necessary. Intestinal parasites are a common cause of diarrhea, and appropriate anthelmintics are administered as dictated by the results of fecal testing. Acute colitis in dogs is frequently caused by whipworms, although confirmation of trichuriasis can be complicated by the inconsistent passage of eggs in the feces. Thus empirical treatment of whipworms using mebendazole (Telminic), butamisole (Styquin), or fenbendazole, is considered when signs of colitis are present, even though multiple fecal flotations are negative. Ascariasis and ancylostomiasis are reliably diagnosed by detection of eggs on fecal flotation; however, routine deworming with pyrantel pamoate (Nemex) is considered in neonates with acute diarrhea and a questionable deworming history.

Systemic antibiotics are administered when pathogenic bacteria are cultured from the feces or when secondary bacterial infections occur, as with parvoviral enteritis or endotoxemia (e.g., HGE).[35] Indiscriminate use of antibiotics is discouraged as they can promote imbalances in normal gut flora. Selection of an appropriate antibiotic is ideally based on results of culture and sensitivity studies; however, general guidelines for treatment include the use of trimethoprim-sulfa, chloramphenicol, or gentamicin for salmonellosis; erythromycin for campylobacteriosis; tetracycline for salmon fluke poisoning (rickettsial infection); and broad-spectrum bactericidal antibiotics for parvoviral enteritis. *Clostridia* spp. has been suspected to play a role in the pathogenesis of hemorrhagic gastroenteritis, and so antibiotics with an anaerobic spectrum may be useful in treating this disease. Metronidazole, a drug with anaerobic activity, is used most frequently for treatment of protozoan infections, e.g., giardiasis.

Symptomatic therapy can be useful whether or not an inciting cause of diarrhea has been identified.[35] Dietary restriction for 12–24 hr is recommended to rest the gastrointestinal tract. This is followed by feeding small amounts of a bland, low-fat diet (e.g., i/d, r/d, boiled rice, lean meat, eggs, or yogurt). Antidiarrheal therapy, including opiates or anticholinergic drugs, can be used to alter motility. Opiates are more effective in treating diarrhea because they increase rhythmic segmentation, thus delaying bowel transit time. Anticholinergic drugs have a very different effect, as peristalsis is inhibited at the expense of segmentation, allowing a generalized reduction of motility that fails to inhibit intestinal flow. Many antidiarrheal preparations are available. Diphenoxylate (Lomotil) 1–5 mg TID is an example of an opiate that is frequently employed in symptomatic antidiarrheal therapy. Locally acting protectorants and adsorbents are commonly administered on an empirical basis. Examples include kaolin and pectin (Kaopectate 1–2 ml/kg QID), aluminum hydroxide (10–30 ml QID), and bismuth subsalicylate (Pepto-Bismol 10–30 ml QID). The effectiveness of bismuth subsalicylate therapy is also attributed to its antisecretory, antiprostaglandin, antienterotoxin, and antibacterial properties.

Imbalances of fluid, electrolyte, and acid-base homeostasis must be managed in patients with severe diarrhea as described in Chapter 4. Supportive fluid therapy is indicated when dehydration is detected on physical examination or when profuse diarrhea is likely to result in hypovolemia. The parenteral route of administration is usually preferable, and lactated Ringer's solution is the fluid of choice. However, when clinical signs are mild and vomiting is absent, oral glucose-electrolyte solutions (Pedialyte) can be effective, as glucose potentiates intestinal absorption of sodium and water.[35] Sodium bicarbonate is administered when acidosis is severe. If parvoviral enteritis is suspected, 50% dextrose is added to the electrolyte solution to make a 2.5–5% solution (25–50 ml/500 ml fluid). This reduces the risk of endotoxemic hypoglycemia. Potassium chloride supplementation is usually based on serum potassium concentrations.

When surgery is needed to treat problems such as foreign bodies and intussusceptions, laparotomy is performed after fluid, electrolyte, and acid-base deficits have been corrected.

Diarrhea associated with systemic disorders, e.g., renal failure or hypoadrenocorticism, is treated symptomatically while primary therapy is focused on correcting the underlying disorder.

Intestinal Obstruction

Intestinal obstruction can be caused by mechanical or functional disorders.[1,10,28,35] Mechanical obstruction of the bowel occurs much more frequently in veterinary medicine and is the focus of the following discussion. Functional obstruction due to paralytic ileus is quite uncommon as a primary problem.

It is commonly accepted that the severity of clinical signs and magnitude of metabolic imbalances in gastrointestinal obstruction are determined by the location, degree (partial versus complete), duration, and acuteness of obstruction.[7,20] Maintenance of mesenteric blood flow is more likely to influence the outcome than is the cause of the obstruction. The definitive treatment of mechanical obstruction is surgery. However, many of the life-threatening clinical manifestations of luminal obstruction are due to fluid, electrolyte, and acid-base disturbances; these should be partially corrected before the animal with intestinal obstruction is taken to surgery.

Etiology and Pathophysiology. Mechanical obstruction of the intestine is due to a wide variety of intraluminal, mural, or extraluminal factors (Table 7-10).[28,36] The etiology of intestinal obstruction may impact on the clinical picture. A sudden onset of clinical signs is expected with volvulus, intussusception, entrapment of bowel in a hernia, and foreign bodies located in the proximal intestine. A more chronic, insidious course is expected with neopla-

Table 7-10. Causes of Intestinal Obstruction

Mechanical ileus
  Foreign bodies
  Bezoars
  Enteroliths
  Fecal impactions
  Parasites
  Intussusception
  Volvulus
  Bowel incarceration (diaphragmatic, inguinal, mesenteric, and abdominal wall hernias)
  Stricture (traumatic or surgically induced)
  Intramural abscess, granuloma, or hematoma
  Neoplasia
  External bowel compression (mass, adhesions)
  Congenital defects (malformation, stenosis, atresia)
Functional ileus
  Paralytic ileus
    Peritonitis
    Spinal cord injury
    Hypokalemia
    Anticholinergic drug therapy
    Secondary to mechanical ileus
    Hypothyroidism
  Intestinal pseudoobstruction
  Mesenteric thrombosis and emboli
  Parvoviral enteritis[a]

[a] This etiology merits special mention owing to its common occurrence.

sia, inflammatory mural lesions, adhesions, strictures, and foreign bodies lodged distally in the intestine or incompletely obstructing the lumen.

The clinical signs and metabolic sequelae of gastrointestinal obstruction are attributable to the course of events that follow luminal occlusion and intestinal ischemia.[7,20] Distention of the bowel proximal to an obstruction is a consistent finding on barium radiography and at surgery. Dilation leads to inhibition of gut motility and accumulation of fluid within the lumen. This fluid accumulation is due to increased secretion and decreased resorption of water and electrolytes. In addition to the extracellular fluid and electrolytes that are sequestered in the gut, vomiting causes further loss and leads to dehydration, disturbed plasma pH, and abnormal electrolyte concentrations. Acid-base imbalance is principally dependent on the site of obstruction. With occlusion of the proximal duodenum, principally gastric juice is lost, leading to metabolic alkalosis. Obstruction distal to this site generally causes loss of sodium and bicarbonate, resulting in metabolic acidosis. The severity of the water and electrolyte loss is greater with more proximal lesions because the jejunum, the major site of fluid and electrolyte resorption, is short-circuited. This is not so with distal ileal or colonic obstructions.

Intestinal ischemia is the other major factor affecting patient survival.[7,20] The most common causes of acute bowel infarction are intussusception, volvulus, and incarceration of the bowel. However, with time, ischemia occurs in the proximal distended portion of bowel even with other types of simple luminal obstruction. In addition, pressure necrosis may occur adjacent to a lodged foreign body. Ischemia causes tissue hypoxia, gut edema, and eventual necrosis of the wall. Necrotic bowel may rupture, causing peritonitis or allowing enteric bacteria or toxins to escape. Ultimately, the sequelae of devitalized intestine are peritonitis, sepsis, endotoxemia, and shock.

Diagnosis. Intestinal obstruction is suspected based on the patient history and physical examination, and is confirmed by radiography. Clinical signs of intestinal obstruction are numerous, with vomiting, anorexia, and lethargy being most consistently present. Diarrhea, abdominal pain, abdominal distention, palpable distention of gut loops, and identification of an intestinal foreign body are all possible findings in intestinal obstruction. When complications of peritonitis, gut perforation, or endotoxemia are present, the clinician may detect fever, collapse, or signs of shock. In general, the more proximal and complete the obstruction, the more severe the clinical signs.[7,20] It must be emphasized that with distal or incomplete obstruction signs are often chronic, vague, and more referable to malnutrition.

Confirmation of GI obstruction is obtained by radiography.[28] Contrast studies may be required. The salient feature of intestinal obstruction is identification of dilated fluid- or gas-filled loops of small bowel. A radiopaque foreign body may be identified in some cases. Contrast studies show delayed transit time, luminal filling defects, and the level of obstruction. Occasionally there is a need to differentiate functional ileus from mechanical obstruction.[1,10,28] This is best achieved with contrast radiography (especially in dogs with parvoviral enteritis).[10] Frequently, one may not know the cause of obstruction, only that it is present. In such cases surgery is usually required for both definitive diagnosis and treatment.

Treatment. Fluid therapy is an essential adjunct to surgery and is best based on laboratory findings. If the blood is alkalotic, use of 0.9% sodium chloride solution and potassium chloride is preferred. If it is acidotic, lactated Ringer's solution or saline with sodium bicarbonate is used. Shock must be treated (Ch. 2), particularly if there is endotoxemia or peritonitis. Broad-spectrum antibiotics are indicated, as peritonitis, endotoxemia, and devitalization of the intestine are anticipated in most cases. Gentamicin (beware nephrotoxicity), ampicillin, and cephalothin are commonly prescribed. Metabolic and fluid deficits are corrected as quickly as possible (3–8 hr) so that surgery is not unduly delayed. Perforation, peritonitis, endotoxemia, and hypovolemic shock may be circumvented with prompt identification, fluid therapy, and early surgical correction.

Gastric Dilatation-Volvulus

Acute gastric dilatation-volvulus (GDV) in the dog is a medical and surgical emergency. This condition is associated with a high mortality rate due to hypovolemic, hypotensive, and neurogenic shock; acid-base and electrolyte imbalances, cardiac arrhythmias, endotoxemia, myocardial depression, and DIC.[23–25,45] Medical management is focused on early recognition of the prob-

lem, gastric decompression, treatment of shock, and control of cardiac arrhythmias.

Etiology and Pathophysiology.   The cause of GDV is unknown. It is most
common in large, deep-chested breeds of dogs.[25,45] Most studies show an increased incidence in mature dogs, and some suggest a male predilection. Factors most frequently implicated in the etiopathogenesis of GDV are overeating,
exercise, and excessive water drinking.[45] Less frequently identified risk factors
include parturition, trauma, vomiting, neoplasia, duodenal obstruction, adynamic ileus, and anesthesia.

Requirements for the development of gastric dilatation are the retention
of gas or fluid in the stomach and the existence of impaired mechanisms for
relieving their accumulation.[45] The source of gas is primarily swallowed air,
although it may be produced by bacterial fermentation, diffusion from the
blood, or chemical reaction of gastric HCl and bicarbonate. Abnormal swallowing of air may be an important factor, inasmuch as GDV is often related
to excitement, eating, and drinking. Mechanical factors that occur secondary
to dilation may prevent eructation or pyloric outflow, or it may be that neurogenic abnormalities are present. When the stomach is dilated, especially
chronically, disruption of ligamentous stability predisposes the animal to gastric
volvulus. This causes mechanical obstruction of both the esophagus and pylorus. Passive rotation of the spleen obstructs venous return and causes splenomegaly and ischemia of this organ.

There are several expected mechanical and physiological sequelae to
GDV.[23,45] The dilated stomach obstructs the caudal vena cava and portal vein,
leading to venous congestion and impaired venous return to the heart. The
resulting decline in cardiac output may also be influenced by neurogenic factors. Regardless, the end result is decreased arterial pressure, compromised
coronary blood flow, and hypovolemic shock. These hemodynamic abnormalities are heralded by tachycardia, weak femoral pulses, pale mucous membranes, slow capillary refill time, and oliguria.

The hemodymamic changes that accompany GDV affect many organs.[45]
Cardiac function is impaired owing to myocardial ischemia and circulating myocardial depressant factors that originate from ischemic pancreatic tissue.[26,45]
Arrhythmias, which are primarily ventricular in origin, i.e., premature ventricular depolarizations, paroxysmal ventricular tachycardia, and sustained
ventricular tachycardia, frequently occur as a result of autonomic imbalance,
electrolyte and acid-base disturbances, or myocardial ischemia.[25] The enlarging
stomach also impinges on the thoracic cavity, leading to hypoventilation. Decreased lung compliance and ventilation-perfusion mismatches have also been
reported. Clinically, one often observes a rapid respiratory rate, and less frequently respiratory acidosis is detected. Respiratory alkalosis may be caused
by pain or increased sympathetic tone, or as compensation for metabolic acidosis.[24] Ischemia of the stomach, pancreas, liver, and spleen occur secondary
to hypotension and impairment of blood flow in the celiac artery.[45] Pancreatic
ischemia is thought to cause release of myocardial depressant factors that are
capable of causing negative inotropy, splanchnic vasoconstriction, and retic-

uloendothelial cell depression. Endotoxemia and septic shock can be caused by compression of the portal vein. Elevations of intragastric pressure cause venous stasis and mural hypoxia, resulting in hemorrhage, edema, necrosis, and ulceration of the gastric mucosa.

The most consistently observed metabolic consequences of GDV are metabolic acidosis and hypokalemia.[24] Metabolic acidosis is caused by inadequate tissue perfusion, arterial hypoxemia, and lactic acid production from anaerobic metabolism. Hypokalemia results from sequestration of potassium chloride in gastric fluids and urinary losses due to aggressive fluid therapy. However, because other combinations of acid-base and electrolyte disturbances have been reported, generalizations can be misleading, thus effective therapy is best guided by laboratory evaluation of these parameters.[24]

Diagnosis.   The diagnosis of acute GDV is suspected from the characteristic historical information and from results of the physical examination. Nonproductive vomiting or retching and progressive abdominal enlargement are frequently observed by the owner. On physical examination the abdomen is tense, tympanic, and distended. Splenomegaly may also be detected. Hyperpnea is common. With deterioration of clinical status, signs of shock develop, including collapse, tachycardia, slowed capillary refill time, and weak femoral pulses.

The diagnosis of GDV is confirmed by radiography; however, films are taken only after emergency gastric decompression and shock therapy have been initiated. Survey abdominal radiographs suffice in most cases. Evidence of gastric volvulus is suggested by the combination of: (1) a large air or fluid distended stomach; (2) displacement of the pylorus to the left and dorsally; and (3) the presence of a tissue-dense line across the stomach indicating compartmentalization of this organ.[23] If the stomach has ruptured, free abdominal air may be detected. Contrast radiography is occasionally required to confirm malposition of the stomach, particularly in chronic GDV.

Treatment.   Initial emergency management of the patient with GDV is directed at relieving gastric distention and treating shock. Gastric decompression is attempted by passing a stomach tube. If resistance to passage occurs, the tube is gently rotated or the animal is moved to a position other than sternal recumbency. Chemical restraint is used cautiously in those animals who resent intubation, inasmuch as cardiovascular stability is precarious. Although phenothiazines may be dangerous tranquilizers in these patients, meperidine HCl (Demerol 0.5 mg/kg IM) has been suggested to be adequate for this purpose.[23] Successful intubation of the stomach does not eliminate the possibility of volvulus, and radiography is performed after the animal has been stabilized. Once the tube has been successfully passed, the stomach is emptied and then repeatedly lavaged with saline.

Intravenous fluid administration is initiated simultaneously with gastric decompression. Rapid infusion (80 ml/kg the first hour) of a balanced electrolyte solution, e.g., lactated Ringer's, is advocated while waiting for results of blood gas and electrolyte determinations. Additional therapy consisting of glucocorticoid and sodium bicarbonate administration may be necessary when shock is present. If the stomach tube cannot be passed, gastrocentesis is performed with an 18-gauge needle introduced on the left side, caudal to the ribs.[23] Temporary gastrotomy has also been recommended to allow time for correction of shock and metabolic imbalances before surgery.[23]

Supportive care prior to surgery consists of continuous intravenous fluid administration and monitoring of blood gases, central venous pressure, capillary refill time, and urine output. Arrhythmias may be observed during the preoperative period but are most frequent 12–36 hr after the initial presentation.[25] Antibiotics, e.g., chloramphenicol, penicillin, cephalothin, or kanamycin, are administered to prevent the complications of septic shock.[23] If endotoxemia is suspected, dextrose may be added to the fluids.

In most instances, surgery is performed expeditiously to reposition the stomach and spleen and to inspect the stomach for areas of necrosis and devitalization.[23] Prophylactic procedures, e.g., tube gastrostomy, gastropexy, and pyloromyotomy, are often performed concurrently to prevent recurrence of GDV. If surgery is to be delayed, the stomach must be kept decompressed, either by performing a temporary gastrostomy or by placing a pharyngostomy tube. The surgical management of GDV is described in the next volume in this series.

Complications of GDV include gastric necrosis and rupture, peritonitis, hemoperitoneum due to torn vessels, endotoxemia, DIC, arrhythmias, and hypokalemia.[23,24,45] However, early recognition of the disease and prompt medical and surgical treatment can result in a successful outcome for many animals with GDV.

SPLENIC EMERGENCIES

Splenic Torsion

Torsion of the splenic pedicle that is unassociated with GDV occurs rarely in dogs.[22,37,38] The etiology of splenic torsion is unknown. It has been hypothesized that partial gastric torsion causes malpositioning of the spleen.[22] When the stomach untwists, the spleen is thought to remain displaced. The observation that both GDV and splenic torsion are most common in large deep-chested dogs may support this theory.[22,37,38]

Diagnosis of splenic torsion can be difficult owing to the lack of specificity of clinical, laboratory, and radiographic findings.[38] The most consistent clinical signs are vomiting, anorexia, and depression.[22,37,38] Polydipsia, polyuria, and abdominal distention have also been noted.[37,38] These signs may be acute or chronic and may progress to collapse and shock. Splenomegaly is usually detected on abdominal palpation. The presence of abdominal pain, though, is inconsistent. Pallor of mucous membranes may be attributed to either hemolytic anemia or shock. Ventricular arrhythmias are occasionally auscultated.

Hemoglobinemia, hemoglobinuria, red blood cell fragments, and mild anemia suggest the presence of intravascular hemolysis.[38] This has been attributed to microangiopathic destruction or red blood cell membrane alterations that result from sequestration of cells in the ischemic spleen.[22,38] DIC may contribute to anemia in some cases and is suggested by the findings of thrombocytopenia, fibrin degradation products, and prolonged OSPT and APTT.[38] Other nonspecific laboratory abnormalities detected in dogs with splenic torsion are neutrophilia with a mild left shift, mildly increased alkaline phosphatase activity, proteinuria, and bilirubinuria.[22,37,38]

Although splenomegaly is usually detected on abdominal radiographs, they rarely confirm a diagnosis of splenic torsion.[38] Marked enlargement of the spleen with a significant increase in density may suggest the diagnosis of splenic torsion.[37] However, in most cases the radiographic distinction between torsion and other causes of splenomegaly cannot be made, and exploratory laparotomy is required to confirm the diagnosis.[38]

If signs of hemolytic anemia or shock are present, treatment is directed toward establishing an effective circulating blood volume by administering a whole blood transfusion or intravenous crystalloid fluids, e.g., lactated Ringer's solution. Ventricular arrhythmias are treated as described in Chapter 2. The surgical aspects of treatment of splenic torsion and splenectomy are discussed elsewhere.[38]

Splenic Rupture

Splenic rupture in the dog is most frequently caused by trauma or angiogenic tumors, e.g., hemangiosarcoma or hemangioma.[8,11,12] Traumatic splenic rupture and its metabolic consequences have been discussed previously in this chapter. The following discussion focuses on splenic hemangiosarcoma.

Etiology and Basis for Diagnosis. Splenic hemangiosarcoma (HSA) occurs most frequently in older dogs, with a median age of 9 years.[12] German shepherd dogs, and possibly males, seem to be at increased risk for this tumor.[11,12] Clinical signs include progressive lethargy, pallor, anorexia, and weight loss. A history of intermittent weakness or collapse that improves after 12–24 hr is common and suggests previous minor episodes of tumor hemorrhage into the abdominal cavity. Animals are often presented on an emergency basis for acute collapse or shock.

Characteristic findings on physical examination include abdominal distention, palpation of an abdominal mass (often quite large), and pallor of the mucous membranes.[11] If acute intraabdominal hemorrhage has resulted from rupture of the splenic hemangiosarcoma, abdominal fluid (blood) may be ballotted and signs of hypovolemic shock detected. Occasionally, concurrent metastatic HSA involves the right atrium, bone, skin, or other organs.[11] Additional physical findings might then include tachycardia, arrhythmias, or muffled heart sounds with cardiac involvement; bone pain or lameness with skeletal metastasis, or mass lesions in other areas of the body.

Abdominocentesis is performed if the presence of abdominal fluid is suspected. Typically, a serosanguineous, nonclotting fluid is obtained with ruptured HSA.[11] Cytologic evaluation of a buffy coat smear from abdominal fluid occasionally reveals exfoliated tumor cells.[11]

The characteristic hematologic finding associated with HSA is regenerative anemia with a disproportionate increase is nucleated red blood cells (RBCs).[11] Anemia may be caused by microangiopathic destruction, splenic sequestration and lysis, or hemorrhage. Increased numbers of nucleated RBCs has been attributed to bone marrow infiltration by malignant cells, extramedullary hematopoiesis, and hypoxia. Later, splenectomy may also contribute to this finding. Hypochromasia, target cells, acanthocytes, and a neutrophilic leukocytosis with a regenerative left shift have also been observed.[11]

Abdominal radiographs usually confirm the presence of a mass, but, its relationship to the spleen is not always obvious. Irregular splenomegaly may be the predominant finding. If free blood or widespread peritoneal metastases are present, intraabdominal contrast is poor. Thoracic radiographs are obtained in dogs with suspected splenic neoplasia. However, radiographic evidence of metastatic pulmonary HSA is infrequently detected because of the small, miliary nature of the metastases.[11]

Although the history, physical examination, hematologic tests, and radiographs are frequently suggestive of splenic HSA, definitive diagnosis requires exploratory laparotomy and splenic biopsy (usually splenectomy).[11,12] HSA without gross metastases can be difficult to differentiate grossly from nodular hyperplasia, hematoma, siderofibrosis, or hemangioma; thus clinical decisions for patient care must be based on results of histopathologic studies.[11] Hemangiosarcoma and hemangioma may be difficult to distinguish histologically, and the presence of gross abdominal metastases may be used to suggest HSA.[11] However, the presence of widespread microscopic metastases is common in HSA, despite gross evidence suggesting isolated splenic involvement.[11,12] Thus the diagnosis of this highly malignant tumor warrants a poor prognosis regardless of the extent of gross involvement.

Treatment.   Animals presented for acute collapse and hypovolemic shock caused by ruptured splenic HSA constitute a life-threatening emergency. Fluid therapy is initiated at shock doses with a balanced electrolyte solution, e.g., lactated Ringer's. Frequently, a blood transfusion is necessary. Electrolyte and acid-base disturbances are detected and treated in anticipation of anesthesia and surgery. Immediate surgical exploration and splenectomy are required when evidence of ongoing blood loss from a ruptured splenic mass is detected. Splenectomy controls the blood loss unless DIC, a common complication, is present. However, the long-term prognosis is poor because of the highly malignant nature of this neoplasm.[11] The effectiveness of chemotherapy in controlling this tumor has not yet been established.

REFERENCES

1. Arrick RH, Kleine LJ: Intestinal pseudoobstruction in a dog. J Am Vet Med Assoc 172:1201, 1978
2. Badylak SF, Dodds WJ, Van Vleet JF: Plasma coagulation factor abnormalities in dogs with naturally occurring hepatic disease. Am J Vet Res 44:2336, 1983

3. Badylak SF, Van Vleet JF: Alterations of prothrombin time and activated partial thromboplastin time in dogs with hepatic disease. Am J Vet Res 42:2053, 1981

4. Blass CE: Surgery of the extrahepatic biliary tract. Compend Contin Educ 5:801, 1983

5. Bunch SE, Castleman WL, Hornbuckle WE, et al: Hepatic cirrhosis associated with long-term anticonvulsant drug therapy in dogs. J Am Vet Med Assoc 181:357, 1982

6. Burrows CF: Metoclopramide. J Am Vet Med Assoc 183:1341, 1982

7. Chambers JN: Diseases of the intestines. In Bojrab MJ (ed): Pathophysiology in Small Animal Surgery. p. 112. Lea & Febiger, Philadelphia, 1981

8. Crane SW: Evaluation and management of abdominal trauma in the dog and cat. Vet Clin North Am 10:655, 1980

9. DiBartola SP: Gastrointestinal problems. In Fenner WR (ed): Quick Reference to Veterinary Medicine. p. 65. Lippincott, Philadelphia, 1982

10. Farrow CS: Radiographic appearance of canine parvovirus enteritis. J Am Vet Med Assoc 180:43, 1982

11. Fees DL , Withrow SJ: Canine hemangiosarcoma. Compend Contin Educ 3:1047, 1981

12. Frey AJ, Betts CW: A retrospective survey of splenectomy in the dog. J Am Anim Hosp Assoc 13:730, 1977

13. Hansen JF, Carpenter RH: Fatal acute systemic anaphylaxis and hemorrhagic pancreatitis following asparaginase treatment in a dog. J Am Anim Hosp Assoc 19:977, 1983

14. Hardy RM: Diseases of the liver. In Ettinger SJ (ed): Textbook of Veterinary Internal Medicine Diseases of the Dog and Cat. 2nd Ed. p. 1372. Saunders, Philadelphia, 1983

15. Hardy RM, Johnson GF: The pancreas. In Anderson NV (ed): Veterinary Gastroenterology. p. 621. Lea & Febiger, Philadelphia, 1980

16. Johnson GF, Zawie DA, Gilbertson SR, et al: Chronic active hepatitis in Doberman pinschers. J Am Vet Med Assoc 180:1438, 1982

17. Kock MD: Peritonitis. Compend Contin Educ 1:295, 1979

18. Kolata RJ: Abdominal trauma. Compend Contin Educ 1:445, 1979

19. Kolata RJ: Diagnostic abdominal paracentesis and lavage: experimental and clinical evaluations in the dog. J Am Vet Med Assoc 168:697, 1976

20. Lantz GC: The pathophysiology of acute mechanical small bowel obstruction. Compend Contin Educ 3:910, 1981

21. MacCoy D: Peritonitis. In Bojrab MJ (ed): Pathophysiology in Small Animal Surgery. p. 142. Lea & Febiger, Philadelphia, 1981

22. Maxie MG, Reed JH, Pennock PW, et al: Splenic torsion in three Great Danes. Can Vet J 11:249, 1970

23. Morgan RV: Acute gastric dilatation-volvulus syndrome. Compend Contin Educ 4:677, 1982

24. Muir WM: Acid-base and electrolyte disturbances in dogs with gastric dilatation-volvulus. J Am Vet Med Assoc 181:229, 1982

25. Muir WM: Gastric dilatation-volvulus in the dog, with emphasis on cardiac arrhythmias. J Am Vet Med Assoc 180:739, 1982

26. Muir WW: Myocardial ischemia in dogs with gastric dilatation-volvulus. J Am Vet Med Assoc 181:363, 1982

27. Mulvany MH, Feinberg CK, Tilson DL: Clinical characterization of acute necrotizing pancreatitis. Compend Contin Educ 4:394, 1982

28. O'Brien T: Small intestine. In O'Brien T (ed): Radiographic Diagnosis of Abdominal Disorders in the Dog and Cat. p. 279. Saunders, Philadelphia, 1978

29. Parent J: Effects of dexamethasone on pancreatic tissue and on serum amylase and lipase activities in dogs. J Am Vet Med Assoc 180:743, 1982

30. Polzin DJ, Osborne CA, Stevens JB, et al: Serum amylase and lipase activities in dogs with chronic primary renal failure. Am J Vet Res 44:404, 1983

31. Roberts KE, Thompson FG, Poppell JW, et al: Respiratory alkalosis accompanying ammonium toxicity. J Appl Physiol 9:367, 1956

32. Rogers WA: Diseases of the exocrine pancreas. In Ettinger SJ (ed): Textbook of Veterinary Internal Medicine Diseases of the Dog and Cat. 2nd Ed. p. 1435. Saunders, Philadelphia, 1983

33. Rogers WA: Liver failure. In Fenner WR (ed): Quick Reference to Veterinary Medicine. p. 535. Lippincott, Philadelphia, 1982

34. Schenker S, Breen KJ, Anastacio MH, Jr: Hepatic encephalopathy: current status. Gastroenterolgy 66:121, 1974

35. Sherding RG: Diseases of the small bowel. In Ettinger SJ (ed): Textbook of Veterinary Internal Medicine, Diseases of the Dog and Cat. 2nd Ed. p. 1278. Saunders, Philadelphia, 1983

36. Sherding RG: Hepatic encephalopathy in the dog. Compend Contin Educ 3:55, 1981

37. Stead AC, Frankland AL, Borthwick R: Splenic torsion in dogs. J Small Anim Pract 24:549, 1983

38. Stevenson S, Chew DJ, Kociba GJ: Torsion of the splenic pedicle in the dog: a review. J Am Anim Hosp Assoc 17:239, 1981

39. Strombeck DR: Hepatic necrosis and acute hepatic failure. In Strombeck DR (ed): Small Animal Gastroenterology. p. 414. Stonegate Publishing, Davis, CA, 1979

40. Strombeck DR: Introduction to diseases of the liver. In Strombeck DR (ed): Small Animal Gastroenterology. p. 362. Stonegate Publishing, Davis, CA, 1979

41. Strombeck DR: Vomiting and its neural control. In Strombeck DR (ed): Small Animal Gastroenterology. p. 73. Stonegate Publishing, Davis, CA, 1979

42. Strombeck DR, Farver T, Kaneko JJ: Serum amylase and lipase activities in the diagnosis of pancreatitis in dogs. Am J Vet Res 42:1966, 1981

43. Suter PF, Olsson S: The diagnosis of injuries to the intestines, gallbladder and bile ducts in the dog. J Small Anim Pract 11:575, 1970

44. Twedt DC, Grauer GF: Fluid therapy for gastrointestinal, pancreatic, and hepatic disorders. Vet Clin North Am 12:463, 1982

45. Wingfield WE: The stomach. In Bojrab MJ (ed): Pathophysiology in Small Animal Surgery. p. 101. Lea & Febiger, Philadelphia, 1981

8 | Hematologic Emergencies

Timothy A. Allen

This chapter focuses on hematologic conditions seen in general or emergency veterinary practice that require immediate therapy or diagnostic intervention. The emphasis is placed on recognition of these emergencies by physical examination and basic laboratory tests.

ANEMIA

The term anemia, as it is used in clinical medicine, refers to a reduction below normal in the number of red blood cells or the hemoglobin concentration of the blood. The "normal" packed cell volume (PCV) and hemoglobin concentration vary depending on age, species, and altitude of residence.

Anemia is not a diagnosis in itself. Rather, it is an objective sign of disease. Usually successful treatment of the anemia requires knowledge of the underlying pathogenesis.

The signs observed in anemic cats and dogs depend on several factors, including the magnitude of reduction in the oxygen-carrying capacity of the blood, the extent of change in total blood volume, the rate at which these changes have occurred, the ability of the cardiovascular and pulmonary systems to compensate for the anemia, and the presence of other manifestations of the underlying disease process. The physiological adjustments that occur with chronic anemia primarily involve the cardiopulmonary system and changes in the oxygen dissociation curve. Red blood cell 2,3-diphosphoglycerate (2,3-DPG) is increased in chronic anemia. This facilitates the delivery of oxygen to the tissues by decreasing the affinity of hemoglobin at the oxygen tension found at the tissue level. The cardiac index generally is increased in anemia. In severe chronic anemia the rate and depth of respiration are increased, and the minute ventilation is increased.

Although there are many causes of anemia, a methodical and systematic approach to the anemic patient yields useful information about pathogenesis and consequently the therapy of the anemia. The clinical evaluation of the patient starts with the careful, detailed medical history and a complete physical examination.

If anemia is present or suspected, it is important to ask certain questions in addition to the routine medical interview. A detailed environmental history is essential. Exposure to drugs and chemicals may produce hemolytic or aplastic anemia. Cleaning fluids, organic solvents, adhesives, insecticides, and paints may produce blood dyscrasias. The dietary history is quite important, although it can be difficult to obtain an accurate one. When considering possible nutritional deficiencies, quantitative information about the foods consumed is vital. It is important to recognize any nutritional idiosyncrasies in the preparation of food or in the use of supplements. A history of anemia in housemates may suggest a common environmental toxin or infectious agent. A familial history of anemia may suggest an inherited problem. The owner should be questioned about discoloration of the urine, as red or orange urine may be a manifestation of a hematologic problem. A history of bruises, epistaxis, melena, or hematochezia may suggest a source of blood loss.

Physical Examination

Pallor is the most obvious sign of anemia. When anemia is present, pallor can be detected most constantly in oral mucous membranes and the conjunctiva. Other areas that should be inspected include the rectal, penile, and vulvar mucous membranes and the external pinnae. Jaundice, cyanosis, pigmentation, and vasodilatation can all mask pallor. Pallor associated with mild icterus suggests hemolytic anemia. Marked pallor associated with petechial hemorrhage suggests anemia and thrombocytopenia.

It is important to emphasize that pallor may be present in the absence of anemia, and conversely anemia may be present without pallor. Therefore detection and confirmation of anemia requires laboratory evaluation.

The general body condition is assessed as a possible indication of disease. Tachycardia and dyspnea at rest or after minimal exertion can be seen with moderate and severe anemias.

Heart murmurs are a common cardiac sign associated with significant anemias. The murmur (anemic bruit) is primarily due to increased blood flow, increased turbulence, and decreased viscosity. The murmurs associated with anemia are usually systolic and heard loudest over the mitral or pulmonic valve areas. Typically the murmurs are moderate in intensity. With chronic anemia, cardiac dilatation may result in mitral and tricuspid insufficiency.

Lymph nodes are systematically checked for palpable enlargement. Peripheral lymphadenopathy may be noted if lymphosarcoma is the underlying cause of the anemia. The spleen, liver, and kidney are carefully palpated. Hepatosplenomegaly may be present with lymphosarcoma or immune-mediated hemolytic anemia. Small, irregular kidneys may indicate that chronic renal failure is the cause of the anemia.

A rectal examination to evaluate the character of the stool is performed to determine if blood is being lost via the gastrointestinal tract. The physical examination also includes a thorough ophthalmologic examination for hyphema and retinal hemorrhage. The compressibility of the cranial thorax is evaluated in cats. If the thorax cannot be compressed, thymic lymphosarcoma is a possibility.

Laboratory Evaluation

The PCV, hemoglobin, and electronically determined red blood cell (RBC) count are useful in evaluating the severity of anemia. Examination of the peripheral blood smear is the single most valuable procedure in evaluating the anemic patient.[48] Correct interpretation depends on proper preparation, staining, and examination. Blood films can be prepared on glass microscope slides or on cover slips.

Several modifications of the Romanowsky method of staining are used for preparing blood films. Two commonly used stains are Wright and Giemsa stains. A properly stained blood film appears pink when viewed with the naked eye. When viewed under the microscope the erythrocytes are pinkish orange in color and the nuclei of the leukocytes purplish blue. Bottles of stain are kept tightly closed to avoid staining problems. In order to prevent precipitation of the stain, the slide is flooded with clear water.

So much information can be obtained from the examination of the stained blood film that it is worthwhile for the veterinarian to examine it personally or submit it to a consulting clinical pathologist.

When evaluating the anemic patient, a systematic approach to the examination of the blood film is important. The blood film is examined under low power to evaluate the distribution of cells and quality of the stain. Indications of a poor film include disruption of leukocytes, overlapping or clumping of RBCs, or areas of the film where there is a uniform loss of central pallor and the presence of polygonal shapes. Next, after switching to high power the RBCs are examined for abnormalities in size (macrocytosis, microcytosis), variations in size (anisocytosis) or shape (poikilocytosis), and changes in staining qualities (hypochromia, polychromasia). The stained smear is also evaluated for RBC parasites and nucleated RBCs. These evaluations are made in the counting area which lies between the feathered edge and the body, or thick part, of the smear.

Polychromasia refers to the relative number of polychromatophilic erythrocytes. These cells stain a light blue gray and represent immature cells that are still undergoing maturation. The light blue gray color is due to the presence of basophilic metabolic debris that has not yet been eliminated and decreased amounts of hemoglobin. Polychromatophilic cells complete the normal maturation process within 1–2 days. Polychromasia is marked if more than five polychromatophilic cells are seen in an average oil immersion field.

Anisocytosis refers to variation in RBC size. Normal canine erythrocytes vary slightly in size. Anisocytosis is more prominent in cat blood smears. The presence of size variation in itself is not significant. However, it does indicate the presence of a hematologic abnormality that should be identified. Anisocytosis may be due to the presence of increased numbers of small cells (spherocytes) or large (megaloblastic) cells.

Hypochromic cells are recognized by the presence of an enlarged area of central pallor that gradually blends with the surrounding pigmented area. Hypochromic cells are not observed in the cat. Spherocytes are small erythrocytes that lack an area of central pallor. Because normal feline erythrocytes have little or no central pallor, it is impossible to reliably detect spherocytes in cat blood smears. Occasional spherocytes are present on a canine blood smear because of normal RBC senescence.

Schistocytes are distorted helmet or triangle-shaped cells or fragmented cells. Fragmented cells result from impact with fibrin strands and damaged vessel walls. Schistocytes have been associated with disseminated intravascular coagulation (DIC), vascular neoplasia, and splenic torsion.

Precipitated stain adheres to erythrocytes and can be confused with intraerythrocyte organisms. Stain can be recognized because it is brightly refractile as the focus is adjusted.

Heinz bodies are clumps of oxidized precipitated hemoglobin. These clumps are most readily demonstrated with supravital stains, e.g., new methylene blue. The Heinz bodies appear as blue bodies at the periphery of the cell. These clumps are very large and may be evident on Wright-stained smears as pale-staining projections from the cell membrane. Heinz bodies are normally plucked from circulating RBCs by the reticuloendothelial system and thus are more prominent in splenectomized patients. Heinz bodies have been called erythrocyte refractile (ER) bodies in the cat. ER bodies may be present in the absence of significant anemia.

Spur cells are cells that have lost their biconcave shapes and have multiple irregular spicules projecting from the surface. They are differentiated from crenated cells by the irregularity of the projections and by the number of cells affected. With artifactual crenation the majority of cells are involved. Spur cell anemia has been reported in a young dog with severe hepatic disease.[42] The exact cause of spur cell formation is not known, but abnormalities in serum lipids and RBC membrane lipids are suspected.

Nucleated red blood cells (NRBCs) associated with polychromasia are considered to be part of the regenerative response of the erythron to anemia. In the absence of polychromasia, NRBCs in the blood film have been associated with a diverse group of hematologic and nonhematologic problems. Extramedullary hematopoiesis, hemangiosarcoma, myelopathies, and lead poisoning can cause increased NRBCs. Nonhematologic causes of increased numbers of NRBCs include hyperadrenocorticism and high-dose immunosuppressive therapy.

The RBC indices are helpful in evaluating the anemic patient. Many electronic blood counting systems include the RBC indices in the routine hemogram. This information is reliable with canine specimens; however, the small size of the feline RBC necessitates modification of most commercial instruments.

Normal mean corpuscular volume (MCV) values are 60–77 femtoliters (10^{-15}) in the dog and 39–55 femtoliters in the cat. If the MCV is decreased, the anemia is considered microcytic. When the MCV is increased, it is usually due to increased numbers of immature erythrocytes in the peripheral circulation. The mean corpuscular hemoglobin concentration (MCHC) is the measure of the hemoglobin concentration in the average RBC. The results are expressed in grams of hemoglobin per deciliter of packed RBCs. The normal MCHC ranges from 32 to 36 g/dl in dogs and cats. An increased MCHC is usually due to hemolysis or laboratory error in the measurement of the PCV or hemoglobin. When the MCHC is decreased, the anemia is considered hypochromic.

The relationship between polychromasia and reticulocytes is a close but imperfect parallelism. The reticulocyte is an immature erythrocyte seen with new methylene blue stain that is equivalent to the polychromatophilic cells seen with Wright's stain. New methylene blue causes the metabolic debris to aggregate and form threads and knots. This collection of matter is called a reticulum and hence the name reticulocyte.

The reticulocyte count is considered the most reliable means of assessing the response of the erythron to anemia. The presence of polychromasia on a stained blood smear is subjective and dependent on such variables as the quality of the stain and the experience of the examiner. Although the reticulocyte count is a valuable determination, the margin of error is great.

The technique for counting reticulocytes is to mix 5 drops of blood with 5 drops of new methylene blue in a small test tube. The mixture is incubated for 10 min, and a routine thin blood film is made from a drop of the mixture.

In making the reticulocyte count, all RBCs that contain blue staining threads or granules are counted. The percentage of reticulocytes among 1,000 red blood cells is counted. An accurate estimate can be made only if the RBCs are evenly distributed without overlapping.

The cat requires special attention when determining the reticulocyte count and interpreting its significance. Three types of reticulocytes have been described in cats based on the degree of reticulation. The lightly reticulated reticulocyte is a better indicator of the magnitude of the erythropoietic response, and the heavily reticulated reticulocyte is most useful in detecting early responses. Stress can increase the reticulocyte count significantly. This increase is probably due to the release of sequestered reticulocytes mediated by epinephrine.

It is very useful to correlate the reticulocyte count with the severity of the anemia. The PCV is used in the following formula to determine the reticulocyte index:

Corrected reticulocyte count (%)

$$= \text{observed reticulocyte count } (\%) \times \frac{\text{patient PCV}}{\text{normal PCV}} \times 100$$

The normal PCV is considered to be 44 in the dog and 35 in the cat. Obviously the presumption that every dog has a normal PCV of 44 and every cat has a normal PCV of 35 is an approximation.

When evaluating an anemic patient, the first step is to determine whether the anemia is regenerative or nonregenerative. This determination is based on the peripheral blood smear, the RBC indices, and the reticulocyte index. By evaluating all these criteria, the veterinarian is less likely to be misled by an aberrant piece of information.

If an anemia is nonregenerative, there is no evidence of polychromasia, the MCV and MCHC are normal, and the reticulocyte index is less than 1 in the cat and 1.5 in the dog. In a regenerative anemia, polychromasia is marked, the MCV is increased, the MCHC is decreased, and the reticulocyte index is greater than 1.0 in the cat and greater than 1.5 in the dog. Of the various criteria cited, the RBC indices are probably the least reliable and therefore should not be evaluated out of context.

When differentiating a regenerative from a nonregenerative anemia, it is important to recall that evidence for regeneration is not detected in the peripheral blood for 2–4 days after acute blood loss. If the anemia is regenerative, the cause is either hemorrhage or hemolysis. If the anemia is nonregenerative, consider the three components required to maintain a normal erythron: nutrients, precursor cells, and an adequate stimulus for production.

Regenerative Anemias

Blood Loss Anemia. Hemorrhage is the suspected cause of the anemia if the physical examination reveals evidence of hematuria, melena, hematochezia, epistaxis, or retinal hemorrhage. If hemorrhage has been detected, it must be determined if it is occurring at single or multiple sites. If there are multiple hemorrhagic sites, a coagulopathy is a possibility. The diagnostic plan therefore includes a platelet count and clotting times. If the hemorrhage is focal in distribution, localized problems are considered first (e.g., cystitis, nasal tumor). If local disease has been ruled out, the diagnostic plan is expanded to include evaluation for a coagulopathy.

Massive hemorrhage can occur following trauma or surgery. Measurement of the PCV can be misleading immediately after acute blood loss because of compensatory vasoconstriction and splenic contraction. The PCV may remain normal for many hours after an acute bleed. As the intravascular volume is restored by the redistribution of body fluids, the PCV decreases. Collectively, the following clinical parameters are better indicators of acute hemorrhage than the PCV alone: depth and rate of respiration, mucous membrane color, capillary refill time, PCV, urine production, central venous pressure, and arterial blood gases.

Hemolytic Anemia. The presence of splenomegaly, abnormal RBC morphology, bilirubinemia, or bilirubinuria in the absence of clinical evidence of hemorrhage suggests hemolysis. The majority of cases of hemolytic anemia have abnormal RBCs on the blood smear.

Hemolytic anemias result from the excessive destruction of erythrocytes within the body. Destruction can be either intra- or extravascular. Extravascular hemolysis occurs when erythrocytes are lysed after they have been phagocytized by cells in the reticuloendothelial system. Extravascular destruction is more common in dogs[20] and cats.

The clinical and laboratory signs associated with hemolysis vary depending on the severity, rate, site, and mechanism of destruction. Erythrocytes can be damaged by a variety of mechanisms. Damaged erythrocytes are less deformable than usual and are removed from the circulation by macrophages located in the reticuloendothelial system. The spleen is the major organ involved in the removal of damaged RBCs. However, the liver and marrow are also sites of destruction. After the macrophages have lysed the RBCs, the hemoglobin is broken down into iron, amino acids, and free (unconjugated) bilirubin. Thus a severe hemolytic crisis results in hyperbilirubinemia. Intravascular hemolysis may occur with immune-mediated or isoimmune hemolytic anemias, vena caval syndrome of dirofilariasis, Heinz body hemolytic anemia, severe hypophosphatemia, and babesiosis. If hemoglobinuria is present in association with hemoglobinemia, intravascular hemolysis should be suspected. Reduced serum haptoglobin levels suggest recent intravascular hemolysis.[22]

Immune-mediated hemolytic anemia may be primary (i.e., autoimmune) or secondary to neoplasia, infectious diseases, or drug administration. Primary immune-mediated hemolytic anemia may be a component of canine systemic lupus erythematosus. In secondary immune-mediated hemolytic anemia, foreign antigens adhere to or alter the surface of the erythrocytes so that antibody production is stimulated. Few cases of drug-induced hemolytic anemia have been documented in veterinary medicine. Levamisole has been incriminated as a potential cause of hemolytic anemia in the dog.[1]

Signs of immune-mediated hemolytic anemia usually develop rapidly. Clinical signs include lethargy, dyspnea, anorexia, pallor, and decreased exercise tolerance. Icterus may or may not be present. In immune-mediated hemolytic anemia, the erythron is generally strongly regenerative. However, it has been suggested that immune-mediated mechanisms may also injure proliferating hematopoietic cells in the bone marrow and thus produce a nonregenerative anemia. Examination of the peripheral blood smear usually reveals spherocytes. The severity of the anemia varies, although it can be quite marked. Typically there is a moderate to marked leukocytosis characterized by an absolute neutrophilia and a left shift. Macroagglutination of erythrocytes on the walls of the glass tube or microscope slide is seen in some cases of immune-mediated hemolytic anemia. In order to differentiate macroagglutination from rouleaux formation, a drop of blood can be suspended in a drop of normal saline on a microscope slide. When mixed, the clumping disappears if it is due to rouleaux formation but persists if due to macroagglutination.

Cold hemagglutinin disease is a form of autoimmune hemolytic anemia caused by cold-acting erythrocyte autoantibodies.[18] Clinical signs of cold hemagglutinin disease are variable and are due to either agglutination within capillaries or anemia. Skin lesions result from abnormalities in the microcirculation. These skin changes are due to exposure to cold and usually involve the extremities (e.g., ears, nose, nailbeds). Anemia is less common than the changes in the extremities. In cold hemagglutinin disease, in vitro agglutination occurs at room temperature and is reversed by warming the blood to 37°C.

Definitive diagnosis of immune-mediated hemolytic anemia requires the demonstration of antibodies coating erythrocytes. This is done by means of the direct antiglobulin (Coombs) test. In the direct antiglobulin test, the patient's washed erythrocytes are tested against antiglobulin serum. RBC agglutinins can be immunoglobulin G (IgG), complement, or less frequently IgM and IgA. Species-specific reagents should be used for the antiglobulin test. False-positive antiglobulin tests have been associated with the use of cephalosporin antimicrobials. False-negative antiglobulin tests may be due to corticosteroid therapy, too weak or too strong antiserum, and too few antibody molecules on erythrocytes.

An alternative technique to the antiglobulin test has been described.[15] The alternative technique involves the combined use of low ionic suspending solution and papain-treated RBCs. The theoretical advantage of this technique is that it increases the uptake of autoantibodies by RBCs and is able to detect low-affinity autoantibodies in the serum.

If immune-mediated hemolytic anemia has been documented, the initial recommended therapy is immunosuppressive doses of corticosteroids. Prednisone or prednisolone are commonly used at the approximate dose of 2–4 mg/kg/day. The dose is divided and given twice per day. After hematologic improvement has been noted, the dose is gradually tapered over a 2- to 3-month period. No further treatment is necessary if the patient remains in remission; however, if anemia recurs, indefinite maintenance therapy is recommended. Maintenance requirements vary; however, prednisolone or prednisone, usually in an approximate dose of 0.5–1 mg/kg, is administered every other day. It must be stressed that immunosuppressive doses of corticosteroids should be utilized initially as lower doses may not only be ineffective but also may make remission more difficult to achieve, even with subsequent higher doses. If a prompt response to corticosteroids does not occur or if severe macroagglutination or intravascular hemolysis is demonstrated, combined immunosuppressive therapy with corticosteroids and cyclophosphamide is considered. The recommended dose of cyclophosphamide is 2 mg/kg administered daily for four consecutive days of each week. The dose is reduced by 25% in dogs greater than 25 kg in body weight and increased by 25% in dogs less than 5 kg. When cyclophosphamide is used concurrently with prednisone or prednisolone, the steroid dose is reduced to a maximum of 1–2 mg/kg/day. The rationale for the immediate use of combined steroid-cyclophosphamide therapy for severe intravascular hemolysis or macroagglutination is that these findings portend a poor response to steroid therapy and a potentially life-threatening situation.

Sterile hemorrhagic cystitis and myelosuppression are untoward effects associated with the use of cyclophosphamide. A CBC and platelet count are performed at weekly intervals. If leukopenia (leukocyte count < 3,000/µl) or thrombocytopenia (platelet count <75,000/μl) develops, cyclophosphamide is discontinued.

Transfusion therapy is reserved for life-threatening situations, as transfused erythrocytes may precipitate or exacerbate the hemolytic process. If transfusion therapy is required, simultaneous administration of immunosuppressive drugs is recommended.

Splenectomy is a very controversial form of therapy; however, it should be considered in patients refractory to therapy or who have developed untoward effects from immunosuppressive therapy.

A congenital hemolytic anemia has been reported in beagles and basenjis that is due to erythrocyte pyruvate kinase deficiency. Pyruvate kinase-deficient RBCs have abnormal glucose metabolism, and subsequently the cells are lysed prematurely. The shortened erythrocyte life span results in anemia. Clinical signs associated with pyruvate kinase deficiency include lethargy and decreased exercise tolerance. Clinical signs are apparent by 1 year of age. Hematologic findings include moderate anemia (PCV between approximately 14 and 28) and marked reticulocytosis. Hyperbilirubinemia is usually not seen because of the insidious nature of the hemolysis. During the second and third years of life, myelofibrosis and osteosclerosis occur, and affected dogs die of hematopoietic failure.

Pyruvate kinase deficiency anemia in basenjis and beagles is an inherited disorder. The trait is transmitted as an autosomal recessive. Homozygous dogs are anemic; heterozygous animals have one-half the normal enzyme activity but do not develop anemia. Definitive diagnosis can be difficult. Pyruvate kinase assays are available in specialized hematologic laboratories; however, the presence of an unstable fetal isoenzyme in affected adults can confuse the diagnosis. Heterozygous (carrier) animals can be recognized because of reduced enzyme activity and thus can be eliminated from breeding programs.

Another hereditary hemolytic disorder has been described in Alaskan malamute chondrodysplastic dogs. The laboratory findings include a normal PCV but reduced hemoglobin content. The erythrocytes are macrocytic and hypochromic, but the reticulocyte count is comparatively low. The characteristic morphologic finding is the presence of stomatocytes, which are erythrocytes with an elongated area of central pallor. The precise metabolic defect that predisposes to premature lysis has not been determined.

Hemolytic anemias can also be due to infectious diseases. The etiologic agent of haemobartonellosis in dogs is *Haemobartonella canis*, a rickettsia. *H. canis* is an epicellular erythrocyte parasite transmitted by ticks. Blood transfusions can be a source of iatrogenic infections.

Most *H. canis* infected dogs are asymptomatic carriers, although severe hemolytic anemia has occurred following splenectomy. Other clinical situations associated with detectable anemia in *Haemobartonella*-infected dogs include splenic neoplasia, concurrent infection with *Babesia canis* or *Ehrlichia canis*, septicemia, and other conditions that produce blockade of the reticuloendothelial system. Diagnosis is based on demonstrating the presence of the etiologic agent in peripheral blood smears. With routine stains the organism appears as a blue-staining coccoid or ring-shaped structure that frequently is in chains. The anemia is characteristically regenerative in nature, and the direct anti-globulin test may be positive. Experimental cases have been successfully treated with thiacetarsamide sodium.

Canine babesiosis is an arthropod-borne disease caused by the protozoa *Babesia canis*. Other species, e.g., *Babesia gibsoni*, have also been implicated. The clinical course of canine babesiosis can be subclinical, acute, or chronic. Frequently the clinical signs are not apparent until infected dogs are subjected to stress factors, e.g., splenectomy and concurrent infection. Pathogenicity varies with different strains of *B. canis*. Babesiosis and ehrlichiosis can occur concurrently. Acute babesiosis occurs more frequently in young dogs. Clinical signs associated with canine babesiosis include weakness, depression, fever, anorexia, icterus, splenomegaly, and pallor. Laboratory changes in canine babesiosis include hemolytic anemia, thrombocytopenia, bilirubinemia, bilirubinuria, hemoglobinuria, azotemia, and cylinduria. Generally, in acute babesiosis the anemia is more severe and the hemolysis is primarily intravascular.

The chronic form of canine babesiosis can be difficult to diagnose because the causative organism frequently cannot be demonstrated in the blood. Definitive diagnosis requires demonstration of the organisms on a blood smear, identification of the parasite after inoculation of suspected infected blood into a test animal, or a positive fluorescent antibody test.

A single subcutaneous injection of the babesiocidal drug diminazene aceturate is reported to be an effective treatment.

Nonregenerative Anemias

When considering nonregenerative anemias, it is important to consider the three components required to maintain a normal erythron: adequate nutrients, a sufficient number of precursors, and the presence of the normal physiological stimuli for RBC production. In dogs, the only nutrient deficiency that results in a clinically significant problem is iron deficiency.[21] If a nonregenerative microcytic hypochromic anemia is recognized, a source or site of chronic external blood loss should be sought. If there are no obvious findings on the surface of the body, e.g., blood-sucking ectoparasites (fleas), the search should turn to the gastrointestinal tract. A fecal flotation test is performed to search for blood-sucking endoparasites. If negative for parasite ova, the stool is evaluated for occult blood loss. A positive occult blood test might indicate neoplasia or a bleeding ulcer in the gastrointestinal tract.

Bone marrow failure results in a nonregenerative anemia. In dogs and cats, marrow failure can be either primary or secondary to systemic disease. Secondary marrow failure is more common; therefore when formulating a diagnostic plan, systemic disease must be ruled out before performing a bone marrow biopsy.

Systemic diseases that can produce a nonregenerative anemia include renal failure, hypothyroidism, neoplasia, feline leukemia virus infection, and any problem that produces chronic inflammation. The degree of azotemia is typically proportional to the severity of the anemia. The pathogenesis of the anemia is complex; decreased production of erythropoietin by the kidneys, decreased responsiveness of the marrow to erythropoietin, and blood loss due to chronic gastrointestinal hemorrhage seem to be the important factors. Hypothyroidism is frequently accompanied by a mild, nonregenerative anemia. Rather than being a true anemia, this may simply reflect decreased demand for RBCs. Neoplasia produces a nonregenerative anemia by chronic blood loss or by producing chronic inflammation. Feline leukemia virus infection can cause a nonregenerative anemia.[7] The mechanism is unknown, although it has been suggested that certain viral strains of the feline leukemia virus have an increased affinity for bone marrow stem cells. Recently macrocytic nonregenerative anemia has been associated with the feline leukemia virus.[24] Chronic inflammation produces anemia by primarily altering ferrokinetics and to a lesser extent reducing RBC survival.[49,50]

Primary marrow failure is infrequent in the dog and cat. Primary marrow failure is suspected if pancytopenia is observed in the routine hemogram. If secondary marrow failure has been ruled out and the cause of the primary failure is not apparent on the peripheral smear (e.g., leukemia), a bone marrow aspirate is performed. Marrow failure has been associated with the following in dogs and cats: estrogen toxicity,[3] phenylbutazone toxicity,[47] thiacetarsamide toxicity,[46] myelotoxicity due to cancer chemotherapeutic agents, feline leukemia virus, *Ehrlichia canis*, myelofibrosis,[45] and chemical toxins such as benzene-ring-containing compounds.

Estrogen-induced myelosuppression can be due to endogenous or exogenous hyperestrogenism. Endogenous hyperestrogenism can occur in the male due to Sertoli cell tumor of the testes.[37] Less frequently it can be due to an interstitial cell tumor of the testes. In the bitch, granulosa cell tumors and adenocarcinoma of the ovaries can produce endogenous hyperestrogenism. Exogenous estrogens are used in a variety of situations, including mismating, prostatic hyperplasia, perianal adenomas, hormone-responsive incontinence in spayed bitches, endocrine alopecia, and pseudocyesis. The pathogenesis of estrogen-induced myelosuppression is unknown, although the effect is presumed to occur at the stem cell level. Androgens seem to act at a different site and consequently do not block the toxic effects of estrogen. When diethylstilbestrol is administered at equivalent estrogenic doses, it is less myelotoxic than estradiol cypropionate. There seems to be species variation on the susceptibility of the marrow to estrogen-induced myelosuppression, cats seeming to be significantly less susceptible than dogs.

In most cases of estrogen-induced myelosuppression, there is an initial thrombocytopenia and granulocytosis followed by granulocytopenia, thrombocytopenia, and anemia. Physical examination may reveal signs of male feminization syndrome. Petechial hemorrhage may be present. Treatment involves eliminating the source of endogenous estrogens. Transfusion therapy may be required as well.

Blood Transfusion

Blood transfusion is an expensive and potentially hazardous form of treatment. Therefore clear indications for its use must be present. The effect of transfusion is temporary; consequently, every effort must be made to identify and correct underlying problems. Severe blood loss is an indication for transfusion therapy. In other types of anemia, indications for transfusion therapy are less clear-cut. The decision to transfuse is based on clinical signs, etiology, and how quickly the cause of the anemia can be corrected, rather than an arbitrarily determined PCV or hemoglobin concentration.

There are eight canine blood groups. Blood groups are designated by the major blood group antigen. The antigens—canine erythrocyte antigens—are numbered 1–8 (e.g., CEA-1, CEA-2). Any of these erythrocyte antigens can stimulate antibody production if they are transfused into a recipient negative for that particular antigen. CEA-1 is the most powerful stimulus for such antibody production. Reactions to CEA-2 are less pronounced, although they can still be of clinical significance. Reactions to the other CEAs are generally clinically insignificant. Antibodies directed against CEA-1 and CEA-2 do not occur naturally; consequently, clinically significant adverse reactions do not occur on initial transfusion. After the first incompatible transfusion, however, destruction of the transfused RBCs occurs 7–10 days later, and the animal becomes sensitized to subsequent transfusion of CEA-1-positive blood. With repeat incompatible transfusions, the previously sensitized dog mounts a more severe immediate reaction.

A CEA-1-positive dog is a universal recipient and can safely receive blood from either CEA-1-positive or CEA-1-negative dogs. A CEA-1-negative dog is a universal donor and can give blood to any dog. A CEA-1-negative dog should receive blood only from another CEA-1-negative dog so as to prevent a transfusion reaction. Transfusion of untyped blood to breeding females is contraindicated because of the possible development of hemolytic disease of the newborn.

Two blood group antigens, A and B, have been reported in the AB blood group system of cats. An immediate fatal reaction following the first transfusion of incompatible RBCs has been reported.[2] Based on the frequency of antigens in the general cat population, the authors of this report estimated that the chance of an incompatible transfusion if untyped blood is transfused is 37.5%. By comparison, another group reported an observed incidence of transfusion reactions of 0.3%.[23] The observed adverse reactions were mild, consisting of vomiting and dyspnea. The clinical experience of others supports the view that transfusion reactions in the cat are infrequent. The most frequent reaction is vomiting, which can be controlled by stopping the infusion of blood for a few minutes and restarting the transfusion at a slower rate. With repeat transfusions of incompatible blood in cats, the survivability of transfused RBCs has been shown to be less than 5 days.[33]

If multiple blood transfusions of untyped blood are necessary, cross-matching is performed to detect donor-recipient incompatibility. A major cross match is performed by combining 2 drops of a 4% suspension of the donor's RBCs suspended in the donor's serum with 2 drops of the recipient serum and incubating in a test tube at room temperature for 15 min. The tube is then centrifuged at 1,000 revolutions per minute for 1 min and the contents examined for hemolysis. If hemolysis is present, the transfusion is incompatible and that donor is not used.

Canine blood donors should be negative for CEA-1 as well as be heartworm-negative. Heartworm disease cannot be transmitted by transfusing blood of infected dogs. The microfilaria of *Dirofilaria immitis* must undergo two molts in the intermediate host (mosquito) before becoming infective. Nonetheless, donors should be microfilaria-negative in order to prevent spread of heartworm disease within the hospital by the bite of mosquitos. Donor cats should be negative for feline leukemia virus and *Haemobartonella felis*. In large blood donor programs, each animal is permanently identified and has a permanent medical record.

Routine periodic laboratory evaluation consisting of a complete blood count, biochemistry panel, urinalysis, and fecal flotation helps to assess the health status of the donors. Routine immunization is performed as required. The donor is fed a good commercial diet and is given a hematinic (vitamin and iron supplement).

Approximately 10 ml of blood per pound body weight may be withdrawn every 3 weeks without excessively stressing the canine donor. In the cat, approximately 60 ml can be withdrawn every 3 weeks without excessive stress to the donor.

The actual method of collection varies depending on the specific situation. The donor is first anesthetized and a surgical preparation of the collection site is performed. Possible collection sites in the dog include the jugular vein, heart, and femoral artery. In the cat the jugular vein and heart are possible sites. In permanent donors the jugular vein is the preferred site. Blood collection is performed rapidly and without interruption, utilizing a single site to avoid excessive activation of the clotting cascade and damage to the RBCs.

Several anticoagulants are available for routine collection of blood. Blood withdrawn into heparin must be used within 24–48 hr. The limited shelf-life is due to the marked increase in pH and subsequent decrease in RBC adenosine triphosphate (ATP) observed when heparin is the anticoagulant. These chemical changes result in rigid RBCs that do not deform and are thus very rapidly removed from the recipient circulation. If blood is to be stored for more than 48 hr, either acid-citrate-dextrose (ACD Evacuated Blood Collection Bottle, Diamond Laboratories, Inc., Des Moines, IA 50304) or citrate phosphate dextrose (CPD Blood Pack Units With Integral Donor Tubes, Fenwall Laboratories, Inc., Deerfield, IL 60015) must be used as the anticoagulant and the blood stored at 1–6°C. The temperature cannot vary by more than 2°C, and if the blood is out of refrigeration long enough to warm to 10°C (approximately 30 min) it must be used immediately. During storage, the blood should be mixed gently periodically. When collected and stored as described, blood drawn in ACD has an effective storage life of approximately 14 days in the dog and 30 days in the cat,[34] and blood drawn in CPD has an effective storage life of approximately 21 days in the dog.[43] Blood stored beyond these limits has reduced posttransfusion survival and reduced oxygen-carrying ability because of a shift to the left of the oxygen dissociation curve during storage.[39] The CPD plastic packs generally require the use of a vacuum collection device. This device provides vacuum-powered negative pressure for quick, efficient filling as well as a means of gently mixing the blood with the anticoagulant. Each pack or bottle is immediately labeled with the donor's name, the expiration date, and the blood type.

Blood is gradually warmed to approximately 37°C prior to administration. Refrigerated blood can be warmed by passing it through a coiled tube in a 48°C water bath or by other appropriate means. Care is exercised to prevent excessive warming (>50°C), which causes hemolysis.

It is essential that strict asepsis be maintained during collection, storage, and administration of blood and blood products. Once a blood storage container has been entered, the stored blood should be used within 24 hr.

Blood is administered through a sterile blood administration kit (Blood Administration Set, Diamond Laboratories, Inc., Des Moines, IA 50204). If the practice has a frequent demand for transfusion therapy, it is desirable to make optimal use of the available blood by separating it into its components and administering only the needed component. Packed RBCs and plasma can be produced by either centrifugation or sedimentation of whole blood. Plasma frozen at less than 20°C has a storage life of greater than 1 year. If frozen plasma is to be used to treat bleeding disorders, the plasma should be frozen within a few hours of collection.

If the major indication for transfusion is decreased oxygen-carrying capability, the patient should receive packed RBCs. These can be administered rapidly with less risk of creating volume overload in a patient with compromised cardiovascular function. The use of packed RBCs also reduces the frequency of transfusion reactions due to plasma protein incompatibilities.

Plasma transfusions are used primarily to expand the extracellular fluid volume. Fresh frozen plasma is a source of coagulation factors, including factors V and VIII.

Complications of blood transfusion can be both immunologic and non-immunologic in origin. Immunologic reactions can result from the transfusion of incompatible blood. Clinical consequences of hemolytic transfusion reactions include the rapid development of tachycardia, hypotension, vomiting, salivation, and muscle tremors. Laboratory changes associated with significant acute hemolysis include hemoglobinemia, hemoglobinuria, and possible acquired coagulation disorders.

Delayed hemolytic reactions sometimes occur after multiple transfusions. Delayed hemolysis is suspected if the PCV drops unexpectedly 2–21 days posttransfusion. The clinical and laboratory signs of acute hemolysis mentioned above may not be detected in delayed hemolytic reaction.

Transfusion reactions may also be caused by immunologic reactions due to leukocyte, platelet, or plasma protein incompatibilities. Reactions between antigen and antibody may activate the complement system and thus release vasoactive substances that may be responsible for trembling, vomiting, and urticaria. Prior transfusion is not required for these reactions to occur. Some authorities have advocated the use of antihistamines approximately 30 min before transfusion to reduce these reactions.

Transfusion-induced fever is caused by the response of the donor to foreign proteins. The initial step in controlling transfusion-induced fever is to slow the rate of transfusion. If no response is noted when the rate is reduced, aspirin is administered. Bacterial contamination of the transfused blood also produces fever.

Nonimmunologic transfusion reactions are principally due to vascular overload. Signs of vascular overload include a cough, dyspnea, and vomiting.

Autotransfusion—the infusion of autologous blood recovered from the site of active bleeding—has been utilized in the management of traumatic hemothorax in the dog.[51] In the cases described, the blood in the chest cavity was collected into an ACD vacuum collection bottle and was infused intravenously through a micropore blood filter (Ultrapor Filtration, Pall Corporation, Glencove NY).

Autotransfusion is contraindicated in cases of infection or malignancy. Possible complications include hemolysis, coagulopathies, and microembolism due to platelet or leukocyte microaggregates. Autotransfusion has several potential advantages over the use of homologous donor blood. These include elimination of the risk of sensitization to transfused antigens, elimination of the risk of transmitting diseases such as haemobartonellosis, and the immediate availability of compatible blood.

METHEMOGLOBINEMIA

Methemoglobin is hemoglobin with an iron atom in the ferric (Fe^{3+}) state rather than the usual ferrous (Fe^{2+}) state. Methemoglobin is not capable of carrying oxygen reversibly.

Excessive accumulation of methemoglobin occurs with certain erythrocyte enzyme deficiencies[29] or with exposure to drugs or chemicals that have oxidative properties. Oxidation of hemoglobin that exceeds the reductive capacity of the erythrocyte metabolic pathways may cause methemoglobinemia, Heinz body hemolytic anemia, or both. Heinz bodies are composed of oxidized hemoglobin. Drugs associated with Heinz body hemolytic anemia in cats include methylene blue, acetaminophen,[16] and phenazopyridine. Onions, benzocaine, and methylene blue have been incriminated as etiologic agents in dogs.

Blood from patients with methemoglobinemia is brownish in color and does not become red when mixed with air.

No treatment is necessary for methemoglobinemia unless the patient is symptomatic. General therapeutic measures include oxygen therapy and elimination of the offending agent by gastric lavage, etc. Severe cases have been treated with ascorbic acid. More recently, acetylcysteine has been shown to be a safe, effective oral antidote for acute acetaminophen toxicosis in cats (Ch. 11).[41]

ERYTHROCYTOSIS AND POLYCYTHEMIA

Relative erythrocytosis refers to the situation in which the hematocrit is elevated because of a decrease in plasma volume. Relative erythrocytosis is due to such things as severe vomiting or diarrhea and other causes of clinical dehydration. Therapy consists of volume expansion and the correction of the underlying cause of the volume depletion.

Absolute erythrocytosis refers to a true increase in the total mass of circulating RBCs. A rapid, transient erythrocytosis may occur in the dog and cat when excitement or stress causes shunting of RBCs into the circulation from the splenic storage pool. Chronic absolute erythrocytosis results from a sustained increase in RBC production. Absolute erythrocytosis can be due to secondary erythrocytosis or polycythemia vera. Secondary erythrocytosis refers to an absolute increase in the RBC mass that is not associated with a myeloproliferative disorder. Causes of secondary erythrocytosis can be classified based on whether the increased levels of erythropoietin are appropriate or inappropriate. Appropriate increases in erythropoietin are due to disorders that produce significant tissue hypoxia (e.g., severe pulmonary disease or right-to-left cardiovascular shunting). Conditions associated with inappropriate elevation of erythropoietin include polycystic kidneys, hydronephrosis, renal cysts, and tumors.[40]

Primary polycythemia (polycythemia vera) is considered a myeloproliferative disorder. Polycythemia vera is presumed to be due to proliferation of a clone of erythroid precursors, independent of erythropoietin levels. Polycythemia vera can progress to myelofibrosis, acute leukemia, or myeloid metaplasia.

Erythropoietin levels are useful in the differential diagnosis of polycythemia. They are low in polycythemia vera and elevated in secondary erythrocytosis.

The clinical manifestations of erythrocytosis are related in part to the underlying disorder. Other manifestations are directly related to the increased blood volume and increased blood viscosity associated with erythrocytosis. These manifestations include hyperemic mucous membranes, neurologic disturbances, and bleeding complications.

The relationship between blood viscosity and hematocrit is characterized by a steep curve. After the hematocrit exceeds 60%, small increases result in substantial increases in blood viscosity. The main emergency therapy for polycythemia vera is phlebotomy and simultaneous intravenous fluid administration.

The optimal long-term therapy for polycythemia vera is unknown. Hydroxyurea has been used successfully to treat primary polycythemia. The recommended therapeutic approach is to first reduce the PCV to less than 60%

by means of phlebotomies and intravenous fluid therapy and then start hydroxyurea.

HYPERVISCOSITY SYNDROME

Viscosity refers to the property of fluid to resist flow. For serum the resistance to flow is a function of both the concentration and types of protein present. The intrinsic viscosity of the serum protein is influenced by its physicochemical properties. Thus increased concentrations of a serum protein with a high molecular weight or a tendency to form aggregates are associated with increased serum viscosity.

The term hyperviscosity syndrome is applied to clinical situations in which serum viscosity increases as a result of greatly increased concentrations of normal or abnormal serum proteins. The clinical manifestations of hyperviscosity syndrome in the dog and cat[25] include neurologic,[4,5] ophthalmologic,[6] hematologic, and rarely cardiac disorders. The associated neurologic signs are seizures, visual disturbances, and alteration of the sensorium. The circulatory disturbances can be graphically visualized in the ocular fundi as alternating bulges and constrictions of the retinal vessels ("boxcar" or "link-sausage" effect). Hemorrhage is associated with hyperviscosity syndrome and results from the formation of complexes between macroglobulins and specific clotting factors. It has also been reported that macroglobulins interfere with platelet function. Rarely, congestive heart failure is associated with hyperviscosity syndrome. This is due to the altered hemodynamic properties of the blood.

A practical means of estimating viscosity of serum is to measure the time it takes the meniscus to fall from above to below the bulb of a blood cell counting pipette. The time measured for serum can be compared with the time measured for water. Normally, the viscosity of serum is approximately 1.5 times the viscosity of water. In animals symptomatic for the hyperviscosity syndrome, the serum is at least four times as viscous as water. Precise measurement of the viscosity of serum requires the use of an instrument such as an Ostwald viscosimeter.

An animal showing signs of hyperviscosity syndrome should undergo phlebotomy and plasmapheresis. Phlebotomy involves the removal of whole blood until a subjective improvement in clinical signs or a decrease in the estimated serum viscosity is achieved. Plasmapheresis refers to the removal of plasma from withdrawn blood and reinfusion of the formed blood elements. The vascular volume is maintained by administering intravenous fluids. Long-term therapy for the hyperviscosity syndrome involves treating the underlying cause of serum protein abnormality.

Cryoglobulins are serum proteins or protein aggregates that undergo precipitation at low temperatures but redissolve when heated. Expected clinical manifestations of cryoglobulinemia include cold sensitivity and peripheral vascular occlusion precipitated by the cold. However, in reported cases of cryoglobulinemia associated with IgA multiple myeloma and macroglobulinemia in the dog, these clinical signs were not present.[6,26]

DISORDERS OF LEUKOCYTES

Leukocyte Response to Acute Infection

Quantitative and qualitative changes in blood leukocytes are associated with most infectious processes. During the initial phase of an acute bacterial infection, neutrophilia, eosinopenia, and lymphopenia are usually present. Neutrophil releasing factor accelerates the rate of release of segmented neutrophils and bands from the bone marrow reserve. The bone marrow reserve consists of as many as 10–15 times the number of neutrophils which are normally present in peripheral blood.

In many bacterial infections, the development of neutropenia is a poor prognostic sign. Neutropenia represents exhaustion of the marrow reserve. Neutropenia can also occur if the marrow reserve is reduced prior to the onset of infection. Neutropenia can result from overutilization or consumption of neutrophils. Neutropenia due to consumption can be recognized by the presence of vacuoles, toxic granules, Döhle bodies, and an increased number of bands in the peripheral smear.

Granulocytopenia

Leukopenia refers to reduction of the total white blood cell (WBC) count to less than 3,500 cells/μl. Neutropenia and granulocytopenia refer to a total neutrophil or granulocyte count of fewer than 1,500 cells/μl. Agranulocytosis refers to the virtual absence of granulocytes in the blood. The risk of infection becomes a serious potential complication when the neutrophil count drops below 1,000 cells/μl, and the risk becomes still greater when the count is less than 500 cells/μl. In addition to the number of WBCs, the rate of decrease seems to be an important factor influencing susceptibility to infection.

A reduced number of peripheral neutrophils may be associated with thrombocytopenia and anemia (i.e., marrow failure) or may involve only the myeloid series. Neutropenia can be due to increased peripheral destruction or utilization, or secondary to decreased production. Potential causes of neutropenia in the dog include ehrlichiosis, parvoviral gastroenteritis, primary bone marrow failure, myelophthisis, myelofibrosis, myelosuppression secondary to drugs or radiation therapy, canine cyclic neutropenia, septic shock, and immune-mediated causes.[32] Additional considerations in the cat include panleukopenia and feline leukemia virus infection. A careful drug history is essential, as drugs are an important potential cause of acute neutropenia.

Bone marrow biopsy is often valuable in the evaluation of leukopenia, especially in determining whether a primary marrow problem is present. The marrow is evaluated for both the number of myeloid elements and the orderly progression of myeloid precursors. Maturation arrest is a condition in which there are adequate numbers of promyelocytes and myelocytes but markedly reduced numbers of more mature forms.

Canine Cyclic Hematopoiesis

Cyclic neutropenia or cyclic hematopoiesis is an inherited syndrome reported only in the gray collie. The mode of inheritance seems to be simple, autosomal recessive. Affected collies have a unique dilution of their hair color that results in a silver gray coat. Whether the color dilution and the hematologic disorder are due to the same genetic defect or merely closely linked is not known.

In affected dogs, neutropenia and thrombocytopenia occur at approximately 11- to 12-day intervals. The nadir can be as low as 0–400 neutrophils/μl and persist for approximately 3 days. During the remainder of the cycle, the neutrophil counts are normal or slightly increased. Experimental evidence suggests that the fundamental defect is at the multipotential hematopoietic stem cell level. The neutrophils from these collies also show metabolic and functional defects that result in decreased bacterial killing.

Typical clinical signs include anorexia, fever, lethargy, diarrhea, epistaxis, and gingivitis. Clinical changes are usually detected within the first 6 months of life. With repeated neutropenic episodes, more severe problems, e.g., septicemia, pneumonia, abscesses, and hemorrhagic enteritis are noted. Coagulopathies, amyloidosis, and anemia may complicate the latter stages of the clinical course.

Pelger-Huët Anomaly

Pelger-Huët anomaly refers to hyposegmentation of the nuclei of neutrophils and eosinophils. The cell size and cytoplasm are normal, but the nuclei are oval or bean-shaped. Although the disorder is rare, it has been reported in a number of dog breeds and in two related cats. Affected animals are clinically normal and are diagnosed by the presence of a persistent left shift with a normal total leukocyte count.

Leukemia

Leukemia may be defined as a group of disorders in which there is widespread neoplastic proliferation of one line of leukocytes that is usually associated with abnormal peripheral WBC counts.

Lymphoproliferative disorders may primarily involve the tissue (i.e., lymphoma), or they may be primarily abnormalities noted in the peripheral blood (i.e., leukemia). It is important to emphasize that between these extremes there is a continuum. In other words, gradations exist between exclusive involvement of the peripheral blood and exclusive involvement of peripheral tissues.

Acute Lymphoblastic Leukemia. Canine acute lymphoblastic leukemia is a progressive proliferation of poorly differentiated lymphocytes (lymphoblasts) that infiltrate the marrow and lymphatic tissues.[35] Clinical signs usually occur suddenly. Some prominent signs are directly related to alteration of normal marrow function (e.g., pallor, fever, and bleeding). Other signs are less specific and include vomiting, diarrhea, lameness, lethargy, and anorexia. Physical examination findings include pallor, fever, lymphadenopathy, splenomegaly, and hepatomegaly. The basis of the clinical diagnosis is the presence of lymphoblasts as the predominant cell type in the peripheral blood smear and bone marrow aspirate. Anemia and thrombocytopenia are frequently associated hematologic problems.

Acute lymphoblastic leukemia is distinct from the advanced stages of lymphosarcoma. In the advanced stages of lymphosarcoma, there may be evidence of neoplastic cells in the peripheral blood.

Chronic Lymphocytic Leukemia.   Canine chronic lymphocytic leukemia is a neoplastic disorder of small mature lymphocytes. Lymphoid cells are present in the marrow, blood, lymph nodes, liver, and spleen. This is a rare disorder seen primarily in middle-aged dogs.[31] Usually the diagnosis of chronic lymphocytic leukemia is made serendipitously when the blood smear is evaluated for a nonrelated problem.

An absolute lymphocytosis is the essential diagnostic criterion. The WBC count varies between 30,000 and 50,000/µl, with 40–80% of these cells being lymphocytes. The predominant cell type in the marrow is the lymphocyte. RBCs and platelet counts may be normal at the time of diagnosis. The presence of severe anemia or thrombocytopenia indicates a poor prognosis.

This form of leukemia may be associated with monoclonal gammopathy and hyperviscosity syndrome.

Chlorambucil administered orally has been effective in controlling this leukemia in the small number of cases that have been treated.[31]

Canine Myelogenous Leukemia.   Myelogenous leukemia is rare in dogs. Typical clinical signs consist of weight loss, weakness, fever, pallor, splenomegaly, hepatomegaly, and lymphadenopathy. The severity of lymphadenopathy and hepatomegaly is variable. Canine myelogenous leukemia is a collective term that refers to granulocytic, monocytic, myelomonocytic, basophilic, and megakaryocytic leukemias. Definitive diagnosis is made by thorough examination of the peripheral smear and bone marrow aspirate. The various forms of myelogenous leukemia may be difficult to differentiate on routine Romanowsky-type stains. Histochemical stains may aid differentiation.

There are few reports describing the treatment of myelogenous leukemia in the dog. Hydroxyurea has been used successfully in treating a dog with basophilic leukemia and a dog with neutrophilic leukemia.[31]

Myeloma

Myeloma is a neoplastic proliferation of plasma cells in various stages of maturity. The proliferating clone of cells behaves as a functional tumor and produces excessive levels of immunoglobulin. The resultant monoclonal gammopathy may produce specific clinical syndromes, e.g., hyperviscosity syndrome or cryoglobulinemia.

Anemia is very common in multiple myeloma. Thrombocytopenia and granulocytopenia may also be present. Evaluation of the serum electrophoretogram reveals a "church spire" peak in the globulin fraction. Rarely, two peaks are noted. One peak may represent an aggregate of the abnormal immunoglobulin.

Plasma cells are rarely observed in the peripheral blood smear, although examination of the bone marrow aspirate reveals an increased number of plasma cells. The presence of plasma cells in the marrow is not specific for myeloma. However, the greater the number and the more primitive the plasma cells, the greater is the likelihood of myeloma. Osteolytic radiographic changes occasionally are present in multiple myeloma. The skull, ribs, pelvis, and vertebrae are the sites most frequently involved.

Diagnosis of multiple myeloma requires that two of the following criteria be met: a diagnostic bone marrow biopsy, radiographic evidence of osteolytic bone lesions, a monoclonal gammopathy, and Bence-Jones proteinuria. Bence-Jones proteins are component polypeptide chains of immunoglobulins that are excreted in the urine because of their small size. The presence of these polypeptides is best detected by electrophoretic techniques. The commercial dipsticks available for the detection of proteinuria are sensitive only to albumin, not to Bence-Jones protein.

Renal failure may be a sequela to multiple myeloma. The precise pathogenesis of the renal failure has not been elucidated, but it has been suggested that the tubules become obstructed with abnormal proteins.

Hypercalcemia and hypercalciuria may also complicate the clinical course of multiple myeloma. Hypercalcemia usually occurs in the absence of osteolysis and is an example of a paraneoplastic syndrome.

Patients with multiple myeloma display an increased susceptibility to infection. The use of immunosuppressive drugs in the treatment of multiple myeloma further impairs host defense mechanisms.

The combination of melphalan and prednisone is effective in treating multiple myeloma in the dog.[30] Clinical improvement is usually noted 3–4 weeks after the start of therapy. A convenient way of monitoring therapy is to evaluate changes in the serum electrophoretogram.

Chlorambucil is recommended for the treatment of IgM (macroglobulin)-producing plasma cell tumors. Cyclophosphamide can be used to treat dogs that have become resistant to melphalan or chlorambucil. A recent report proposes that the failure to respond to therapy and aggressive behavior of the tumor suggest a diagnosis of plasma cell leukemia rather than multiple myeloma.[9] Cats with multiple myeloma seem to be less responsive to therapy.

BLEEDING DISORDERS

The diagnosis and emergency treatment of bleeding disorders can be simplified by briefly reviewing the components of hemostasis.

Platelets are essential for sealing defects in vessel walls and providing the platelet phase of primary hemostasis. The sequence of platelet function is adhesion, primary aggregation, release reaction, secondary aggregation, and contraction.

When the endothelial surface is disrupted, platelets adhere to the exposed collagen. Platelet membrane complex, calcium, fibrinogen, von Willebrand factor, and a portion of coagulation factor VIII are required for normal platelet adhesion. Primary platelet aggregation is mediated by a number of factors including adenosine diphosphate (ADP) and a glycoprotein receptor. The release reaction requires a different glycoprotein receptor and ionized calcium within the platelet. The platelet release reaction involves the release of vasoactive substances, ADP and prostaglandins, from storage granules. These released substances enhance secondary platelet aggregation and contraction. Secondary platelet aggregation results in the release of platelet factor 3.

The clotting cascade includes a complex series of proteolytic reactions involving various enzymatically activated coagulation factors. Activation of coagulation results in the formation of thrombin, an enzyme capable of converting fibrinogen into fibrin. The fibrin is deposited within and around the primary hemostatic plug. The fibrin increases the strength of the clot and helps bind it to the vessel wall.

The clotting cascade can be divided into the intrinsic, extrinsic, and common pathways. The origin of the term intrinsic is that all the factors required for this pathway are present in the circulating blood. The intrinsic pathway is initiated when factor XII is activated by injury to the vessel wall. Phospholipids and calcium are required at several points in the pathway. The extrinsic pathway is more rapid and is activated by the release of tissue thromboplastin from damaged cells or vascular endothelium. Although called extrinsic, this pathway is intravascular and contributes to the activation of the common pathway along with the intrinsic pathway. The final product of the common pathway is insoluble fibrin polymer.

The final component of hemostasis is the fibrinolytic system, which is responsible for remodeling, dissolution, and organization of the fibrin thrombus. Plasmin is the enzyme responsible for the proteolytic breakdown of fibrin, fibrinogen, and factors V and VIII into fibrinogen/fibrin degradation products (FDPs). Fibrinogen/FDPs possess antithrombin action, inhibit fibrin polymerization, and inhibit platelet aggregation. Excessive fibrinolytic activity can lead to a bleeding disorder that resembles a coagulation defect.

The platelet count, prothrombin time, and activated partial thromboplastin time are recommended as the minimum data base if a hemostatic defect is suspected. The venipuncture should be as atraumatic as possible, as elaboration of tissue thromboplastin artifactually activates the clotting cascade and initiates platelet adhesion.

The number of platelets can be counted directly by using a hemocytometer chamber or an electronic cell counter. An indirect way of approximating the platelet count is to multiply the average number of platelets per oil immersion field in 10 fields by 15,000. More simply, if there are more than 10–20 platelets per oil immersion field the count is probably normal.

The one-stage prothrombin time measures the biologic activity of the extrinsic and common pathways of the clotting cascade (factors VII, X, V, II, and I). If the time is more than 3–6 sec longer than the control, it is considered significant.

The activated partial thromboplastin time measures the biological activity of the intrinsic and common pathways (factors XII, XI, IX, VIII, X, V, II, and I). A significant prolongation is 10–15 sec longer than the control time.

The activated coagulation time (ACT) is a simple, relatively reproducible test of the intrinsic and common coagulation pathways.[36] This test is more likely to be available to veterinarians on an emergency basis than the activated partial thromboplastin time. Because of variations in technique and materials, each hospital must establish normals.

Fibrin/FDPs are detected with a macroscopic slide agglutination test. In this test, antibodies to human fibrinogen, fibrin monomer, and fibrin fragments are adsorbed to latex particles, and dilutions of serum are mixed with the latex particle suspension. The test is positive if agglutination occurs. Positives at specific dilutions have quantitative equivalents. Increased levels of FDPs are associated with excessive fibrinolysis or liver disease.

Thrombocytopenia

When evaluating thrombocytopenia it is important to differentiate decreased production of platelets by the bone marrow from increased peripheral destruction or sequestration of platelets.[10] An aspiration biopsy of the bone marrow is important when evaluating thrombocytopenia. If thrombocytopenia is due to increased peripheral destruction, the bone marrow contains normal or increased numbers of megakaryocytes. If the thrombocytopenia is due to decreased production of platelets by the marrow, the bone marrow aspirate will reveal hypoplasia of the megakaryocytic series.

Increased peripheral destruction, sequestration, or consumption of platelets can be due to immune or nonimmune etiologies. Nonimmune causes include hypersplenism, septic shock, and DIC. The spleen normally acts as a reservoir for about one-third of the peripheral platelet pool, but with splenomegaly this proportion increases to three-fourths. Splenomegaly can be due to neoplasia, immune stimulation, or hemolytic crisis. In septic shock platelet margination is increased. DIC is an acquired bleeding diathesis in which platelets are consumed in the formation of thromboemboli.

Immune-mediated thrombocytopenia is due to the production of antiplatelet antibodies. The types of immune-mediated thrombocytopenia that have been recognized include autoimmune, transfusion-related, drug-induced, and idiopathic forms. Autoimmune thrombocytopenia is frequently associated with other forms of autoimmune disease, e.g., autoimmune hemolytic anemia and systemic lupus erythematosus. Posttransfusion purpura syndrome is a poorly understood process that results in the destruction of autologous platelets 7–10 days post transfusion. Drug-induced thrombocytopenia can occur when a drug or hapten directly binds to the platelet membrane and stimulates antibody production or when antigen-antibody complexes are adsorbed onto platelet membranes. If the thrombocytopenia is drug-induced, it disappears within 2 weeks after withdrawal of the drug. The idiopathic disease is the most commonly diagnosed form of immune-mediated thrombocytopenia. The diagnosis is confirmed by a positive platelet factor 3 test. The test is an indirect method of detecting antiplatelet antibody.

Decreased production of platelets has been associated with marrow failure. In addition to the etiologies mentioned earlier, treatment with chloramphenicol, dapsone,[28] and gold salts[13] have been incriminated in animals.

When the platelet count drops below 50,000/µl, spontaneous, life-threatening hemorrhage can occur. Therefore in severe thrombocytopenia, surgery, intramuscular injections, and medications that interfere with platelet function (e.g., aspirin) should be avoided. Whole blood, platelet-rich plasma, or platelet concentrates can be used for platelet replacement therapy. If whole blood is used, it should be collected in plastic bags and be less than 8 hr old. A transfusion of 250 ml of whole blood supplies approximately 50 million platelets to the recipient. This may increase the platelet count above the critical level and control spontaneous hemorrhage. Platelet-rich plasma is prepared by the centrifugation of blood withdrawn in plastic bags at 1,500 rpm for 3–5 min. The platelet-rich plasma is separated immediately and infused.

In cases of thrombocytopenia, stimulation of marrow thrombopoiesis is attempted. Corticosteroids are reported to increase platelet production and release from megakaryocytes. Vincristine has been recommended for the treatment of thrombocytopenia.[19] Vincristine seems to increase platelet numbers by increasing megakaryocyte fragmentation. The vincristine can be repeated or combined with corticosteroids to derive the maximal response.

Corticosteroids are used in the treatment of immune-mediated thrombocytopenia because of the following effects: decreased production of antiplatelet antibody, decreased sequestration and destruction of platelets in the spleen and liver, and decreased consumption of platelets because of stabilization of vascular membranes. Immunosuppressive levels of prednisolone (1–2 mg/kg divided twice per day) are recommended until the platelet count exceeds 100,000/µl. At this point the dose of prednisolone can be tapered over a period of 4–6 weeks. The platelet count must be monitored frequently as the dose is tapered because of the high incidence of recurrence. A therapeutic response is generally observed within 7–10 days unless the patient is refractory. If the patient is refractory to corticosteroids, another immunosuppressive drug is added to the regimen. Cyclophosphamide and azathioprine have been used for this purpose. Cyclophosphamide is preferred because of its more rapid onset of action. When this agent is added, the dose of prednisolone is reduced. If the thrombocytopenia is still refractory, splenectomy is considered. The spleen is the major site of production of antiplatelet antibody and of platelet sequestration and destruction.

Disseminated Intravascular Coagulation

DIC is a paradoxical problem that involves both the coagulation pathways and the opposing fibrinolytic system. Coagulation factors and platelets are depleted because of activation of the clotting cascade. The fibrinolytic system causes lysis of fibrin and fibrinogen and elaborates FDPs, which impair fibrin polymerization and platelet aggregation. A number of conditions have been associated with DIC in animals, including heat stroke, acute pancreatitis, intravascular hemolysis, dirofilariasis, bacteremia, infectious canine hepatitis, severe trauma, and various neoplasms.

DIC ranges in severity from very subtle petechial hemorrhage to severe life-threatening hemorrhage. There are no rigid laboratory criteria for the diagnosis of DIC.[12,14] It has been suggested that DIC be divided into three arbitrary stages based on the severity of clinical signs and the degree of alteration of laboratory parameters.[17] The main purpose in staging DIC is to provide more rational therapy. In the early, mild or chronic stages of DIC, the major laboratory finding is thrombocytopenia. In the acute stage, thrombocytopenia is accompanied by moderate prolongation of the prothrombin time, activated partial thromboplastin time, and activated coagulation time. In the acute stage there is also a moderate increase in FDPs and a marked decrease in antithrombin III levels. In end-stage DIC there is severe thrombocytopenia, marked prolongation of the coagulation tests, a significant increase in FDPs, and tremendously reduced antithrombin III levels. In the mild early stage or the chronic stage of DIC, a platelet inhibitor, e.g., aspirin or low-dose heparin (canine dose: 150–250 units/kg SC t.i.d.) therapy, is indicated. In the acute stage an intermediate dose of heparin (500 units/kg SC t.i.d.) is recommended. In end-stage DIC, low-dose heparin therapy is combined with replacement therapy using whole blood (10–20 ml/kg/24 hr) or fresh frozen plasma. In patients with DIC superimposed on liver disease, the response to heparin therapy is poor.

Correction or elimination of the underlying condition is the most important factor in the successful treatment of DIC. Supportive measures that are frequently indicated include vigorous fluid therapy to correct volume deficits and hypotension, oxygen therapy to correct hypoxemia, bicarbonate therapy to correct acidosis, and antimicrobial therapy to eliminate sepsis.

Primary fibrinolysis is a rare disorder that may be difficult to differentiate from the secondary fibrinolysis that occurs in DIC. When compared with DIC, primary fibrinolysis tends to have normal platelet numbers, no schistocytes on the peripheral smear, and increased clot lysis. Because of the difficulty in differentiating primary from secondary fibrinolysis and the possibility of thrombotic complications, epsilon-aminocaproic acid is infrequently used in veterinary medicine.

Hereditary Coagulation Factor Deficiencies

Hereditary coagulation factor deficiencies have been reported in both dogs[27] and cats.[8] Because of the common practice of selective inbreeding, these deficiencies are most prevalent in rare breeds or breeds where certain animals are used extensively as foundation breeding stock.

Hereditary coagulation abnormalities are probably the least common of the bleeding disorders described in this section. Because the coagulation factors are required for the generation of fibrin, deficiencies in any of the coagulation factors results in a fragile clot. Consequently, delayed bleeding following surgery or trauma is characteristic of coagulation factor deficiencies. In mildly affected patients, bleeding may not be apparent until an acquired hemostatic defect is superimposed on the inherited defect. An example of such a situation is when acquired platelet dysfunction develops after administration of aspirin or modified live virus vaccines.

The prothrombin time and the activated partial thromboplastin time are the most useful tests in the initial characterization of suspected inherited coagulation defects. However, specific and specialized tests are necessary to confirm the diagnosis. Excellent reviews on the diagnosis and treatment of inherited coagulation deficiencies are available.[11,27]

Anticoagulant Rodenticide Poisonings

Warfarin and other anticoagulant rodenticide poisonings are one of the more common intoxications in dogs. These rodenticides interfere with the function of vitamin K in the formation of factors II, VII, IX, and X. Typically, in cases of anticoagulant rodenticide poisoning the activated coagulation time and the activated partial thromboplastin time are moderately prolonged and the prothrombin time is severely prolonged.

Most of the anticoagulant rodenticide products are not highly toxic on a single-dose basis. Recently, new rodenticides have been introduced that are effective against warfarin-resistant rodents. Brodifacoum has been reported to be 10–20 times more potent than warfarin. Brodifacoum may have single-dose toxicity, and secondary toxicity may occur when small dogs or cats eat poisoned rodents.[44] Diphenadione belongs to the indandione class of anticoagulants. This toxin is more potent and has a longer duration of effect than warfarin.[38]

Clinical signs vary; however, pallor, dyspnea, weakness, hematemesis, hematochezia, and epistaxis occur frequently. Scleral, conjunctival, and subcutaneous ecchymotic hemorrhage may be noted on physical examination. Acute death has been associated with massive intrathoracic hemorrhage or hemorrhage into the pericardial sac or central nervous system.

If exposure to an anticoagulant rodenticide is probable and clinical and laboratory findings are consistent with toxicosis, treatment with vitamin K is started immediately. The most effective therapeutic form of vitamin K is vitamin K_1 (phytonadione or phylloquinone), given by intramuscular or subcutaneous injection. The recommended dose is 5 mg/kg body weight using the smallest possible needle. If hemorrhage is severe, vitamin K_1 can be given intravascularly. It should be diluted in a small volume of 5% dextrose in water and administered slowly. If hemorrhage is severe or the anemia profound, transfusion with fresh whole blood (less than 24 hr old) is indicated.

If an animal has just ingested an anticoagulant rodenticide, absorption can be decreased by inducing emesis (Ch. 11). An injection of vitamin K_1 is administered immediately, and oral vitamin K_1 (5 mg/kg) is prescribed for 2–3 weeks.

REFERENCES

1. Atwell RB, Johnstone L, Read R, et al: Haemolytic anemia in two dogs suspected to have been induced by levamisole. Aust Vet J 55:292, 1979
2. Auer L. Bell K, Gates S: Blood transfusion reactions in the cat. J Am Vet Med Assoc 180:729, 1982
3. Bland-Van Den Berg P, Bomzon L, Lurie A: Oestrogen-induced bone marrow aplasia in a dog. J S Afr Vet Assoc 49:363, 1978
4. Braund KG, Everett RM, Albert RA: Neurologic manifestations of monoclonal IgM gammopathy associated with lymphocytic leukemia in a dog. J Am Vet Med Assoc 172:1407, 1978
5. Braund KG, Everett RM, Bartels, JE, et al: Neurologic complications of IgA multiple myeloma associated with cryoglobulinemia in a dog. J Am Vet Med Assoc 174:1321, 1979
6. Center SA, Smith JF: Ocular lesions in a dog with serum hyperviscosity to an IgA myeloma. J Am Vet Med Assoc 181:811, 1982
7. Cotter SM: Anemia associated with feline leukemia virus infection. J Am Vet Med Assoc 175:1191, 1979
8. Cotter SM, Brenner RM, Dodds WJ: Hemophilia in three unrelated cats. J Am Vet Med Assoc 172:166, 1978
9. Couto CG, Ruehl W, Muir S: Plasma cell leukemia and monoclonal (IgG) gammopathy in a dog. J Am Vet Med Assoc 184:90, 1984
10. Davenport DJ, Breitschwerdt EB, Carakostas MC: Platelet disorders in the dog and cat. II. Diagnosis and management. Comp Contin Educ Pract Vet 4:10, 788, 1982
11. Dodds WJ: Bleeding disorders. In Ettinger SJ (ed): Textbook of Veterinary Internal Medicine. p. 1679. Saunders, Philadelphia, 1975
12. Drazner FH: Clinical implications of disseminated intravascular coagulation. Comp Contin Educ Pract Vet 4:12, 974, 1982
13. Fadok VA, Janney EH: Thrombocytopenia and hemorrhage associated with gold salt therapy for bullous pemphigoid in a dog. J Am Vet Med Assoc 181:261, 1982
14. Feldman BF: Disseminated intravascular coagulation. Comp Contin Educ Pract Vet 3:1, 46, 1981
15. Feldman BF: Use of low ionic strength solution in combination with papain treated red blood cells for the detection of canine erythrocyte autoantibodies. J Am Anim Hosp Assoc 18:653, 1982
16. Finco DR, Duncan JR, Schall WD, et al: Acetaminophen toxicosis in the cat. J Am Vet Med Assoc 166:469, 1975
17. Greene CE: Management of DIC and thrombosis. In Kirk RW (ed): Current Veterinary Therapy VIII. p. 401. Saunders, Philadelphia, 1983
18. Greene CE, Kristensen F, Hoff EJ, et al: Cold hemagglutinin disease in a dog. J Am Vet Med Assoc 170:505, 1977
19. Greene CE, Scoggin J, Thomas JE, et al: Vincristine in the treatment of thrombocytopenia in 5 dogs. J Am Vet Med Assoc 180:140, 1982
20. Harvey JW: Canine hemolytic anemias. J Am Vet Med Assoc 176:970, 1980

21. Harvey JW, French TW, Meyer DJ: Chronic iron deficiency anemia in dogs. J Am Anim Hosp Assoc 18:946, 1982

22. Harvey JW, Gaskin JM: Feline haptoglobin. Am J Vet Res 39:549, 1978

23. Hayes A, Mastrota F. Mooney S, et al: Safety of transfusing blood in cats (letter to editor). J Am Vet Med Assoc 181:4, 1982

24. Hirsch V, Dunn J: Megaloblastic anemia in the cat. J Am Anim Hosp Assoc 19:873, 1983

25. Hribernik TN, Barta O, Gaunt SD, et al: Serum hyperviscosity syndrome associated with IgG myeloma in a cat. J Am Vet Med Assoc 181:169, 1982

26. Hurvitz AI, MacEwen EG, Middaugh CR, et al: Monoclonal cryoglobulinemia in a dog. J Am Vet Med Assoc 170:511, 1977

27. Johnstone IB: Inherited defects of hemostasis. Comp Contin Educ Pract Vet 4:483, 1982

28. Lees GE, McKeever PJ, Ruth GR: Fatal thrombocytopenic hemorrhagic diathesis associated with dapsone administration to a dog. J Am Vet Med Assoc 175:49, 1979

29. Letchworth GJ, Bentinick-Smith J, Bolton GR, et al: Cyanosis and methemoglobinemia in two dogs due to a NADH methemoglobin reductase deficiency. J Am Anim Hosp Assoc 13:75, 1977

30. MacEwen EG, Hurvitz AI: Diagnosis and management of monoclonal gammopathies. Vet Clin North Am 7:119, 1977

31. MacEwen EG, Patnaik AK, Wilkins RJ: Diagnosis and treatment of canine hematopoietic neoplasms. Vet Clin North Am 7:105, 1977

32. Maddison JE, Hoff B, Johnson RP: Steroid responsive neutropenia in a dog. J Am Anim Hosp Assoc 19:881, 1983

33. Marion RS, Smith JE: Survival of erythrocytes after autologous and allogeneic transfusion in cats. J Am Vet Med Assoc 183:1437, 1983

34. Marion RS, Smith JE: Posttransfusion viability of feline erythrocytes stored in acid-citrate-dextrose solution. J Am Vet Med Assoc 183:1459, 1983

35. Matus RE, Leifer CE, MacEwen EG: Acute lymphoblastic leukemia in the dog: a review of 30 cases. J Am Vet Med Assoc 183:85, 859, 1983

36. Middleton DJ, Watson ADJ: Activated coagulation times of whole blood in normal dogs and dogs with coagulopathies. J Small Anim Pract 19:417, 1978

37. Morgan RV: Blood dyscrasias associated with testicular tumors in the dog. J Am Anim Hosp Assoc 18:970, 1982

38. Mount ME, Feldman BF: Mechanism of diphacinone rodenticide toxicosis in the dog and its therapeutic implications. Am J Vet Res 44:2009, 1983

39. Ou D, Mahaffey E, Smith JE: Effect of storage on oxygen dissociation of canine blood. J Am Vet Med Assoc 167:56, 1975

40. Peterson ME, Aznjani ED: Inappropriate erythropoietin production from a renal carcinoma in a dog with polycythemia. J Am Vet Med Assoc 179:995, 1981

41. St. Omer VV, McKnight ED: Acetylcysteine for treatment of acetaminophen toxicosis in the cat. J Am Vet Med Assoc 176:911, 1980

42. Shull RM, Bunch SE, Maribei J, et al: Spur cell anemia in a dog. J Am Vet Med Assoc 173:978, 1978

43. Smith JE, Mahaffey E, Board P: A new storage medium for canine blood. J Am Vet Med Assoc 172:701, 1978

44. Stowe CM, Metz AL, Arendt TD, Schulman J: Apparent brodifacoum poisoning in a dog. J Am Vet Med Assoc 182:817, 1983

45. Thompson JC, Johnstone AC: Myelofibrosis in the dog: three case reports. J Small Anim Pract 24:589, 1983

46. Watson ADJ: Bone marrow failure in a dog. J Small Anim Pract 20:681, 1979
47. Watson ADJ, Wilson JT, Turner DM, et al: Phenylbutazone-induced blood dys-crasias suspected in three dogs. Vet Rec 107:239, 1980
48. Weiser MG: Correlative approach to anemia in dogs and cats. J Am Anim Hosp Assoc 17:286, 1981
49. Weiss DJ, Krehbiel JD: Studies of the pathogenesis of anemia of inflammation: erythrocyte survival. Am J Vet Res 44:1830, 1983
50. Weiss DJ, Krehbiel JD, Lund JE: Studies on the pathogenesis of anemia of in-flammation: mechanism of impaired erythropoiesis. Am J Vet Res 44:1832, 1983
51. Zenoble RD, Stone A: Autotransfusion in the dog. J Am Vet Med Assoc 172:1411, 1978

9 | Medical Emergencies of the Central Nervous System

William Fenner

This chapter deals with those central nervous system (CNS) dysfunctions for which rapid and appropriate therapy is the key to both preserving life and minimizing sequelae. These situations arise when patients are presented manifesting active seizures (in status epilepticus), coma, acute meningitis/encephalitis, brain injury, or spinal cord injury. This chapter presents a brief discussion of the pathophysiology of these disorders as well as their differential diagnoses and treatment. The pathophysiology is essential because understanding the mechanisms of injury allows the veterinarian to be more flexible in this era of rapidly developing and changing therapy. It is essential to remember that in all of the disorders under discussion overtreatment may result in serious complications or even death. For this reason, vigor in treatment must be tempered with caution.

THE ACTIVELY SEIZURING PATIENT

An animal may be presented to the veterinarian actively seizuring from: (1) a variety of metabolic and toxic processes which may affect the CNS; (2) some organic cerebral insult; or (3) an exacerbation of (or initial presentation for) functional epilepsy. A clinical seizure represents an uncontrolled, abnormal electrical discharge from the cerebrum which manifests as a clinical abnormality.[30] It holds therefore that any process which is capable of disrupting cerebral homeostasis, whether chemical or mechanical, may result in seizures or other evidence of cerebral dysfunction.[5,6] To facilitate the diagnosis of the patient with seizures, it helps to consider the etiologies of seizure disorders as falling into three broad categories.

Etiologic Classification

The first category is extracranial epilepsy. In these cases the seizures are caused by some metabolic, nutritional, or toxic process which is affecting the animal. The animals are often systemically ill in addition to having CNS dysfunction. Generally, animals with extracranial epilepsy have a normal neural examination between seizures, although they may have abnormalities of mentation, e.g., personality and behavioral disorders. The diagnosis here rests primarily on history, physical examination, and general laboratory screening, e.g., serum biochemistries and urinalysis. Specific neurodiagnostic tests, e.g., cerebrospinal fluid (CSF) analysis, electroencephalography (EEG), and skull radiographs, are usually either normal or show nonspecific abnormalities. The major disorders to be considered in this category include hypoglycemia, hypocalcemia, lead intoxication, thiamine deficiency, organophosphate intoxication, liver disease, and ethylene glycol intoxication. Treatment requires correcting any underlying metabolic defect as well as correcting or treating the seizures themselves. The diagnosis and treatment of these disorders are discussed later and are presented in Figure 9-1.

The second major etiologic category contains those epilepsies of intracranial, structural etiology. These are patients who have some physical or organic brain injury that results in the seizure disorder, including encephalitis, tumors, vascular accidents, and brain injury. Patients in this category typically have a persistently abnormal neurologic examination. Thus even when the patient is between seizures, one should be able to find cranial nerve deficits, mentation abnormalities, deficits of gait and stance, or spinal reflex changes that support the presence of some organic cerebral disease. The diagnosis of these patients tends to rest on specific neurodiagnostic testing. CSF evaluation, EEG, computerized axial tomography (CAT scans), and skull radiographs, frequently yield valuable information that, when combined with the history and neurologic examination, allows one to arrive at a highly accurate clinical diagnosis. The treatment of these disorders is aimed at treating the etiology as well as regulating the seizures themselves. Seizures are often very difficult to control in these patients, and frequently the animals carry a more guarded prognosis than those with extracranial or functional epilepsy.[13,18]

The final etiologic category consists of animals with functional epilepsy. These are animals for which no underlying etiology for the seizures can be detected. For this reason, such patients are diagnosed as having a functional disorder of cerebral physiology which manifests solely by recurrent paroxysms of spontaneous abnormal cerebral electrical discharges (seizures). These animals are also known as idiopathic epileptics, inherited epileptics, or simply epileptics. The diagnosis of functional epilepsy is one of exclusion, and the

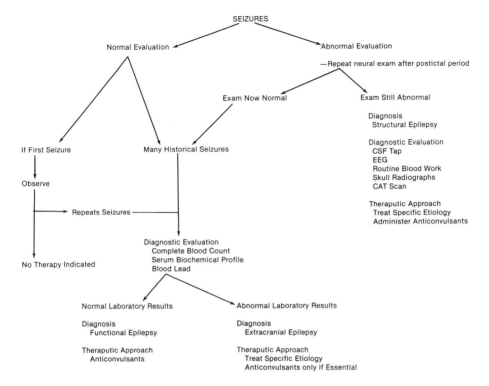

Fig. 9-1. Evaluation of the epileptic. (Adapted from Fenner WR: Seizures and head trauma. p. 31. In Wingfield WE (ed): Symposium on Emergency Medicine. Veterinary Clinics of North America. W. B. Saunders, Philadelphia, 1981, Vol. 11.)

treatment is aimed at treating the seizures themselves as well as the metabolic effects of those seizures.

Pathophysiology

It is not appropriate in this chapter to present an in-depth discussion of the pathophysiology of epilepsy per se. Rather, emphasis is placed on the effects seizures have on the animal and the implications they have for therapy. The reviews by either Holliday[18] or Russo[30] are recommended for the reader who wishes a more detailed discussion of the mechanisms of epileptogenesis.

An actively seizuring patient undergoes a variety of metabolic and systemic derangements. Some of these changes are confined to the CNS, whereas others are more generalized.[7] These abnormalities can result in progression of the epilepsy to a more severe and intractable disease, or they may result in the death of the patient. Discussion begins with the effects confined to the CNS and then progresses to the systemic effects.

Those metabolic changes which occur in the CNS include an increase in cerebral blood flow and an increase in the cerebral rate of oxygen consumption.[7,27] As a by-product of the increased rate of oxidative metabolism in the CNS, there is an increase in CO_2 production within the CNS which can potentiate CNS acidosis.[2] As the seizures persist, there is a gradual decrease in cerebral partial pressure of oxygen, an increased level of calcium within the neurons, and accumulations of toxic levels of metabolic by-products, e.g., arachidonic acid and prostaglandins. Brain edema may result, and an increase in CSF pressure may be seen. Eventually neuronal death occurs from the excessive increase in metabolic demands.[23] The destruction of neurons may cause abnormal mentation and behavior change that can render the animal unacceptable as a pet. If severe enough, the neuronal change may result in brain death.

A variety of systemic effects also contribute to neuronal toxicity. These systemic effects include an initial hyperglycemia that is eventually followed by hypoglycemia if the seizures persist. There is an elevation of body temperature that may result from intense muscular activity, dysfunction of the thermoregulatory centers, or both. Cardiac arrhythmias, including potential life-threatening ventricular arrhythmias, may occur. Neurogenic pulmonary edema may be seen which can cause respiratory failure and death. As a result of the tremendous muscular exertion, a state of lactic acidosis may develop which can result in a blood pH of 7.1 and lower.[7,26]

A further effect on the CNS is the phenomena of kindling and the development of mirror foci. In these phenomena the bombardment of normal neurons by abnormal electrical discharges results in the development of more abnormal neurons and therefore more epileptic neurons. This results in a progression of the seizure disorder to a more intractable and less easily controlled state. The clinical significance of kindling can be summarized as the creation of more epileptic neurons which results in a progressive refractoriness to anticonvulsants that eventually may lead to total failure of therapy. This process occurs over months or years.[18,30]

In summary, the seizuring patient undergoes a variety of systemic and neural derangements during the event. The systemic sequelae include lactic acidosis that if severe enough may be life-threatening, hyperthermia which may be profound, hypoglycemia, pulmonary edema, and ventricular arrhythmias. The sequela to all these events is the potential for death of the patient. The neural sequelae include neuronal death, brain edema, and increased epileptogenesis. Thus immediate vigorous treatment of active seizures is indicated.

Treatment

The treatment of the actively seizuring animal or one in status epilepticus must begin simultaneously with, and take precedence over, the diagnostic effort. This begins with a historical evaluation that is brief but complete as well as physical and neurologic examinations in an attempt to rule out acute vestibular disease or narcolepsy from the differential diagnosis. The animal with acute vestibular disease has constant pathologic nystagmus, and the animal with narcolepsy generally has a stress-associated loss of consciousness with absence of motor movement.

Once it has been established that the animal is seizuring, everything possible is done to stop the seizures without harming the patient. An intravenous line is established to allow rapid delivery of anticonvulsant drugs, and supportive therapy is initiated. Blood samples are submitted to the laboratory for glucose evaluation and, if the seizures have persisted more than 30 min, for analysis of serum electrolytes and acid-base status. The patient is maintained in a high-oxygen atmosphere or intubated if necessary to prevent the development of hypoxia. The patient's head is elevated above the level of the rest of his body to prevent increases in intracranial pressure and to help prevent brain edema. Infusion of a maintenance dose of a balanced electrolyte solution, e.g., lactated Ringer's, is started. The animal is also given intravenous dextrose, generally a 50% dextrose solution 1 g/kg as a slow intravenous bolus. If the animal responds to this and stops seizuring, a maintenance intravenous drip of 5% dextrose is used to prevent further seizures. This patient would not require intravenous anticonvulsant drugs.

Seizures unresponsive to dextrose infusion are controlled initially by the administration of diazepam. Diazepam is given slowly to effect at a dosage of 0.25–0.5 mg/kg IV. A demonstrable effect should be seen in 3–5 min. If in that time the seizures stop, the patient is observed for recurrence of seizures for 10–15 min. Seizures may recur this rapidly because of the short half-life for distribution of diazepam in dogs, which results in a rapid lowering of serum levels as the drug is distributed through tissue stores. If the animal remains seizure-free after that period, the next time when exacerbation of seizures is likely is at 6–8 hr, as both dog and cat have an approximately 7-hr half-life for elimination of diazepam. If the initial dose of diazepam does not stop the seizures within 5 min, the dose can be repeated every 5 min until a total of three doses has been given. If at the end of three diazepam doses there has been no clinical improvement, it is probable that the drug will not work.

At this point, phenobarbital is administered intravenously at the rate of 2–4 mg/kg. The additive effects of phenobarbital and diazepam may cause respiratory depression. Therefore, if phenobarbital is added, close monitoring of respirations is necessary. If after 10–15 min the initial dose of phenobarbital has not successfully abated the seizures, the dose is repeated until a maximum phenobarbital dose of 20 mg/kg has been reached. If the patient's seizures have not been stopped within 1 hr or after the maximum level of phenobarbital has been given, whichever comes sooner, the patient is anesthetized. During anesthesia, it is vital to monitor respiration and to maintain the patient on supplemental oxygen. The preferred anesthetic is a long-acting barbiturate, as all of the gas anesthetics currently in use in veterinary medicine potentiate or cause elevated intracranial pressure.

Maintenance fluids are continued throughout the treatment period, and any biochemical or electrolyte disturbances detected are treated. Treatment of the acidosis is usually not necessary; once the seizures are controlled, the blood

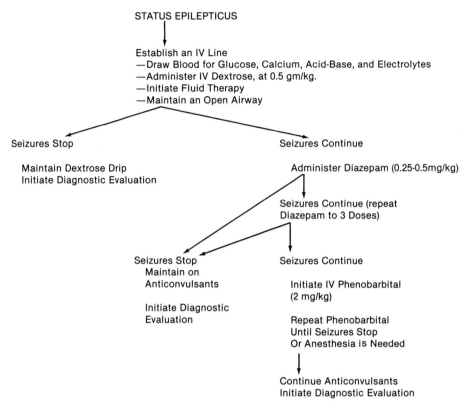

STATUS EPILEPTICUS

Establish an IV Line
—Draw Blood for Glucose, Calcium, Acid-Base, and Electrolytes
—Administer IV Dextrose, at 0.5 gm/kg.
—Initiate Fluid Therapy
—Maintain an Open Airway

Seizures Stop

Maintain Dextrose Drip
Initiate Diagnostic Evaluation

Seizures Continue

Administer Diazepam (0.25-0.5mg/kg)

Seizures Continue (repeat
Diazepam to 3 Doses)

Seizures Stop
Maintain on
Anticonvulsants

Initiate Diagnostic
Evaluation

Seizures Continue

Initiate IV Phenobarbital
(2 mg/kg)

Repeat Phenobarbital
Until Seizures Stop
Or Anesthesia is Needed

Continue Anticonvulsants
Initiate Diagnostic Evaluation

Fig. 9-2. Therapy of active seizures. (Fenner WR: Seizures and head trauma. p. 31. In Wingfield WE (ed): Symposium on Emergency Medicine. Veterinary Clinics of North America. W.B. Saunders, Philadelphia, 1981, Vol. 11.)

pH will rapidly return to normal. Treatment of the acidosis may be indicated to facilitate the treatment of seizures that are difficult to regulate. In addition, the patient is monitored with an electrocardiogram (ECG) to detect life-threatening arrhythmias. Arrhythmias must be treated as they may produce hypoxia, which can compound the potential for brain injury. The basic protocol for the treatment of the actively seizuring patient is reviewed in Figure 9-2.

After control of the seizures, the animal is worked up to determine the etiology of the seizures (Fig. 9-1). Any patient who presents in status epilepticus warrants a complete neurologic evaluation and a vigorous diagnostic work-up consisting of a thorough history, physical examination, and neurologic examination. Note that the drugs used in treating status epilepticus may cause persistent depression, dementia, and abnormalities of the neurologic examination for several days after cessation of the seizures. In addition, the seizures themselves may result in a variety of abnormalities on the neurologic examination as postictal phenomena. Only those neurologic abnormalities that are persistent and consistent in the days following cessation of the seizure activity are considered significant. Neurologic abnormalities that are constantly changing or cannot be demonstrated on repeated examinations are considered the effects of either the postictal state or the anticonvulsant medications. In addition to the physical and neurologic examinations, a complete biochemical profile is performed to look for evidence of metabolic disease. In the patient with persistent neurologic abnormalities, CSF is collected, and, if available, skull radiographs, EEG, and CAT scans are performed. If the results of this testing are normal, a diagnosis of functional epilepsy is made. Long-term treatment with anticonvulsants should be strongly considered in any dog who has initially presented in status epilepticus. Complete descriptions of the diagnostic approach and long-term maintenance treatment for epileptics may be found in several texts[3,4,12,13,24,25] and are summarized in Figure 9-1.

Complications

Complications of status epilepticus include neuronal death with resultant organic cerebral disease clinically manifested as dementia and personality changes. The author has also observed persistent postictal blindness. Enhancement of cerebral neuronal excitability also occurs which tends to make the animal less responsive to long-term anticonvulsant medication and to worsen the prognosis for long-term therapy. There are several potentially life-threatening systemic complications, including CSF and serum acidosis, neurogenic pulmonary edema, ventricular arrhythmias, and hypoglycemia.[2,7,18,26,27] The latter, when it occurs, follows the initial hyperglycemia generated by epinephrine release.

PATIENTS WITH ABNORMALITIES OF CONSCIOUSNESS

Etiology

The patient presented with abnormal consciousness forms one of the most challenging diagnostic and therapeutic problems in veterinary neurology. Any disease process that affects the cerebrum diffusely or one which affects the rostral brainstem either focally or diffusely is capable of causing an abnormality in consciousness. A variety of metabolic disturbances, including hypoxia, profound hypovolemia, hypoglycemia, and hepatic disease, as well as a variety of toxic disturbances, e.g., lead poisoning, are all capable of causing abnormalities in the level of consciousness. In addition to metabolic disturbances, organic brain diseases, e.g., tumors, infarcts or hemorrhages, inflammatory diseases, and traumatic injuries of the brain, are also capable of causing alterations in consciousness. Finally, altered consciousness may be seen as a sequela of status epilepticus.[28]

The regulation of consciousness requires interaction between the brainstem and cerebrum. The sleep-wake cycles seem to be controlled by the as-

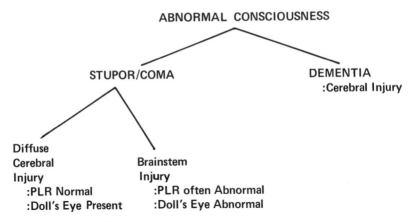

Fig. 9-3. Evaluation of abnormal consciousness. (Fenner WR: Head trauma and nervous system injury. In Kirk RW (ed): Current Veterinary Therapy VIII—Small Animal Practice. W.B. Saunders, Philadelphia, 1983.)

cending reticular activating system located in the rostral brainstem, specifically the rostral one-third of the pons and the midbrain. The reticular activating system is responsible for activating and alerting the cerebrum in response to noxious or potentially harmful stimuli. One interesting clinical observation in man is that it seems to require lesions rostral to the level of cranial nerve V to cause coma, suggesting that deafferentation from painful sensory stimuli may play a significant role in the development and maintenance of altered states of consciousness.[28] Alerted by the brainstem reticular activating system, cerebral health is also essential in the maintenance of consciousness. However, for cerebral disease to cause an abnormality in consciousness, the disease must be both bilateral and diffuse, as the cerebrum has greater redundancy of function than the brainstem. Any patient with an abnormality in consciousness must have a dysfunction of either the cerebrum or brainstem. That dysfunction may be either organic or metabolic in nature.

Clinical Signs and Neurologic Examination

Disorders of consciousness may be manifested as an abnormal content of consciousness, an abnormal level of consciousness, or both (Fig. 9-3). The content of consciousness is regulated by the cerebrum, and patients with abnormalities in content of consciousness are described as demented. These patients appear disoriented, are often very fearful, may be hyperirritable, and are frequently startled by or misjudge stimuli. Dementia is often a major sign in metabolic diseases of the CNS, although it can be seen with cerebral disease of any etiology.

Abnormalities in the level of consciousness may be described as obtundation, stupor, and coma. The obtunded patient is one who has a mild to moderate reduction in alertness, has increased number of hours of sleep in the day, often appears drowsy, but is easily aroused. Stupor is a condition characterized by deep sleep and environmental unresponsiveness from which the patient can be aroused only by vigorous or painful stimuli. When the stimulus is removed, the patient relapses back into the sleep-like state. The comatose patient is in a state of total unresponsiveness. He cannot be aroused even with repeated vigorous and painful stimuli. All of these abnormalities—obtundation, stupor, and coma—may arise from a bilateral and severe cerebral disease or from any brainstem dysfunction that affects the reticular activating system.

When evaluating the patient with coma, the initial step is to distinguish organic from metabolic disease and focal from multifocal disease. It is critical in the evaluation of patients with coma that several neurologic examinations are performed, findings are recorded accurately, and special attention is paid to the pupils, eye movements, muscle tone, and respiratory patterns. The centers for eye movement and pupillary constriction are in the brainstem; therefore changes in pupil size and eye movement may allow one to differentiate between brainstem and cerebral disease. The different motor pathways that go to the limbs to regulate muscle tone originate at separate levels of the brainstem and cerebrum. Thus lesions in selective levels may cause specific variations in muscle tone that help in evaluating the comatose patient. In addition, there are certain respiratory patterns that suggest a metabolic versus an organic disease, although this is not common in veterinary medicine.

When performing the evaluation, first look for symmetry and consistency of signs. Neurologic abnormalities that are asymmetrical (worse on one side of the body than the other) are called lateralizing signs and suggest that an organic or structural disease process is producing the neurologic signs. Examples of lateralizing signs include asymmetry in spinal reflex activity, i.e., reflexes on one side being either more exaggerated or depressed than another, differences in proprioception or pain perception from one side to another, loss of voluntary movement on one side versus another, asymmetery in pupil size from one side to another, and loss of eye blink reflex on one side versus another. Any of the various reflexes or responses tested in the nervous system may become asymmetrical, and that asymmetry may allow localization of the disease process. With cerebral disease the clinical signs are usually worse opposite the diseased hemisphere, and with brainstem diseases they should be worse on the same side as the lesion.

In addition, the consistency and persistence of the neurologic abnormalities are evaluated. One of the hallmarks of metabolic disease is constantly changing or shifting clinical signs. If there are neurologic abnormalities, even focal ones, that are not consistent but seem to constantly shift, be suspicious of the presence of a nonorganic or metabolic disorder.[28]

When evaluating the pupillary light response (PLR), remember that the pupillary constrictor muscle is innervated by cranial nerve III, which arises in the brainstem midbrain. The sympathetic innervation to the eye (pupillary dilator) has fibers traveling from the hypothalamus caudally to the thoracic spinal cord, where they exit to return to the eye via the sympathetic trunk. Lesions at different levels of the CNS may cause different pupillary abnormalities de-

ABNORMAL PUPIL SIZE

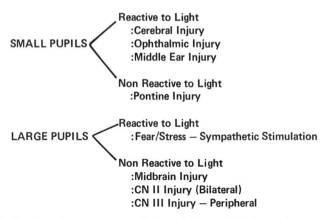

SMALL PUPILS
  Reactive to Light
    :Cerebral Injury
    :Ophthalmic Injury
    :Middle Ear Injury

  Non Reactive to Light
    :Pontine Injury

LARGE PUPILS
  Reactive to Light
    :Fear/Stress — Sympathetic Stimulation

  Non Reactive to Light
    :Midbrain Injury
    :CN II Injury (Bilateral)
    :CN III Injury — Peripheral

Fig. 9-4.   Evaluation of abnormal pupil size. (Fenner WR: Head trauma and nervous system injury. In Kirk RW (ed): Current Veterinary Therapy VIII—Small Animal Practice. W.B. Saunders, Philadelphia, 1983.)

pending on the combination of sympathetic/parasympathetic involvement (Fig. 9-4).[3,4,25] Generally cerebral diseases do not cause pupillary abnormalities, although occasionally an animal is seen with an acute cerebral injury and smaller-than-normal pupils. The small pupils of cerebral injury are usually reactive to light. Diencephalic disease may cause a first-order Horner's syndrome in which the pupils are smaller than the normal pupil and yet still responsive to light. Lesions at the level of the midbrain affect both the sympathetic and parasympathetic innervation to the eye, causing a fixed and midrange pupil that is nonresponsive to light and does not dark-adapt; that is, the pupil gets neither larger in the dark nor smaller when a penlight is directed into it. A lesion outside the midbrain affecting the peripheral cranial nerve III, such as may be seen in the early stages of cerebral herniation, paralyzes the pupillary constrictor muscle without involvement of the sympathetic nerve. In this injury the result is a fixed and dilated pupil that is nonresponsive to light. Lesions in the pons occur caudal to the level of cranial nerve III and involve predominantly the sympathetic fibers. Patients with pontine lesions frequently have pinpoint pupils that are nonresponsive to light. Metabolic disorders which affect the CNS generally do not affect the pupils significantly. If they do, the pupils usually become smaller than normal but remain reactive to light.

When evaluating eye movements, it must be remembered that voluntary eye movements are under cerebral control, and involuntary eye movements are under vestibular and brainstem control. In patients with abnormal consciousness, there is usually no opportunity to test voluntary eye movement. Thus the emphasis is on evaluating the resting ocular position and the involuntary eye movements. At rest, both eyeballs should be facing in the same direction or have what is known as conjugate gaze. Deviation of one eye away from or toward the other eye is known as strabismus. Strabismus may result from either a vestibular imbalance in muscle tone or paralysis of one of the extraocular muscles. Primary ophthalmic disease, e.g., retrobulbar masses, glaucoma, or other primary orbital disease, may also result in strabismus. Most ocular deviations of neural origin are either medial or ventrolateral. A medial deviation occurs with paralysis of cranial nerve VI, and a ventrolateral deviation with either cranial nerve III injury or vestibular injury.[3,4,25] After noting the presence or absence of strabismus and its direction, if present, the Doll's eye maneuver (creating physiological nystagmus) is performed by moving the animal's head from side to side. In a normal animal nystagmus is generated, the fast component of which is in the direction the head is turned. In animals with cerebral disease, the initial or slow component of this nystagmus is generated but not the fast or completing component. In these patients the eyes deviate away from the direction the head is being turned and remain there. When the head motion is stopped, the eyes return to the midline. This is known as the Doll's eye phenomena and suggests cerebral dysfunction. If on turning the head from side to side there is no movement at all (neither a fast nor a slow component), a brainstem injury or bilateral peripheral vestibular disease is suspected. If the Doll's eye phenomenon is present in one eye but not in the other, it suggests paralysis of the extraocular muscles in the involved eye. If the Doll's eye movement is present and normal in all respects in a patient with an abnormality in the level of consciousness, a primary cerebral disease is indicated.

After performing the Doll's eye maneuver, the patient is evaluated for the presence of spontaneous or pathologic nystagmus. This is evidence of vestibular dysfunction, which suggests that the patient has a brainstem or cerebellar injury. A normal animal at rest demonstrates no nystagmus. If nystagmus is present, it is called pathologic nystagmus.

The remainder of the cranial nerve examination as outlined in any text of neurology and the spinal reflex examination are completed. Other features that are of critical importance when evaluating patients with altered consciousness are posture and muscle tone, respiratory pattern, and nuchal rigidity. Generally patients with alterations of consciousness have an increase in muscle tone because of involvement of the upper motor neurons. With certain lesions, however, there may be variations on this typically increased muscle tone. A selective lesion in the midbrain may cause decerebrate posturing. In this situation there is total release of all of the vestibulospinal and reticulospinal facilatory pathways to the antigravity muscles of the body, which then creates an opisthotonic posture where the head is extended, and there is severe extensor rigidity in all four limbs. This opisthotonic posture may also be seen in cerebellar disease, although these diseases are not typically associated with abnormalities in consciousness. Lesions in the pons may selectively destroy the vestibular apparatus and allow the inhibitory motor system to predominate over the facilatory fibers. These animals with pontine destruction may have a hypotonic muscle paralysis, yet because the lesion involves the upper motor neuron, reflexes are normal or exaggerated.[28] These reflex changes allow one to separate the hypotonic upper motor neuron paralysis from the hypotonic lower motor neuron paralysis. Occasionally an animal with a diffuse cerebral injury or an acute spinal cord injury also has a hypotonic upper motor neuron paralysis by an unknown mechanism.

The respiratory pattern is evaluated next, remembering that in veterinary medicine specific respiratory patterns are not of much value. However, animals with cerebral disease generally have normal respirations if the disease is organic in nature. Metabolic cerebral diseases, on the other hand, may cause either hyper- or hypoventilation, depending on the specific disease, which can also lead to certain acid-base changes. (See discussion in Chapter 4.) Animals with brainstem disease frequently have ataxic or irregular respirations (Chapter 3). These patients seem to breathe in response to no particular stimulus, such that they may breathe rapidly for a while, not breathe at all for a while, breathe slowly for a while, and so forth.

Finally, the animal is evaluated for neck pain or nuchal rigidity. A variety of inflammatory diseases of the CNS may cause neck pain and marked increases in the tone of the neck muscles, resulting in typical nuchal rigidity. The finding of meningeal irritation is of tremendous value in differentially diagnosing the disorder causing the coma in an animal.

Diagnosis

The diagnosis of the patient with coma requires a history for toxins and metabolic disease, a neural examination looking for lateralizing signs, etc., and a complete laboratory work-up. The latter consists of a complete biochemical profile as well as an evaluation of the acid-base status. A complete hematologic screen may indicate the presence of severe inflammatory disease as well as lead poisoning. An ophthalmoscopic examination may reveal evidence of increased intracranial pressure, e.g., papillitis or papilledema, or the presence of inflammatory lesions that may support the diagnosis of encephalitis and meningitis.

Patients with coma can be divided into three basic etiologic groups (Table 9-1). The first of these is comprised of patients with a structural mass lesion that causes the coma. These patients frequently have abnormal and asymmetrical signs on the neurologic examination as well as abnormal pupils and eye movements. Moreover, because there is a primary CNS disease the spinal fluid, the CAT scan, and the EEG are frequently abnormal. Etiologic considerations in this group include CNS hemorrhage or infarction, brain trauma, neoplasia, focal encephalomyelitis, and granulomatous diseases which may cause focal lesions.

The second group contains patients who have a diffuse or multifocal disease rather than a mass causing the coma. These are representative of the inflammatory diseases of the CNS. The animals generally show symmetrical or inconsistently asymmetrical motor signs. Frequently the neurologic examination does not show abnormalities of the pupils, but the animals often have

Table 9-1. Classification of Coma

Neurologic Findings	Etiologic Considerations
Structural mass lesions[a]	
Asymmetrical motor signs	CNS hemorrhage secondary to systemic
Abnormal pupils	bleeding disorders
Abnormal eye movements	CNS infarction due to thrombosis or embolism
Signs progress in an orderly fashion	(hypothyroidism, feline ischemic
CSF often abnormal	encephalopathy)
	Epidural and subdural hemorrhage secondary
	to brain trauma
	CNS neoplasia
	Focal encephalomyelitis
	Granulomatous disease (granulomatous
	meningoencephalitis, fungal infections,
	parasite migration)
	Reticulosis
Structural generalized lesions[b]	
Neck pain present	Encephalitis
Abnormal CSF	Toxoplasmosis
Abnormal reflexes	Cryptococcosis
	FIP
	Canine distemper
	Other infections
	Meningitis
	Subarachnoid hemorrhage
Metabolic disorders[c]	
Usually normal reflexes	Intoxication
Normal pupils	Metabolic disturbances (diabetic acidosis,
Normal CSF	uremia, addisonian crises, hepatic coma,
	hypoglycemia, hypoxia)
	Severe systemic infections
	Circulatory collapse (shock) from any cause
	Epilepsy—postictal behavior
	Hyperthermia or hypothermia
	Concussion

[a] With or without changes in the CSF, often have focal or lateralizing signs.

[b] With blood or excess of white blood cells in CSF; usually without focal or lateralizing signs, often have meningismus.

[c] No alteration of cellular count of CSF, no focal or lateralizing signs.

Adapted from Fenner WR: Quick Reference to Veterinary Practice. Lippincott, Philadelphia 1982.

nystagmus or other abnormal eye movement. Animals in this group may also be febrile, have neck pain, and show abnormal CSF. Inflammatory disease processes in this group are toxoplasmosis, cryptococcosis, feline infectious peritonitis (FIP), and canine distemper. Patients with subarachnoid hemorrhage are also included in this group.

The final group contains patients with metabolic diseases. These patients generally have normal neurologic examinations except for altered consciousness. They have no focal or lateralizing signs. This etiologic group includes all the various intoxications and metabolic disturbances. Severe systemic infections may produce coma of metabolic origin as a result of shock or endotoxemia. Postictal epileptic patients and those with head trauma may also have nonorganic coma.

Treatment

Treatment of the patient with altered consciousness centers around diagnosis and treatment of the underlying disorder (Table 9-1). Nonspecific, supportive treatment of the comatose patient is provided. The animal is maintained in a high-oxygen environment with the head elevated above the rest of the body. The oxygen helps prevent CNS acidosis and hypoxia, which potentiates CNS edema. These patients are intubated and placed on a respirator if depression of their respiratory centers is seen. The head is elevated to help decrease intracranial pressure and prevent passive venous congestion of cranial venous sinuses.[14] The animal is turned frequently to prevent body sores, and the bladder and bowels are evacuated on a regular basis. Both decubital sores and urinary infections from inadequate evacuation of the bladder are frequently seen in comatose patients. Decubital ulcers can be prevented by maintaining the patient on a soft padded bed or on a water bed. Urinary tract infections and pyelonephritis are best prevented by frequent sterile intermittent catheterization or manual expression of the bladder. Indwelling urinary catheters tend to promote urinary tract infections as well as urethritis and are to be avoided if possible.

As patients with coma do not drink adequately, they frequently develop dehydration and electrolyte abnormalities. They lose water in excess of electrolytes through the respiratory tract and become markedly hypernatremic. Thus acid-base or electrolyte disturbances that arise during a prolonged state of abnormal consciousness must be corrected. Body temperature is monitored and hypo- or hyperthermia is corrected as rapidly and as effectively as possible. Aspiration of normal pharyngeal and oral secretions may serve as a source of aspiration pneumonia. In addition, patients with underlying metabolic disease may be vomiting; if so, special care is needed to prevent aspiration pneumonia from the vomitus. Pulmonary congestion from failure to turn frequently and aspiration pneumonia are major complications in patients with abnormal consciousness that can often be prevented by frequent turning and proper airway management. Septicemia from infection of decubital wounds can occur, and so any decubital sores are vigorously treated in an attempt to prevent this complication. The patient with abnormal consciousness is both a diagnostic and a therapeutic challenge but one that is not considered a hopeless cause without a complete and thorough evaluation. After determination of the etiology and institution of proper therapy for that condition, the patient should begin to improve quickly. Patients who persist in coma for greater than 3–4 days despite therapy generally have a very guarded prognosis for recovery.

MENINGITIS/ENCEPHALITIS

Etiology and Pathophysiology

Encephalitis and meningitis are inflammations of the nervous system or adjacent tissues. Specifically, encephalitis refers to inflammation of the brain; it may also involve the supporting structures, e.g., the vessels and meninges, or it may involve only the parenchyma. Meningitis is an inflammation of the meninges, not involving the nervous tissue primarily. Because there is such a close and intimate relationship between the brain parenchyma and its supporting structures, e.g., meninges, most cases of inflammation of the nervous system involve both meninges and neural parenchyma and are therefore called meningoencephalitis, or meningoencephalomyelitis if they involve the spinal cord as well as brain.

Inflammations and infections of the CNS may be caused by a variety of etiologies that include viral diseases (e.g., canine distemper, feline infectious peritonitis, rabies, and pseudorabies), protozoal diseases (e.g., toxoplasmosis), mycotic infections (e.g., cryptococcosis, blastomycosis, and histoplasmosis), parasitic diseases (e.g., *Cuterebra*), rickettsial diseases, bacterial diseases, and a variety of unclassified inflammations of the CNS, especially granulomatous meningoencephalomyelitis of dogs and cats and polioencephalomyelitis of cats.[1,16,17,20–22]

Inflammation of the CNS tends to produce patchy lesions that are disseminated throughout the CNS. For this reason they frequently produce multifocal signs because they produce a number of lesions in different parts of the nervous system. Each of those lesions causes a set of signs referable to that anatomic location. While performing the neurologic examination, combinations of abnormalities are found as well as historical complaints that cannot be explained by a lesion in one anatomic location, thus leading to a diagnosis of a multifocal disease process.

Infections of the CNS may produce a variety of pathologic changes that result in clinical signs. Predominant among these is necrosis of gray matter, which results in destruction of neurons and sometimes neurologic deficits, e.g., weakness, visual deficits, or epilepsy. Proliferation of astrocytes to form scar tissue may also damage the CNS, resulting in further neurologic deficits. Injury to oligodendroglia causes white matter demyelination, resulting in even further loss of functional integrity of the CNS. In addition to the inflammatory changes noted in the nervous system itself, there may be a primary inflammation of the blood vessels (vasculitis) or vasculitis secondary to the meningitis, either of which may result in infarction of CNS parenchyma.[1,4]

Infections of the CNS characteristically produce a variety of inflammatory cells that may be located within the infected tissue itself, in necrotic areas, or around blood vessels (perivascular cuffs). In encephalitis alone without inflammation of the meninges or the ependyma, there may be no cells shed into the CSF.[14] On the other hand, if the animal has ventriculitis, ependymitis, or meningitis, cells are shed into the CSF. A determination of the cell type provides etiologic information after CSF collection. These inflammatory cells may be mononuclear cells, e.g., lymphocytes or macrophages, or they may be polymorphonuclear leukocytes (neutrophils). Predominantly neutrophilic pleocytosis is expected in severe acute viral infections and bacterial infections. A mixed mononuclear/polymorphonuclear infiltrate is seen in chronic granulomatous diseases, parasitic diseases, and protozoal diseases. A primarily or purely mononuclear infiltrate is most frequently seen in conjunction with viral infections or chronic or resolving infections of other etiologies.[4,14]

Clinical Syndromes

Clinically inflammatory and infectious diseases of the CNS may be categorized as progressive diseases usually having an acute or subacute onset. They are typically multifocal or diffuse in distribution; however, some may form local abscesses or granulomas and thus result in predominantly focal signs. If meningitis is a component of the disease, significant neck pain is usually seen. A careful neurologic examination can uncover the diffuse nature of the disease. Many of these disease processes have an associated fever, and they are often associated with retinal abnormalities, demonstrated by careful ophthalmoscopic examination. The diagnosis of meningitis/encephalitis in dogs and cats requires a thorough history: for prior respiratory disease (which suggests canine distemper encephalomyelitis), for previous exposure to other animals with infectious diseases, for association with herds of cattle and/or swine (which may serve as a source of pseudorabies virus infection), and for free-roaming with animals (placing them in high-risk categories for exposure to toxoplasmosis, fungal diseases, rabies, etc). The neurologic examination may reveal systemic illness in cats with feline infectious peritonitis, in dogs or cats with toxoplasmosis or systemic fungal infections, and in dogs with canine distemper. Cats with cryptococcosis frequently have chronic rhinitis and a mucopurulent nasal discharge.

Diagnostic tests of importance in patients with inflammatory diseases of the CNS include CSF collection and analysis, EEG, and serologic studies. The most significant infections in canine neurology are canine distemper encephalomyelitis, toxoplasmosis, cryptococcal meningoencephalitis, granulomatous meningoencephalitis, and rabies. Of these, probably the most prevalent and the most severe is canine distemper encephalomyelitis. This disease seems to produce several fairly distinctive clinical syndromes which appear to have distinct predilections based on the age of the animal.

Canine Distemper Virus. The young animal is most likely to suffer from a gray matter disease caused by canine distemper virus that affects predominantly the cerebrum and brainstem. The clinical signs include acute onset of seizures, profound vestibular disease, distemper myoclonus (chorea), and visual abnormalities. The animals with the neuronal or gray matter form of canine distemper frequently have systemic illness concomitantly with the CNS disease. This includes primarily gastrointestinal and respiratory disease but may also include ocular disease as well. These animals may have chorioretinitis, and their CSF frequently reveals a nonsuppurative pleocytosis, with mild to moderate protein elevations. Moreover, they are most likely to be positive serologically for canine distemper virus infection.

The second form of canine distemper virus infection occurs in mature dogs and is a multifocal white matter demyelinating disease. These animals tend to have predominantly brainstem, cerebellar, and vestibular signs. They may also display spinal cord signs, e.g., caudal paresis or monoparesis. They have gradual progression of their clinical signs, eventually culminating in death. These animals generally do not have evidence of cerebrocortical disease (i.e., dementia and/or seizures). The majority of these animals do not have any concomitant clinical systemic illness, although they may have a history of suffering canine distemper virus infection when they were puppies. Retinal examination may reveal old chorioretinitis or an active exudative lesion. CSF examination may reveal a nonsuppurative cellular pleocytosis, or it may be totally normal. Serology may be performed on these animals to test for canine distemper virus infection.

The third clinical subgroup of neurologic canine distemper virus infection also occurs in mature animals and is known as "old dog encephalitis." This is another subacute progressive disease but is limited primarily to the cerebrum and rostral brainstem. These animals display profound abnormalities in mentation, vision, and gait, and they often have marked personality changes, e.g., failure to recognize the owner or head pressing. Seizures are rarely reported in animals with "old dog encephalitis." The CSF in these animals is usually normal, and immunofluorescence testing of the conjunctiva may be negative. The primary differentiating feature between the chronic demyelinating encephalomyelitis (CDE) of distemper and old dog encephalitis (ODE) is the predominance of cerebral signs in ODE and the predominance of brainstem/cerebellar signs in dogs with CDE.[1,4,25] Both seem to be manifestations of canine distemper, and both carry grave prognoses.

Postvaccinal canine distemper encephalitis may be seen as well. It usually occurs in younger animals and is characterized primarily by personality changes and other mentation abnormalities. Clinical signs usually begin within a couple of weeks of vaccination and progress rapidly. These animals generally have minimal systemic signs of illness, and the diagnostic work-up may be normal.

Granulomatous Meningoencephalitis/Reticulosis. The second major cause of encephalitis in dogs is granulomatous meningoencephalomyelitis (GME), also called inflammatory reticulosis. This is a disease of unknown pathogenesis that may affect animals at any age although it is generally seen in adults. The disease has a predilection for brainstem and cerebellum; therefore ataxia, pathologic nystagmus, head tilt, weakness of limbs, and cranial nerve deficits are the most common signs. They occur asymmetrically and reflect a multifocal disease process. Because of the meningitis, these animals may have remarkable neck pain and persistent fever. They may also have papillitis or optic neuritis, although many have a normal fundic examination. Animals with GME usually do not have any evidence of systemic illness. The signs in GME typically wax and wane and frequently are steroid-responsive. The CSF often shows a mixed mononuclear/polymorphonuclear pleocytosis with a very high white blood cell (WBC) count accompanied by a moderate to marked elevation of CSF protein as well. The disease carries a guarded to grave prognosis, although steroids may cause temporary remissions.

Feline Infectious Peritonitis. The most common encephalomyelitis in cats is that of feline infectious peritonitis (FIP). This disease causes a vasculitis with an associated pyogranulomatous inflammation of ependyma and meninges. These animals show predominantly cerebellar and vestibular signs, but they may have associated brainstem, spinal cord, and occasionally cerebral signs as well. Animals with FIP frequently have vascular lesions in the eyes, causing anterior uveitis and chorioretinitis. They also may have evidence of systemic illness associated with weight loss, depression, and mild anemia. Occasionally animals have the pleural and peritoneal effusions that are typical of "wet" FIP; however, the majority with nervous system involvement have the noneffusive or "dry form" of FIP. Cats with FIP frequently have marked serum globulin elevations and occasionally have hyperviscosity syndrome with sludging of blood and thus vascular accidents. CSF collection and analysis on these animals reveals a pyogranulomatous inflammation consisting of mixed mononuclear and polymorphonuclear leukocytes in the CSF with moderate to marked elevation of protein. Currently, treatment of FIP has limited success.[1]

Feline Polioencephalomyelitis. Polioencephalomyelitis has also been reported in cats. It is a slowly progressive disease process that affects cats of any age. The signs tend to revolve around the vestibulocerebellar system and result in ataxia, tremor, and head tilt. The animals may develop paresis of limbs as well. Seizures have also been reported with this disorder. These animals frequently are systemically ill with nonspecific bone marrow suppression, including leukopenia, myeloid hypoplasia, and anemia. The disease is progressive and does not seem to respond to medical treatment.[1]

Rabies. Those infectious disease processes of the CNS which affect both dogs and cats include rabies, pseudorabies, fungal diseases, and toxoplasmosis. Rabies is a viral disease affecting the CNS that may infect all warm-blooded animals. The disease has a variable incubation period depending on the route of inoculation, the size of inoculum, and the location of the wound. After the development of clinical signs, rabid animals usually have a short clinical illness that lasts less than 2 weeks and results in profound brainstem paralysis and death. Rabid animals generally show nonspecific cerebral signs first, including personality changes, aggression, dementia, and excitability. These signs then progress to the brainstem signs or to "dumb rabies." In the dumb form of rabies there is profound brainstem paralysis with involvement of multiple cranial nerves. This includes pharyngeal and laryngeal paralysis (which causes excessive salivation), paralysis of cranial nerve V (which paralyzes the jaw), and facial paralysis. As a result of pharyngeal and laryngeal paralysis, there is a decrease in the strength of the vocal muscles and therefore a change in the voice. The severe brainstem involvement causes paralysis of the limbs as well as of the cranial nerves. These animals generally die of respiratory failure within a few days of the development of the brainstem signs.

Animals begin shedding rabies virus up to 3 days before clinical signs are exhibited and continue to shed them throughout the course of the clinical illness. Therefore animals suspected of having rabies are treated with caution because of the potential for human infection. Diagnosis of rabies is based on postmortem examination of tissues and documentation by fluorescent antibody tests. Mouse inoculation and serology have also been used, and currently there is promise of antemortem diagnosis available with fluorescent antibody staining of hair follicles. CSF collection in patients with rabies tends to show a mild to moderate nonsuppurative cellular inflammatory response and mild protein elevation. The CSF in rabies may be normal as well.

A clinical syndrome following vaccination for rabies has been reported in dogs and cats; it is characterized by progressive lower motor neuron paralysis beginning in the hind limbs. Generally, these animals have progression of weakness and loss of reflexes in all limbs, beginning in the vaccinated limb and progressing to the front. The signs usually begin 12–14 days after vaccination. Clinical recoveries have been reported with this condition, and the animals are not believed to be infectious.

Pseudorabies. Pseudorabies is a viral infection of the CNS caused by a herpes virus. Animals usually become infected after ingestion of contaminated meat from pigs. For this reason, it is usually seen in animals from rural and/or farm environments. The clinical signs of pseudorabies are characterized by intense pruritus, brainstem signs, seizures, and acute death. The clinical illness is usually acute in onset, rapid in progress, and fatal. Animals may be found dead with no antecedent clinical illness. The hallmark of this disease is an intense and severe pruritus that results in profound self-mutilation. If the virus travels up cranial nerve V, the pruritus is predominantly around the head and/or face and results in a syndrome similar to tic douloureaux. The CSF reveals an increase in WBCs and protein.

Toxoplasmosis. Toxoplasmosis is a protozoan disease caused by *Toxoplasma gondii*. Infected animals are frequently free-roaming and therefore have access to rodents and/or birds, which are a major source of infection. Cat feces may also serve as the inoculum for the disease. Toxoplasmosis is associated with multifocal necrosis and hemorrhage in the CNS and may occur in any region of the CNS. The signs are unpredictable but generally are acute in onset and progressive. The animals may have evidence of a systemic illness, especially respiratory disease, and may have a granulomatous chorioretinitis. The CSF may contain an increase in both WBCs and protein, although it may also be normal. The treatment for toxoplasmosis consists of folic acid inhibitors, e.g., pyrimethamine, in combination with sulfonamides.

Cryptococcosis. Cryptococcosis is the most common fungal infection of the CNS of dogs and cats, and is discussed as the representative fungal infection of the CNS. Fungal infections primarily cause a granulomatous meningitis and ependymitis, with secondary involvement of the brain parenchyma. The clinical signs are variable depending on the area of greatest involvement, and they may reflect involvement of any portion of the CNS. There may be cranial nerve involvement if the granulomas involve the cranial nerves as they exit the brainstem. Generally, the clinical signs are gradually progressive. The animals frequently have systemic illness, especially respiratory disease. Other dissemination sites include bone, skin, lymphoid tissues, liver, and gastrointestinal tract. Granulomatous chorioretinitis is frequently seen with all of the fungal infections, and many of the patients have anterior uveitis as well.

CSF examination in these animals reveals a granulomatous inflammation with both mononuclear and polymorphonuclear leukocytes and mild to moderate elevations of protein. Fungal infections sometimes cause an eosinophilic CSF pleocytosis as well. The fungal organisms may be seen in CSF, especially with cryptococcal infections. The organisms can often be demonstrated on smears of nasal exudate or draining fistulas from skin infections. The use of serology may be beneficial in the diagnosis of this disease.

Treatment of fungal infections currently consists of the use of either intravenous amphotericin B or oral ketoconazole. Ketoconazole has proved to be an effective treatment for the various systemic fungal infections, and although expensive it has less severe side effects than amphotericin B.

Bacterial Meningitis.   Bacterial meningitis has been reported in the dog.[22] Although an uncommon disease, it is one that should be in the differential diagnosis of an animal who presents with acute neck pain, fever, and nuchal rigidity. Signs of CNS parenchymal involvement are not common, although weakness and ataxia may occur with bacterial meningitis. Occasionally cranial nerve dysfunction is found, especially in animals who develop an abscess at the site of involvement.

The diagnosis of bacterial meningitis is based on finding large numbers of WBCs, predominantly polymorphonuclear neutrophils (PMNs), in CSF, high CSF proteins, and organisms either phagocytized with PMNs or free in the CSF. The diagnosis is further confirmed by positive bacteriologic culture. *Staphyloccocus* spp. and *Pasteurella* are the predominant organisms in bacterial meningitis in the dog. Treatment consists of administering high levels of an antibiotic that is known to cross the blood-brain and CSF-brain barriers. Such drugs include chloramphenicol, the sulfonamides, trimethoprim, and cephalosporins. In addition, penicillin and ampicillin usually cross the blood-brain barrier adequately in the face of inflammation. The majority of patients respond well to treatment.

Nonbacterial Suppurative Meningitis.   A nonbacterial suppurative meningitis has been reported in young dogs, especially beagles, that by CSF cytology could be confused with bacterial meningitis.[16,17,20,21] These animals are febrile and have severe neck pain. The meningitis is not antibiotic-responsive. The disease normally waxes and wanes, so initially it may seem to be partially antibiotic-responsive. The underlying lesion is vasculitis, which in most cases seems to be steroid-responsive. Patients suspected of having this condition should not be treated with steroids until the CSF cultures are confirmed as being negative.

Treatment and Prognosis

Overall, the therapy of meningitis and encephalitis is geared to the underlying disorder. Certain common themes run through the therapy of all infectious disorders of the CNS: adequate supportive therapy, anticonvulsants for the seizuring patient, and treatment of secondary infection. Other than that, there is no effective therapy for a viral infection. The protozoal and fungal disorders may be treated with appropriate antimicrobials; however, success seems to be limited. Bacterial diseases should be treated vigorously with antibiotics. The success rate is higher in these disorders.

Long-term sequelae of CNS infections include seizure disorders which are often refractory to anticonvulsants, permanent mental or personality disorders, weakness, ataxia, and sensory disturbances. It is impossible to predict during the acute illness which of the clinical signs are from actual destruction of neural parenchyma and which represent loss of function because of edema or some other reversible process. Thus even in the treatable infections of the CNS, the prognosis remains uncertain through much of the clinical course of the illness.

THE BRAIN-INJURED PATIENT

Brain injury may arise from a variety of causes, including automobile accidents, falls from apartments, and missiles. Of these, the most common are automobile accidents. Many patients suffer head injury that does not create brain injury.[10,11] All patients with head injury should have a careful historical, physical, and neurologic evaluation to search for brain injury, and only those in whom brain injury is present are treated.

Pathophysiology

The patient with brain injury suffers a variety of direct and indirect effects on its nervous system that may result in neurologic or systemic clinical signs. Direct effects include skull fractures, cerebral contusions cerebral lacerations, etc. Secondary effects include brain edema with elevation of intracranial pressure, bleeding, hypoxia.[19] The secondary effects may rapidly follow the injury and so may be present at the time the animal is seen. Because these secondary effects are the most amenable to treatment, they are emphasized in the following discussion.

The brain is a complex and living organ enclosed within a rigid space. It is permeated with blood vessels and is surrounded and perfused by CSF. The relative volumes of these three components are in balance, and any increase in the volume of one is at the expense of the others. An increase in volume of one greater than the ability of the other two components to compensate results in elevations of intracranial pressure. These pressure increases can result in shifts of a brain component with further destruction of neural tissue.[14,19] The major secondary effects of brain injury that the veterinarian must try to treat or prevent are hypoxia/ischemia, brain edema, and elevations of intracranial pressures. Intracranial hematomas are an uncommon finding in veterinary medicine and generally are not treated as there are few ways to accurately diagnose them.

Brain hypoxia or ischemia is a major contributor to brain damage in traumatic brain injury. The brain is able to store only limited amounts of glucose and O_2; therefore a constant supply of both is required to prevent ischemic or hypoxic brain damage. A fall in blood pressure leads to decreased tissue perfusion. Decreases in O_2 saturation of the blood also cause tissue hypoxia. The result of this hypoxia/ischemia is a progressive impairment of neuronal function and the generation of CNS acidosis. This further diminishes neural function as well as promotes brain edema. Methods that have been promoted to prevent the deleterious effects of hypoxia include hypothermia, barbiturates, and steroids. The most beneficial effect comes from restoration or preservation of blood flow.[14,19]

Brain edema may result from vasogenic or cytotoxic mechanisms. In vasogenic edema there is leakage from vessels into the extracellular space, primarily affecting white matter. Cytotoxic edema is primarily a gray matter disorder consisting of increases of fluid within neurons. With head trauma the principal form of edema is vasogenic. The edema creates an increase in intracranial pressure, which may potentiate brain herniation. Edema also promotes further hypoxic injury. This edema may be resorbed through the vessels or pass via bulk flow into CSF where it is cleared. There is some feeling that steroids may help prevent vasogenic edema and improve its rate of clearance. Raising the arterial pressure is known to potentiate formation of vasogenic edema, whereas decreasing arterial pressure decreases its formation.[14]

Elevations of intracranial pressure result in a number of clinical events, both systemic and neural. Systemic effects of elevated intracranial pressure include cardiac arrhythmias, subendocardial hemorrhage, arterial hypertension, neurogenic pulmonary edema, and gastrointestinal hemorrhage. Many of these events are potentially life-threatening in their own right, and the sum of them, i.e., pulmonary edema, cardiac arrhythmias, and arterial hypertension, may compound CNS hypoxia, edema, or both.[14,19]

The first neural response to elevated intracranial pressure is a decrease in CSF volume as a compensatory mechanism. If CSF outflow from the skull into the spinal column is interfered with, or if there is brain edema or venous engorgement, this compensatory mechanism is ineffective. A second compensatory mechanism is compression of venous sinuses, which results in a decrease in total intracranial blood volume. Finally, the brain attempts to compensate by decreasing extracellular fluid volume. Obviously edema or venous engorgement would block the last two compensatory mechanisms. As the pressure continues to increase, the brain around the expanding lesion(s) shifts, compressing other adjacent areas of brain. This shift, called herniation, may result in compression of vital cardiorespiratory centers and culminate in the death of the patient.

Treatment of the brain-injured patient is directed at preventing hypoxia, decreasing intracranial volume, and relieving elevations of intracranial pressure. Hypoxia may best be prevented by keeping the patient in a high-oxygen atmosphere and maintaining the systemic circulation. Decreasing the intracranial volume requires decreasing (or blocking increases in) CNS elastance, brain edema, CSF volume, and blood volume. Factors that increase intracranial elastance—and so in effect increase pressure responses to changes in brain volume—are increased CO_2, hypoxia, gas anesthetics (they are vasodilating), fever, and nitrous oxide. Agents which decrease elastance are decreased CO_2, increased O_2, hypothermia, and barbiturates. The reduction in elastance decreases the intracranial pressure responses to changes in volume.[14]

Brain edema is more difficult to treat; osmotic agents require an intact blood-brain barrier which is not present in vasogenic edema. Steroids are of debatable efficacy, and other drugs are unproved. Reducing the CSF may be done by decreasing its rate of production with drugs, e.g., carbonic anhydrase inhibitors. The elevation in pressure itself promotes more rapid CSF absorption. Decreasing blood volume may be accomplished by elevating the head to prevent engorgement of venous sinuses. Some drugs, e.g., morphine, diazepam, and pentazocine, increase intracranial pressure by increasing blood flow to the cerebrum.[14] As this may also help prevent hypoxia, their use provides a mixed blessing. In addition, they alter mentation, making further evaluation of the patient difficult.

Clinical Evaluation

In light of these principles regarding the pathogenesis of signs and symptoms seen with brain injury, what is the best clinical approach and treatment? It must be stated here that the author practices a conservative philosophy of therapy for brain-injured patients.[10,11,13]

Treatment is initiated by evaluating the life-threatening nonneural injuries and treating them appropriately. Special attention is paid to the cardiovascular and respiratory systems, as failure to rapidly and completely correct cardiac or respiratory insufficiency may result in exacerbation of CNS signs. After the patient is stabilized, a rapid but complete neurologic examination is performed, combined with a careful examination of the skull for fractures and evaluation of the eye and orbit for local injuries that would confound the neurologic examination. During the neurologic examination special attention is paid to the level of consciousness, pupil size and symmetry, eye movement, and spinal reflexes (refer to the section on abnormal consciousness for added discussion). The information gained from this examination assists in determining if the patient has a peripheral or a central injury and allows early assessment of severity for prognostic purposes. It is very important to record all findings to allow accurate assessment of changes in neural status.[3,4,25]

Many of the patients with head trauma have peripheral nervous system (PNS) injury without, or in combination with, brain injury. Except in the case of vestibular injury, these abnormalities are easy to recognize as a PNS injury, as loss of function of a cranial nerve is present with no other signs. PNS injuries generally do not require therapy. Vestibular injury, on the other hand, causes disorientation, rolling, falling, nystagmus, and ataxia. For these reasons, in the absence of a critical neural examination, vestibular injury may be confused with a brain injury. The features which allow it to be recognized as a PNS vestibular injury include the preservation of consciousness, a normal physiological nystagmus, normal pupillary light reflexes (there may be a Horner's syndrome, which does not affect pupil responsiveness), and preserved strength and reflexes. These patients may have hemorrhage in or rupture of the tympanic membrane on otoscopic examination.[4] Most of these animals do not require therapy, but light restraint may be needed to prevent further self-inflicted injury. In summary, PNS injuries are usually complete (i.e., total loss of function of the involved nerve); they rarely require treatment; and with the exception of vestibular injuries, they rarely cause signs beyond the focal loss of function.[10,11,13]

In the brain-injured patient, the neural examination may show an altered consciousness. If the patient is demented or delirious, it indicates a cerebral injury. If the patient is in a stuporous or comatose state, the injury may be either a diffuse cerebral disorder or a focal brainstem injury. The brainstem injury carries a much worse prognosis in general than the cerebral injury.[4,10] Pupil size, responsiveness, and eye movements help separate the patients with cerebral injury from those with brainstem injury (Figure 9-4).

First, one should see if the pupils are larger or smaller than normal and then test for light-responsiveness. If the pupil is small but still responds to light, the veterinarian should be concerned about a cerebral injury, a middle ear injury, or iritis secondary to a primary ophthalmic injury. If the pupil is small but does not respond to light, it is more likely a sign of a brainstem-pontine injury. If the pupils are large but still responsive to light, they are probably simply reflecting stress with high levels of sympathetic stimulation. If they are large and nonresponsive to light, however, it could reflect a cranial nerve III (CN III) injury (either midbrain or peripheral) or a bilateral optic nerve injury. After pupil size has been evaluated, the patient is checked for strabismus at rest. A ventrolateral strabismus may be seen with lesions of CN III or CN VIII; it may also be seen with retrobulbar hematomas. A medial strabismus may reflect CN VI injury or injury to the lateral rectus nerve. If the animal has resting nystagmus, whether spontaneous or induced it represents a vestibular system injury, which could include injuries to peripheral CN VIII, brainstem, or cerebellum. Next, the doll's eye response (or physiological nystagmus) is tested. If a doll's eye phenomenon can be obtained in both eyes, the brainstem vestibular system is intact, as well as CN III, IV, and VI. If nystagmus cannot be obtained and the abnormality is confined to only one eye, a lesion of either CN III, IV, or VI is suspected in the affected eye, or a lesion of the globe itself and its muscular attachments. The absence of eye movement in both eyes indicates either a lesion of peripheral CN VIII that is bilateral or a lesion of the brainstem.

When testing posture, the concern is the presence or absence of opisthotonic or decerebrate posturing. If the animal has spasms of extensor rigidity of all four legs with arching of its back and hyperextension of the neck, he has one of these two postures. Opisthotonus represents a cerebellar injury, so this patient has normal consciousness. Decerebration represents a midbrain lesion, which is associated with coma and abnormal pupils. Decerebrate posturing usually suggests a very severe injury with a grave prognosis.

Table 9-2. Evaluation of Spinal Reflexes in Spinal Cord Injury

Site of Injury	Reflexes	Signs
C1–C4 vertebrae C1—C5 spinal segments	UMN all four limbs	Tetraparesis
C5–T1 vertebrae C6–T1 spinal segments	LMN front UMN rear	Tetraparesis Possible Horner's syndrome
T2–L2 vertebrae T2–L2 spinal segments	Normal front UMN rear	Rear-limb paralysis
L3–L6 vertebrae L3–S3 spinal segments	Normal front LMN rear	Rear-limb paralysis Loss of anal reflex
L7–S2 vertebrae Cauda equina	Normal front Normal patella LMN sciatic LMN perineal	Can stand Decreased withdrawal Decreased anal tone

(UMN) upper motor neuron. (LMN) lower motor neuron.
Adapted from Fenner WR: Quick Reference to Veterinary Practice. Lippincott, Philadelphia 1982.

Spinal reflexes are also tested (Table 9-2). These help to separate peripheral from central injuries to cranial nerves, as well as allow detection of multiple injuries, i.e., spinal cord trauma in combination with brain injury.[3,4,25]

Treatment

After performing an examination and localizing the area of nervous system injury, therapy is instituted. The goals are to decrease the size of the intracranial mass, provide nutrient substrate (especially O_2), and if possible decrease the metabolic needs of the remaining neurons. A flow chart for evaluation and treatment of the head injury patient is depicted in Figure 9-5.

Although not proved beneficial, animals with brain injury are usually placed on corticosteroids. The author uses dexamethasone in a dose of 0.2 mg/kg body weight given as a single bolus. The same drug is then continued at the same dose level on a daily basis divided two or three times daily for 5 days. This dose is lower than many recommend, and the clinician must be guided by his own judgment in regard to steroid doses.[3,4,10–13,19,25] The animal is kept with the head elevated and is preferably maintained in a 40% O_2 atmosphere to prevent hypoxia and venous engorgement. Efforts to improve ventilation may be needed to prevent hypercarbia. Maintenance or slightly submaintenance intravenous fluids are given, but overhydration must be prevented. If there is significant neural dysfunction with no evidence of hemorrhage in middle ears or evidence of epistaxis, mannitol may be given to decrease cerebral edema and to decrease intracranial pressure. Mannitol 15–20% in a dose of 1 g/kg IV is given slowly. If the blood-brain barrier (BBB) is intact, this may cause significant reduction of intracranial pressure for 3–8 hr. If bleeding or a severely damaged BBB is present, the mannitol could worsen the brain

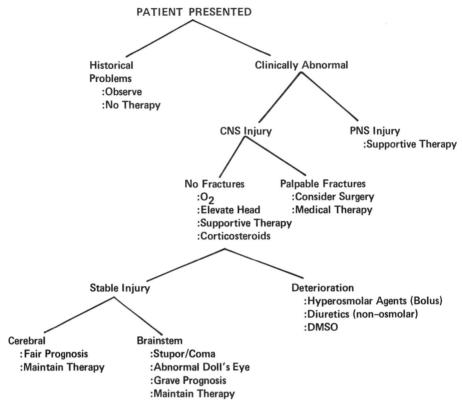

PATIENT PRESENTED

Historical
Problems
:Observe
:No Therapy

Clinically Abnormal

CNS Injury

PNS Injury
:Supportive Therapy

No Fractures
:O_2
:Elevate Head
:Supportive Therapy
:Corticosteroids

Palpable Fractures
:Consider Surgery
:Medical Therapy

Stable Injury

Deterioration
:Hyperosmolar Agents (Bolus)
:Diuretics (non-osmolar)
:DMSO

Cerebral
:Fair Prognosis
:Maintain Therapy

Brainstem
:Stupor/Coma
:Abnormal Doll's Eye
:Grave Prognosis
:Maintain Therapy

Fig. 9-5.   Evaluation and treatment of the patient with head injury. (Fenner, WR: Head trauma and nervous system injury. In Kirk RW (ed): Current Veterinary Therapy VIII— Small Animal Practice. Saunders, Philadelphia, 1983.)

injury. The mannitol may be repeated every 4 hr at 0.5 g/kg, but there is some evidence that only the first dose is effective.[14]

Light restraints may be necessary if the animal is delirious; and mild sedation may be used for chemical restraint when needed. If possible, the use of sedative drugs is to be avoided.

If the animal is seizuring, it is treated according to the protocol outlined earlier in this chapter, remembering that the anticonvulsant drugs may depress respiration, exacerbating CNS hypoxia.

The patient is continually monitored and reevaluated. If deterioration occurs, as evidenced by sudden changes in heart rate, consciousness, pupillary responsiveness, or loss of the doll's eye phenomenon, hypertonic agents are given. Deteriorating patients are also candidates for surgical exploration to look for removable hematomas. In the author's experience, surgery has generally been unrewarding or has not improved the final outcome.

Complications

The immediate sequelae of head trauma include cardiac arrhythmias and pulmonary edema. If these occur, they are usually transient and respond well to appropriate therapy. Long-term sequelae include epilepsy, hydrocephalus, and permanent neural deficit. The epilepsy may occur at the time of the brain injury, or its onset may be delayed for days or months. Posttraumatic epilepsy is usually amenable to maintenance anticonvulsant therapy. Hydrocephalus is not commonly seen but is associated with a rapid deterioration days or weeks after the injury. This condition may be managed with steroids or may require a shunting operation. The permanent neural deficits after brain injury may be compensated for over time, but they may be severe enough to make the animal an unacceptable pet.

SPINAL INJURY

Pathophysiology

Spinal cord injury is frequently associated with some form of external trauma to the body. It may be seen without injury to supporting structures or in association with intervertebral disk disease, vertebral fractures, or luxations of vertebrae. After the injury, there is an immediate hemorrhage and necrosis of both gray and white matter that spreads both cranial and caudal to the site of trauma. This is followed by a period of cord ischemia and loss of autoregulation of spinal cord blood flow. The ischemia promotes cord edema, which may result in local vascular compression, further compounding the ischemia.[29,31] In addition to these events within the cord, there is the possibility of external cord compression from bone, ligament, or disk material. There have also been some reports of compression by hematomas arising within the spinal canal secondary to the trauma.

Clinical Signs

Animals with spinal injury usually present with weakness or ataxia of limbs without evidence of head involvement. If the lesion is in the cervical cord, a Horner's syndrome may be seen. If fractures have occurred, severe neck or back pain is usually present. With cervical cord injuries there may be disruption of the pathways controlling respiration, and so hypoventilation may be seen. Animals with thoracic injury may have Schiff-Sherrington syndrome with release of front limbs from lumbar inhibition. This causes increased tone, with rigidity in the front limbs and retention of both normal reflexes and normal voluntary movement in front. This may lead to incorrect localization of signs to the cervical spine or an incorrect diagnosis of cervical as well as thoracic injury. The use of spinal reflexes in the diagnosis of spinal cord injury is described in Table 9-2.

Diagnosis and Treatment

Clinical management of these patients begins with treatment of life-threatening nonneural injuries. This is followed by a neural evaluation concentrating on the spinal reflex and the sensory examination. Spinal radiographs are obtained to determine the type of injury. If lumbar or sacral spinal injuries are present, the patient is carefully evaluated for rupture of the bladder. The patient is immobilized using external support. If there are no head injuries, mild sedation may be used if needed.

Therapy is directed at relieving the edema and compression, which are the two potentially reversible factors. Edema currently is treated by corticosteroids (dexamethasone 0.2–2 mg/kg/day). Use of DMSO and mannitol have been advocated, but their effectiveness is unproved. Experimentally, opiate receptor antagonists, antiprostaglandins, and β-blockers have been tried with promising results.[8,9,15,29,31,32] As yet, they are not well enough understood for us to advocate their routine use in clinical practice. Compression may be reduced by stabilization or reduction of fractures or luxations when present. Dorsal laminectomies are needed for some compressive lesions.

Nursing care is also vital in these patients. The bladder is emptied at least four times daily, and urinary antibiotics are administered if urinary tract infection develops. The patient is assisted to defecate, and mild bulk laxatives or stool softeners are sometimes needed in constipated patients. Soft bedding and frequent turning helps prevent decubital sores.

Many of these patients require surgical correction of their disease, the discussion of which is beyond the scope of this text. Surgery attempts to relieve spinal cord compression while stabilizing unstable lesions; but most importantly, procedures with a high risk of worsening the patient's condition are avoided.

Prognosis

The prognosis in spinal injury is determined by both the location and the severity of the injury. Cervical cord injuries frequently respond better than lumbar cord injuries. Gray matter injuries in general have a worse prognosis than white matter injuries. Injuries to the gray matter that directly innervates a limb are more severe than injuries which affect the tracts to a limb. A rapid way of using the clinical examination to judge the severity of a lesion is by using the preservation of voluntary movement and pain perception. An animal who is ambulatory and has preservation of voluntary movement usually has only a mild injury and a good prognosis. An animal who is nonambulatory but still has sensation and preserved voluntary movement has a moderate injury with fair prognosis. The paralyzed animal who has no voluntary motion but in whom pain sensation is intact has a major injury with a guarded prognosis. The animal who has loss of both voluntary motion and pain sensation has a very severe injury and a grave prognosis. One of the most common reasons for failure to determine the prognosis of spinal injury patients properly is the tendency to base the opinion on radiographs. An adequate prognosis requires a complete neural examination and an understanding of the location and severity of injury. Therapy also fails if spinal injuries are treated as pure orthopedic cases, as unnecessary reduction of fractures may exacerbate spinal cord injury.

REFERENCES

1. Braund KG: Encephalitis and meningitis. p. 31. In Crane SW (ed): Symposium on Trauma. Veterinary Clinics of North America. W.B. Saunders, Philadelphia, 1980, Vol. 10.
2. Brooks BR, Adams RD: Cerebrospinal fluid acid-base and lactate changes after seizures in unanesthetized man. Neurology 25:935, 1975
3. Chrisman CL: Problems in Small Animal Neurology. Lea & Febiger, Philadelphia, 1982
4. De Lahunta A: Veterinary Neuroanatomy and Clinical Neurology. Saunders, Philadelphia, 1983
5. Delgado-Escueta AV, Treiman DM, Walsh GO: The treatable epilepsies. Part one. N Engl J Med 308:1509, 1983
6. Delgado-Escueta AV, Treiman DM, Walsh GO: The Treatable Epilepsies, Part two. N Engl J Med 308:1576, 1983
7. Delgado-Escueta AV, Wasterlain C, Tremain DM, et al: Management of status epilepticus. N Engl J Med 306:1337, 1982
8. Faden AI, Jacobs TP, Holaday JW: Thyrotropin-releasing hormone improves neurologic recovery after spinal trauma in cats. N Engl J Med 305:1063, 1981
9. Faden AI, Jacobs TP, Mougey E, et al: Endorphins in experimental spinal injury: therapeutic effect of naloxone. Ann Neurol 10:326, 1981
10. Fenner WR: Diagnosis and treatment of traumatic injuries to the brain. In: Proceedings of The Kal Kan Symposium for the Treatment of Dog and Cat Diseases, Kal Kan Foods, Inc., Vernon, California, 1978
11. Fenner WR: Head trauma and nervous system injury. In Kirk RW (ed): Current Veterinary Therapy VIII, Saunders, Philadelphia, 1983
12. Fenner WR: Quick Reference to Veterinary Practice. Lippincott, Philadelphia, 1982
13. Fenner WR: Seizures and head trauma. p. 31. In Wingfield WE (ed): Sumposium on Emergency Medicine. Veterinary Clinics of North America. W.B. Saunders, Philadelphia, 1981, Vol. 11
14. Fishman RA: CSF in Diseases of the Nervous System. Saunders, Philadelphia, 1982
15. Hoerlein BF, Redding RW, Hoff EJ, et al: Evaluation of dexamethasone, DMSO, mannitol, and solcoseryl in acute spinal cord trauma. J Am Anim Hosp Assoc 19:216, 1983
16. Harcourt RA: Polyarteritis in a colony of beagle dogs. Vet Rec 102:519, 1978
17. Hoff EJ, Vandevelde M: Necrotizing vasculitis in the central nervous systems of two dogs. Vet Pathol 18:219, 1981
18. Holliday TA: Seizure disorders. Vet Clin North Am 10:3, 1981
19. Jennett B, Teasdale G: Management of Head Injuries. Davis, Philadelphia, 1981
20. Joshua JO, Ishmael J: Pain syndrome associated with spinal hemorrhage in the dog. Vet Rec 83:165, 1968
21. Kelly DF, Grunsell CS, Kenyon CJ: Polyarteritis in the dog. Vet Rec 92:363, 1973

22. Kornegay JN, Lorenz MD, Zenoble RD: Bacterial meningoencephalitis in two dogs. J Am Vet Med Assoc 173:1334, 1978
23. Montgomery DL, Lee AC: Brain damage in the epileptic beagle dog. Vet Pathol 20:160, 1983
24. Oliver JE: Protocol for diagnosis of seizure disorders in companion animals. J Am Vet Med Assoc 172:822, 1978
25. Oliver JE, Lorenz MD: Handbook of Veterinary Neurologic Diagnosis. Saunders, Philadelphia, 1983
26. Orringer CA, Eustace JC, Wunsch CD, et al: Natural history of lactic acidosis after grand-mal seizures. N Engl J Med 297:796, 1977
27. Plum F, Howse DC, Duffy TE: Metabolic effects of seizures. Res Publ Assoc Nerv Ment Dis 53:141, 1974.
28. Plum F, Posner J: The Diagnosis of Stupor and Coma. Davis, Philadelphia, 1980
29. Rawe SE, Lee WA, Perot PL: The histopathology of experimental spinal cord trauma. J Neurosurg 48:1002, 1978
30. Russo ME: The pathophysiology of epilepsy. Cornell Vet 71:221, 1981
31. Senter HJ, Venes JL: Altered blood flow and secondary injury in experimental spinal cord trauma. J Neurosurg 49:569, 1978
32. Young W, Flamm ES, Demopoulos HB, et al: Effect of naloxone on posttraumatic ischemia in experimental spinal contusion. J Neurosurg 55:209, 1981

10 | Ocular Emergencies

Carol M. Szymanski

Ocular or adnexal conditions which are acute or painful or may result in blindness or loss of ocular function are considered to be emergencies. Most ocular problems which present as emergencies are due to trauma—mainly contusions or lacerations of the globe, eyelids, or both. Many of these traumatic lesions require surgery. Unfortunately, medical ophthalmic emergencies, e.g., acute glaucoma, acute uveitis, or acute blindness due to optic neuritis or exudative retinal detachment, are often not perceived to be urgent. Thus these conditions are frequently presented too late in their course for therapy to be beneficial. This chapter is limited to the medical treatment of ocular emergencies.

ACUTE EXOPHTHALMOS—DISEASES OF THE ORBIT

Exophthalmos is defined as forward displacement of the globe. Any space-occupying lesion within the orbit, e.g., hematoma, abscess, pterygoid and extraocular muscle swelling of eosinophilic myositis, neoplasia, and zygomatic sialocele, may result in protrusion or displacement of the globe. Orbital trauma or infection are the most common causes of acute exophthalmos.

The signs of space-occupying orbital lesions include exophthalmos, protrusion of the nictitating membrane, chemosis, impairment of ocular motility, swelling of the eyelids, and lagophthalmos (inability to close the eye) with resultant corneal drying and ulceration. Pain upon opening the mouth, a sign of orbital cellulitis/abscess or eosinophilic myositis, has been attributed to pressure of the coronoid process of the mandible on the inflamed orbital contents.

Orbital Cellulitis/Abscess

Cellulitis or abscesses of the orbit may be due to oral or conjunctival foreign bodies, dental disease, or extension of nasal or frontal sinusitis. Infected bite wounds are a common etiology of orbital cellulitis in cats.

An acute onset of protrusion of the nictitating membrane, inflammation of the eyelids and conjunctiva, and variable degrees of exophthalmos are observed with orbital cellulitis. Lagophthalmos may be present, which results in corneal drying and predisposes to corneal ulceration. Systemic signs include depression and difficulty or reluctance in eating. The periocular area is warm and painful, and the patient resists opening of the mouth. Orbital cellulitis is generally but not invariably unilateral.

Diagnosis is based on the combination of signs of orbital inflammation and tenderness, oral pain, and a swollen erythematous area caudal to the last upper molar. Fever and leukocytosis are frequently present. General anesthesia is usually required for oral examination.

Treatment consists of providing ventral drainage of the orbital abscess. The erythematous area caudal to the last upper molar is lanced with a No. 15 Bard-Parker blade. A closed hemostat is inserted through the incision for a distance of approximately 2 cm and then opened. Purulent material may or may not drain from the incision, depending on whether an abscess or cellulitis is present. A swab may be inserted into the incision to obtain material for bacterial culture and antibiotic sensitivity tests. Smears obtained for cytology usually demonstrate degenerating polymorphonuclear leukocytes and bacteria (septic purulent inflammation). The drainage wound is swabbed with dilute providone-iodine (Betadine) solution. The oral cavity is also examined for foreign bodies, e.g., bones or sticks, and any infected teeth are extracted. In cats, periorbital abscesses may be drained over the site of maximum swelling, which is often at the dorsolateral rim of the orbit. Orbital abscesses in dogs and cats sometimes communicate with the conjunctival fornix. Such tracts may be probed to locate more abscess pockets or foreign bodies.

A parenteral broad-spectrum antibiotic is used initially for 2–4 days until the oral pain subsides, then oral antibiotics are given for an additional 7–10 days. Warm compresses are applied over the involved globe for 3–4 days. A soft diet is prescribed until the animal can masticate without pain. Clinical improvement is noted after ventral drainage has been established and appropriate antibiotic therapy instituted.

Eosinophilic Myositis

Eosinophilic myositis (masticatory muscle myositis) causes variable degrees of acute exophthalmos in dogs. Many breeds may be affected, but a higher incidence has been reported in German shepherds, golden retrievers, and Labrador retrievers[8]; it is characterized by exophthalmos, protrusion of the nictitating membranes, and chemosis. Lagophthalmos may be partial or complete, resulting in conjuctival and corneal exposure and drying. Exophthalmos has been reported to be due to involvement of pterygoid and extraocular muscles.[1] Accompanying involvement of temporal and masseter muscles causes marked pain upon opening the mouth. The etiology of masticatory muscle myositis is unknown, although an immune-mediated mechanism has been proposed.[4]

Diagnosis is based on the above signs and leukocytosis with or without eosinophilia. Serum concentrations of gamma globulin and creatinine phosphokinase (CPK) may be elevated.[4] Biopsy of the temporal or masseter muscle discloses infiltration with macrophages, lymphocytes, plasma cells, and eosinophils.

Acute eosinophilic myositis is treated with antiinflammatory doses of corticosteroids. Prednisolone acetate is used at 2 mg/kg IM BID for the first 48 hr until oral medication is possible. Oral prednisolone is used at 2 mg/kg for 5–7 days, then reduced gradually over 2 weeks. Response to corticosteroids is marked, but recurrence may be seen after 7–21 days, necessitating a repeated course of corticosteroid treatment. Complications include gradual fibrosis and atrophy of the muscles of mastication resulting in an inability to open the mouth and enophthalmos.

Proptosis

Traumatic proptosis is defined as forward displacement of the eye to the extent that the eyelid margins are posterior to the equator of the globe. Trauma associated with automobile accidents or dog fights are the most common causes. Brachycephalic breeds are predisposed to traumatic proptosis because of their shallow orbits and prominent globes.

Signs of proptosis are extreme anterior displacement of the globe, subconjunctival edema and hemorrhage, and lagophthalmos resulting in corneal dryness, ulceration, or both. The medial rectus muscle may be torn resulting in a laterally deviated globe. The presence of hyphema indicates damage to the uveal tract.

Traumatic proptosis is a true emergency; treatment is surgical and consists of replacing the globe within the orbit followed by a temporary tarsorrhaphy. A thorough description of this technique has been reported.[11] Medical therapy after surgical replacement of the globe and tarsorrhaphy consists of systemic corticosteroids and antibiotics. Prednisolone (2 mg/kg divided BID) is given for 2–4 days then 1 mg/kg for an additional 2–4 days or longer, depending on the extent of inflammation. A systemic broad-spectrum antibiotic is also given for 7–10 days.

The cornea and anterior segment must be assessed prior to replacement of the globe into the orbit. If corneal ulceration and secondary iritis are present, topical antibiotic and atropine ointments are placed three to four times daily between the tarsorrhaphy sutures at the medial canthus. If anterior uveitis is present and the cornea is not ulcerated, an antibiotic/corticosteroid ointment and atropine can be used. The injection of drugs into the retrobulbar area is not recommended as the orbit is already distended by retrobulbar edema and hemorrhage. Warm compresses may be applied 24 hr after the injury. Tarsorrhaphy sutures are generally removed in 10–14 days.

The potential complications of proptosis are dorsolateral deviation of the eye, keratitis sicca, lagophthalmos, and blindness. The globe may be deviated laterally and dorsally when the medial rectus and ventral rectus and oblique muscles are traumatized or avulsed. These muscle avulsions may be repaired surgically; however, the globe often slowly assumes a straight position without surgery within 4–6 months.

Keratitis sicca, which may be temporary or permanent, is another complication. Schirmer tear tests should be monitored after tarsorrhaphy sutures have been removed. Artificial tears, e.g., povidone (Adapt) or a petrolatum, lanolin, or mineral oil ointment (Duratears), are used to treat dry eye. Palsy of cranial nerve V may be present and predisposes to the development of keratitis sicca and corneal ulceration.

Temporary lagophthalmos may be due to orbital swelling, which subsides with time. Lagophthalmos in cases where orbital swelling is not present has been attributed to a temporary orbicularis (cranial nerve VII) palsy. Slight or partial lagophthalmos may be treated with artificial tears to prevent corneal drying. A temporary tarsorrhaphy may be reapplied for an additional 1–2 weeks if lagophthalmos is pronounced.

Blindness after proptosis may result from avulsion of or traction on the optic nerve. Intraocular damage, e.g., retinal detachment, lens luxation, or uveitis with subsequent intraocular fibrosis, may also result in blindness. A particularly poor prognosis for vision is associated with complete hyphema as this indicates damage to the iris, ciliary body, or both. Phthisis bulbi (atrophy of the globe) is frequently a sequel to complete hyphema.

EYELID LACERATIONS

Eyelid lacerations are not genuine emergencies but should be repaired promptly. One of the prime considerations when presented with an eyelid laceration is to determine if the underlying globe has been lacerated or otherwise injured. Lacerations of the globe itself warrant immediate surgical repair.

Full-thickness eyelid lacerations are repaired as soon as is feasible, provided the animal is stable for general anesthesia. Débridement of the laceration should be minimal, as extensive tissue loss from the eyelid compromises lid function. The eyelid margin must be carefully aligned. The reader is directed elsewhere[10] for a discussion of complete surgical management of eyelid lacerations, as these details are beyond the scope of this chapter.

CONJUNCTIVA

Subconjunctival Hemorrhage

Etiologies of subconjunctival hemorrhage are trauma (including over-zealous restraint) and bleeding disorders, e.g., thrombocytopenia, platelet dysfunction, widespread vasculitis, inherited coagulopathies, and warfarin poisoning. Therefore the animal is examined for extraocular petechiae or ecchymoses of the skin and mucous membranes so systemic bleeding disorders are not overlooked. The fundus is examined in cases of trauma or spontaneous hemorrhage.

Simple subconjunctival hemorrhage is not truly an emergency, but its appearance frequently alarms owners such that they present animals to emergency clinics. Subconjunctival hemorrhage due to trauma gradually resorbs without treatment within 7–14 days.

Subconjunctival hemorrhage is occasionally so extensive the conjunctiva balloons out between the eyelids, preventing their closure and resulting in corneal and conjunctival drying. Artificial tears in an ointment base (Duratears) are given every 2 hr. If the cornea is ulcerated, a topical broad-spectrum antibiotic ointment containing neomycin/polymyxin B/bacitracin (Neosporin) is indicated. An alternative treatment is a temporary tarsorrhaphy to close the eyelids over the protruding conjunctiva until the hemorrhage has resorbed.

Conjunctival Foreign Bodies

Conjunctival foreign bodies are most frequently plant material, e.g., grass awns, thorns, or seeds, which may lodge within the conjunctival fornices or behind the nictitating membrane. This is seen most commonly in dogs who have been running in fields.

Ocular pain results in the acute clinical signs of blepharospasm, epiphora, and rubbing of the eye. A careful examination is performed after instillation of a topical anesthetic, e.g., proparacaine HCl (Alcaine). A bright light source and magnifying loupe are extremely useful examination aids. The eyelids and the nictitating membrane are everted with a blunt Adson tissue forceps and a strabismus hook.

A conjunctival foreign body usually may be wiped away with a cotton swab. If the foreign body is embedded, ophthalmic forceps may be used to extract it, or the tip of a 25-gauge needle may be used to flick it out of the conjunctiva. Conjunctival inflammation resolves rapidly after removal of a foreign body. If corneal ulceration is present, a topical broad-spectrum antibiotic ointment is used until corneal epithelialization occurs.

CORNEA

Corneal Foreign Bodies

Foreign material, e.g., grass awns, thorns, wood splinters, and seed hulls, may become embedded in the cornea. Inorganic foreign bodies, e.g., glass or metal, are less frequently encountered. Signs are those of severe pain manifested as blepharospasm, tearing, and rubbing at the eye.

Topical anesthesia with proparacaine is sufficient to permit visualization and removal of most superficial corneal foreign bodies. Irrigation with eyewash or normal saline dislodges foreign bodies adhering to the corneal surface. If the foreign material cannot be dislodged with irrigation, it may be lifted from the cornea with the tip of a 25-gauge needle.

Foreign bodies which are embedded within the corneal lamellae may also penetrate the anterior chamber. Removal of such foreign bodies requires general anesthesia. In many cases the protruding end of the foreign body may be gently extracted from the cornea with a small pair of forceps.

If the foreign body is embedded entirely within the cornea, a small incision is carefully made with a No. 11 Bard-Parker blade over the foreign body so it can be grasped and withdrawn. If the anterior chamber has been entered, aqueous humor will leak from the wound opening after the foreign body has been extracted. In some instances, a small corneal wound has a beveled edge and seals spontaneously. If the corneal wound is larger, the edge must be sutured with 6-0 to 7-0 absorbable suture material.

Treatment after removal of a corneal foreign body consists of topical and systemic broad-spectrum antibiotics. Anterior uveitis is generally present and is treated with 1% atropine ophthalmic solution. Treatment continues until the cornea has epithelialized and inflammation has resolved.

Corneal Lacerations

Full-thickness corneal lacerations with or without iris prolapse require prompt surgical management. A description of the surgical technique can be found elsewhere.[10]

Superficial Corneal Ulcers

Uncomplicated (noninfected) corneal ulceration denotes loss of corneal epithelium and may be due to trauma, soap burns, chemicals, or corneal foreign bodies. Superficial ulcers are common in dogs and cats.

The presenting signs include acute, intense blepharospasm, epiphora, and conjunctivitis. Superficial ulcers are more painful than deep ulcers because the sensory nerve supply to the cornea (cranial nerve V) lies within the superficial one-third of the cornea.

Loss of corneal epithelium is easily demonstrated with fluorescein dye. A superficial, uncomplicated ulcer has distinct edges without cellular infiltration. A drop of 0.5% proparacaine facilitates examination of an acutely painful eye. Conjunctival or corneal foreign bodies are also looked for, especially if an ulcer is adjacent to the nictitating membrane.

Uncomplicated superficial ulcers heal within 72 hr. A topical broad-spectrum antibiotic is recommended to prevent bacterial infection. An ointment containing neomycin/polymyxin B/bacitracin (Neosporin) is instilled three or four times daily until the ulcer has epithelialized. Comparable antibiotic solutions may be used instead of ointments, but they need to be given twice as often.

Anterior uveitis, characterized by a miotic pupil, aqueous flare, and photophobia, may occur secondary to a superficial corneal ulcer. The anterior uveitis is treated with 1% atropine sulfate ophthalmic ointment two or three times daily until the pupil is dilated, then once daily.

Corticosteroids are contraindicated in corneal ulceration because they inhibit epithelial regeneration.[7] The prognosis for superficial, noninfected corneal ulcer is good; healing usually occurs with minimal scarring.

Deep Corneal Ulcers

Ulcers which involve one-third or more of the corneal thickness are considered to be serious, as progression of this type of ulcer may result in corneal perforation. The etiologies of deep or complicated ulcers are the same as for superficial ulcers, but microbial infection is also present. Bacterial keratitis may be due to *Streptococcus*, *Staphylococcus*, *Pseudomonas*, or *Proteus*. *Pseudomonas* is the most devastating bacterial pathogen because it may result in corneal perforation within 48 hr. Brachycephalic dogs with lagophthalmos or keratitis sicca are predisposed to corneal ulceration. Mycotic keratitis is uncommon in dogs and cats. Herpes virus is a cause of severe, often chronic corneal ulceration in cats.

Signs of bacterial keratitis are mucopurulent ocular discharge and variable degrees of blepharospasm. The ulcer is usually axial and crater-like and is characterized by rapid progression. The edges of the ulcer are edematous with white stromal infiltrates. A descemetocele, the deepest of corneal ulcers, appears as a clear membrane at the bottom of a crater-like defect. It may indicate impending corneal perforation. The elastic properties of Descemet's membrane allow it to lie flat or to bulge outward. A descemetocele does not retain fluorescein dye.

Hypopyon, sterile polymorphonuclear leukocytes within the anterior chamber, arises from the leukotactic stimulus of certain bacterial exotoxins, particularly those derived from *Pseudomonas*. Secondary uveitis is usually present with deep corneal ulcerative keratitis.

A "melting" ulcer is an acute severe corneal ulcer which is complicated by liquefactive necrosis (keratomalacia) of the corneal stroma due to the presence of destructive enzymes. Lysozymes and hydrolases are derived from degranulating polymorphonuclear leukocytes, mononuclear phagocytes, and damaged corneal epithelial and stromal cells.[3] These enzymes digest the corneal ground substance. Collagenase, derived from necrotic corneal stroma, lyses collagen, the major structural component of the cornea. In addition, certain bacteria, particularly *Pseudomonas aeruginosa*, may produce a protease which lyses the corneal ground substance.[2] The combined effect of these enzymes is liquefactive necrosis of the cornea, which may progress to perforation within 24–48 hr. A "melting" ulcer has a characteristic gelatinous, edematous appearance and is frequently accompanied by hypopyon.

Treatment of deep "melting" ulcers depends on the cause; laboratory confirmation is needed to select appropriate antimicrobials. Corneal culture is done with a moistened cotton-tipped applicator or calcium alginate swab (Calgiswab). Topical anesthetics are not put into the eye as they contain preservatives which may inhibit bacterial growth. The swab is gently rubbed against the edge and base of the ulcer. The specimen is placed in transport medium and submitted to a commercial laboratory or directly streaked onto blood agar, MacConkey agar, or thioglycollate broth.

After instillation of a topical anesthetic, the edge of the corneal ulcer may be gently scraped with a Kimura platinum spatula or a Bard-Parker blade handle. Material from the scraping is spread across a glass slide and stained with gram stain.

Initial selection of antibiotics is aided by use of the gram stain. If gram-negative rods are obvious, *Pseudomonas* is assumed to be present unless another organism is cultured. Dogs with "melting" ulcers are ideally hospitalized to provide intensive treatment and to evaluate response to therapy, as progression to corneal perforation may occur rapidly. Among the antibiotics commercially available for topical ophthalmic use, only gentamicin, polymyxin B, and tobramycin are effective against *Pseudomonas*. Treatment is applied every 2 hr if an ointment is used and twice as frequently if a solution is chosen. One percent atropine ointment is used every 2–4 hr for the secondary anterior uveitis and to alleviate deep ocular pain associated with ciliary spasm. Equal parts of acetylcysteine 20% (Mucomyst 20%) and povidone (Adapt) are combined in an eyedropper bottle, and this solution is used every 2–4 hr as a protease-collagenase inhibitor.[3] The solution is kept refrigerated to prevent oxidation. After 60 days, a refrigerated solution of Adapt/Mucomyst retains 60% of its activity (G. Severin, personal communication, 1981).

Once it is determined that the ulcer has not increased in circumference or depth, and that the keratomalacia is resolving, the dog may be sent home with the topical antibiotic, topical atropine, and the Adapt/Mucomyst mixture to be given every 3–4 hr. Reevaluation is essential within 24 hr. Treatment with the antibiotics continues for 5–7 days after the ulcer has epithelialized to eliminate bacteria from the corneal stroma.

If a descemetocele is present initially, or if a deep ulcer worsens despite medical therapy, surgery is indicated. A thin bulbar conjunctival flap or a corneoscleral conjunctival transposition provides support and fibrovascular tissue to aid corneal healing.[13]

ANTERIOR UVEA

Acute Uveitis

Acute uveitis is an emergency, as it is a painful condition which may result in permanent blindness. Inflammation of the iris and ciliary body is referred to as anterior uveitis. Inflammation of the choroid is termed posterior uveitis or choroiditis. Panuveitis refers to inflammation of the entire uveal tract.

Etiologies of uveitis are multiple (Table 10-1). In clinical practice, however, the precise etiology of many cases of uveitis is never determined. Immune-mediated mechanisms are prominent factors in many types of uveitis regardless of etiology. A thorough history and physical examination are essential when attempting to elucidate the etiology of uveitis. Complete blood counts, appro-

Table 10-1. Etiology of Uveitis

Bacterial
    Leptospirosis
    Brucellosis
    Tuberculosis
Viral
    Canine adenovirus type 1 (CAV-1)
    Feline infectious peritonitis
    Feline lymphosarcoma
Parasitic
    Toxoplasmosis
    Rocky Mountain spotted fever (*Rickettsia rickettsii*)
    Dirofilaria immitis (aberrant migration)
    Ehrlichiosis
Mycotic
    Blastomycosis
    Cryptococcosis
    Histoplasmosis
    Coccidiomycosis
Neoplasia
    Lymphosarcoma
    Primary or metastatic intraocular tumor
Traumatic
Secondary to corneal ulcers

priate serologic tests, and, in cases of severe inflammation, aqueous or vitreous culture and cytologic studies may aid diagnosis.

Pain and blepharospasm are nonspecific signs of uveitis. Specific signs include miosis, photophobia, aqueous flare, injection of perilimbal vessels (ciliary flush), iris edema, and ocular hypotony. Hyphema and inflammatory cells may be present within the anterior chamber. Blindness may be the presenting sign in cases of severe uveitis.

Treatment of uveitis consists of cycloplegics, corticosteroids, and antiprostaglandins. Atropine (1% or 2%) is the cycloplegic agent of choice in all cases of uveitis.[7] This drug relieves ciliary spasm, pain, and photophobia; it also dilates the pupil and minimizes the likelihood of synechia formation. Atropine is administered every 2–4 hr until the pupil is dilated and then once or twice daily thereafter. Severe anterior uveitis in which the pupil is resistant to dilation with atropine may be treated with a combination of scopolamine and phenylephrine (Murocoll-2) every 4–6 hr.

A potent topical corticosteroid, dexamethasone ointment (Maxidex), is used every 2–4 hr. Exceptions to the use of corticosteroids are corneal ulceration and mycotic disease. If posterior uveitis or panuveitis is present, the corticosteroid must be given systemically as topical medication does not reach the posterior segment. Oral prednisolone is used at a dosage of 2 mg/kg initially and gradually tapered. Some authors recommend subconjunctival medication, but in this author's opinion the systemic route is more readily controllable and thus the preferred route.

Aspirin is beneficial in all cases of uveitis for its antiprostaglandin effect. The dosage of aspirin in the dog is 10–25 mg/kg every 8 hr.[14] Flunixin meglumine (Banamine), although not approved for use in dogs, has been used as a prostaglandin inhibitor for uveitis at a dosage of 0.125 mg/kg IV every 24 hr for up to three doses (M. Wyman, personal communication, 1983).

Hyphema

Hyphema, blood within the anterior chamber, has multiple etiologies, including trauma, bleeding disorders, anterior uveitis, hypertension, lymphosarcoma, chronic glaucoma, intraocular tumors, and congenital intraocular anomalies. The most common cause of hyphema in dogs and cats is trauma. The usual source of hyphema is bleeding from the iris or ciliary body; less frequently it is choroidal or retinal bleeding.

The opposite eye should always be examined for: (1) retinal hemorrhage, which may incriminate a systemic bleeding disorder, vasculitis, or hypertension; or (2) congenital anomalies, e.g., optic nerve colobomas or retinal dysplasia. In addition, a thorough history and general physical examination may aid in determining the etiology of hyphema.

The treatment of hyphema depends on its etiology, extent, and duration. If anterior uveitis is not present, 1% pilocarpine may be given two or three times daily for 2–3 days to facilitate the outflow of red blood cells through the iridocorneal angle.[11] In many cases, an iridocyclitis accompanies hyphema, particularly traumatic hyphema. Pilocarpine is not used in these cases as it would intensify ciliary spasm and increase the likelihood of synechia formation with a miotic pupil. Hyphema with concomitant uveitis is treated with topical 1% atropine ophthalmic ointment and a topical corticosteroid. Intraocular pressure is monitored daily because of the danger of complicating glaucoma. Daily observation determines the duration of treatment. Sedation and cage rest or restriction of exercise is recommended to minimize the possibility of rebleeding.

Secondary glaucoma is a serious but infrequent complication of hyphema and may result from iris bombé, peripheral anterior synechiae, or red blood cells or inflammatory debris occluding the drainage angle. This is not an acute development. These cases are treated with dichlorphenamide (Oratrol), a carbonic anhydrase inhibitor which reduces aqueous production, and a topical adrenergic drug, e.g., epinephrine borate (Eppy 1%).

Phthisis bulbi (atrophy of the globe) may occur after extensive hyphema and is a sequela to severe intraocular trauma and fibrosis.

Acute Glaucoma

Glaucoma, an elevation of intraocular pressure above the normal range of 15–27 mm Hg, is a complex disease, and its discussion in this chapter is confined to acute congestive glaucoma in the dog.

Acute congestive glaucoma is a true ocular emergency that is seen in dogs, particularly in those breeds predisposed to primary glaucoma—basset hounds, beagles, cocker spaniels, norwegian elkhounds, poodles,[5] and others. It is generally a unilateral problem, although the opposite eye usually becomes affected at a later date in predisposed breeds. Acute congestive glaucoma is uncommon in cats.

Signs of elevated intraocular pressure are corneal edema, episcleral congestion, a dilated pupil, and reduced vision or blindness. The eye is painful, and affected animals are frequently lethargic or exhibit behavior changes, e.g., hiding or irritability. Intraocular pressure in acute congestive glaucoma frequently exceeds 50 mm Hg.

The diagnosis is made by the determination of intraocular pressure with a tonometer. The most available type of tonometer for a small animal practice is the Schiötz tonometer. Although this instrument has been calibrated for the human eye and underestimates pressure in the dog eye, it can, with practice and proper positioning on the center of the cornea, be valuable in the diagnosis of glaucoma.

The goal of the medical management of acute glaucoma is to rapidly reduce intraocular pressure so that vision is restored and pain is alleviated. Treatment must be prompt and aggressive as permanent damage to retinal ganglion cells may occur if intraocular pressure remains elevated above 40 mm Hg for 24 hr or more. Treatment of acute glaucoma consists of the use of three drug groups which reduce intraocular volume, decrease aqueous formation, and increase aqueous outflow.

Systemic hyperosmotic agents are indicated in acute glaucoma as the initial step to rapidly reduce intraocular pressure. The mechanism of action is the increase of serum osmolarity and subsequent dehydration of the vitreous, which is 98% water.

Two types of hyperosmotic agents are available: glycerol and mannitol. Glycerol may be given orally at a dosage of 1–2 ml/kg.[5] Vomition due to gastric irritation is a common side effect. Mannitol 20%, which is more effective than glycerol, is given intravenously at a dosage of 1–2 g/kg.[5] The maximum effect of hyperosmotics occurs within 1 hr after administration, and the duration of action is 4–8 hr. Water is withheld from the dog for 3–4 hr after the administration of mannitol or glycerol.

A carbonic anhydrase inhibitor, e.g., dichlorphenamide or acetazolamide, is given immediately after administration of the hyperosmotic drug to maintain lowered intraocular pressure. These drugs decrease the formation of aqueous humor by 20–30%.[5] Dichlorphenamide (Oratrol) is preferred because it has minimal side effects in the dog. The dosage is 2–5 mg/kg daily in two or three doses.[12] Acetazolamide (Diamox; 6–10 mg/kg BID–TID) is also an effective carbonic anhydrase inhibitor, but side effects (acidosis, depression, and emesis) limit its long-term use. It must be stressed that furosemide (Lasix), although an excellent diuretic, is not a carbonic anhydrase inhibitor and has no effect on aqueous humor production.

Topical miotics, the cholinergic and anticholinesterase drugs, increase the outflow of aqueous and may be used alone or with a carbonic anhydrase inhibitor. Pilocarpine, a direct-acting parasympathomimetic agent, is the most frequently used cholinergic drug. The 2% solution is considered to be the most effective in the dog and is used three or four times a day initially right after the administration of the hyperosmotic drug.[5,10] Higher concentrations are no more effective and are much more irritating. Some ophthalmologists use the potent, irreversible anticholinesterase miotics, e.g., demecarium bromide, isoflurophate, and echothiopate, for long-term maintenance therapy of certain glaucomas.

Intraocular pressure is measured 45–60 min after administration of the hyperosmotic drug and again in 4–6 hr, at which time the miotic and the carbonic anhydrase inhibitor should have begun to exert their effects. Once the intraocular pressure is close to the normal range, maintenance therapy may consist of a miotic, a carbonic anhydrase inhibitor, or other drugs alone or in combination.

If minimal or no response is obtained with medical therapy, a variety of surgical procedures, including cyclocryotherapy may be required. Surgical management of glaucoma is described elsewhere.[5,10]

ACUTE BLINDNESS

There are a variety of etiologies of acute blindness: glaucoma, uveitis, retinal detachment, and optic neuritis. Acute glaucoma and uveitis have been previously discussed.

Acute Exudative Retinal Detachment

A syndrome of sudden bilateral blindness in healthy dogs has been observed as a result of idiopathic retinal detachment.[6] Signs are an acute onset of bilateral blindness with dilated or sluggish pupils and exudative retinal detachments. The detached retinas may be observed through the dilated pupils and appear as elevated, grayish veils. A mild anterior uveitis and/or optic neuritis are occasionally present. The retinal detachment results from exudation of fluid from the choroid, which elevates and detaches the overlying retina. The etiopathogenesis is unknown.

The differential diagnosis of retinal detachment in general includes mycotic disease, lymphosarcoma, toxoplasmosis, myeloproliferative disease, multiple myeloma, and protothecosis. These diseases are generally accompanied by systemic signs, and vision loss usually develops gradually and may not be bilateral. Diagnosis is based on the combination of sudden bilateral blindness in otherwise healthy dogs due to exudative retinal detachments. A complete physical examination, complete blood count, and biochemical profile are recommended to rule out systemic disease.

Treatment is prednisolone 2 mg/kg for 5–7 days, then 1 mg/kg for an additional 5–7 days or longer. Clinical improvement should be noted after 4–5 days of treatment as the subretinal fluid resorbs, the retinas reattach, and the dog regains vision. Systemic antibiotics and furosemide have also been used,[6] and corticosteroids alone can be effective. Prognosis is considered to be good.

Optic Neuritis

Optic neuritis is a clinical syndrome characterized by acute onset of blindness and dilated pupils which are nonresponsive or minimally responsive to light stimulation. Optic neuritis is not common, but it is an occasional cause of acute blindness in dogs. Etiologies include peracute canine distemper, lead poisoning, reticulosis, granulomatous meningoencephalitis (GME), cryptococcosis, and lymphosarcoma.[9] Acute optic neuritis is rare in cats and has been observed with lymphosarcoma. Many cases of optic neuritis in animals are idiopathic.

The presenting signs of optic neuritis are sudden bilateral blindness and dilated pupils with minimal or absent pupillary light reflexes. Ophthalmoscopic examination may disclose a swollen optic disk with indistinct margins, which is referred to as papillitis. Frequently blindness occurs when only the retrobulbar portion of the optic nerve is involved even though the optic disk may appear normal. The retina is uninvolved in cases of optic neuritis.

The diagnosis depends on the presenting signs of acute blindness, dilated or sluggish pupils, normal retinas, and either normal disks or papillitis. A thorough physical examination with emphasis on the neurologic examination are important, as dogs with reticulosis or GME frequently have other neurologic deficits. If neurologic abnormalities are present, skull radiographs and cerebrospinal fluid analysis may aid in diagnosis. A complete blood count and biochemical profile are also recommended.

Optic neuritis is treated with high levels of systemic corticosteroids. Prednisolone 2 mg/kg is given for 5–7 days; then 1 mg/kg is given for an additional 5–7 days or longer, depending on the response. Alternate-day therapy may be used if vision improves. Corticosteroids are discontinued if vision does not improve after 2 weeks.

Many cases of optic neuritis are idiopathic, and response to corticosteroids is variable. Reticulosis may initially improve with corticosteroid treatment, but progression of the disease is the usual outcome. The prognosis of optic neuritis is guarded, and optic atrophy often results.

Atypical Retinal Degeneration

Dogs occasionally present with a history of sudden blindness and normal-appearing retinas. The history is suggestive of optic neuritis, but treatment with corticosteroids is unsuccessful. Electroretinograms are extinguished, indicating retinal degeneration which has developed without the typical ophthalmoscopic signs of choroidal furrowing, tapetal hyperreflectivity, or vascular attenuation. The etiology is unknown.

REFERENCES

1. Bistner SI, Aguirre G, Batik G: Atlas of Veterinary Ophthalmic Surgery. Saunders, Philadelphia, 1977
2. Brown SI, Bloomfield SE, Wai-fong T: The cornea-destroying enzymes of Pseudomonas aeruginosa. Invest Ophthalmol Vis Sci 13:174, 1974

3. Brown SI, Hook, CW, Tragakis MP: Presence, significance, and inhibition of lysosomal proteoglycanases. Invest Ophthalmol Vis Sci 11:149, 1972

4. Duncan JD, Griffiths JR: Inflammatory muscle disease in the dog. In Kirk RW (ed): Current Veterinary Therapy. pp. 779–782. Saunders, Philadelphia, 1980

5. Gelatt KN: The canine glaucomas. In Gelatt KN (ed): Veterinary Ophthalmology. pp. 390–434. Lea & Febiger, Philadelphia, 1981

6. Gwin RW, Wyman M, Ketring K, Winston S: Idiopathic uveitis and retinal detachment in the dog. J Am Anim Hosp Assoc 16:163, 1980

7. Havener WH: Ocular Pharmacology. Mosby, St. Louis, 1978

8. Koch S: Diseases of the orbit. In Kirk RW (ed): Current Veterinary Therapy. p. 583. Saunders, Philadelphia, 1980

9. Nafe L, Carter J: Canine optic neuritis. Comp Contin Educ 3:976, 1981

10. Slatter DH: Fundamentals of Veterinary Ophthalmology. Saunders, Philadelphia, 1981

11. Wyman M: Ocular Emergencies. In Kirk RW (ed): Current Veterinary Therapy. p. 545. Saunders, Philadelphia, 1980

12. Wyman M: The eye. In Catcott EJ (ed): Canine Medicine. p. 1317. American Veterinary Publication, Santa Barbara, CA, 1979

13. Wyman W: Ophthalmic surgery for the practitioner. Vet Clin North Am 9:328, 1979

14. Yeary RA, Brant RJ: Aspirin dosages for the dog. J Am Vet Med Assoc 167:63, 1975

11 | Toxicologic Emergencies

Debra S. Barrett
Frederick W. Oehme

There are literally hundreds of potential toxicoses that a small-animal practitioner may encounter during the course of his daily routine. Although a few of these may be easily identified and treated, many poisonings are difficult to define and treatment must be initiated before a definitive diagnosis has been reached. Fortunately, there are basic guidelines which may be followed to prolong the animal's life until laboratory or other assistance is available.

GENERAL EMERGENCY MANAGEMENT OF INTOXICATIONS

First Aid

The first contact a veterinarian may have with a possible poisoning case occurs via the telephone. Careful questioning to determine the onset and progression of clinical signs, as well as the presence and accessibility of rodenticides, pesticides, drugs, paints, and other potential sources, may provide enough circumstantial evidence to suggest a tentative diagnosis. However, often the most essential aspect of successfully treating a poisoning case is admitting the animal to the hospital as quickly as possible; detailed questions must be left for a later time. It depends on the professional judgment of the veterinarian, based on the clinical facts and the client's attitude, which of the following *first aid instructions* should be given over the telephone:

1.   Remove the possible source of the poisoning. The clients are cautioned to protect both themselves and their animal from further contamination.

2.   Induce vomiting (syrup of ipecac 1–2 ml/kg orally, 5 ml hydrogen peroxide orally every 5 min, or 1 teaspoon of salt in the back of the mouth).[2] Any vomitus should be placed in a clean container and retained by the client as an aid in later identifying the poison involved. Vomiting should not be initiated if the animal has consumed a strongly acidic or alkaline substance, or a petroleum product, tranquilizer, or other antiemetic. It is probably wise not to recommend this type of first aid unless the poison is known, the animal is asymptomatic and has not yet vomited, and the owner is calm.

3.   Administer egg whites or milk in cases where strong acids or alkalis are involved.

4.   In cases of skin or eye contact with a toxic or corrosive material, wash the area with large quantities of water.

5.   If the animal is excited, avoid as much additional harm to the animal and the people involved as possible. Wrapping in a blanket or even muzzling may be required.

6.   Proceed to the hospital without delay. The sample or container of suspected poison and any vomitus should be brought along as diagnostic and treatment aids.

Treatment Principles

Upon arrival of a poisoning case, the first priority is *establishment and maintenance of vital signs.*[7] It may be necessary to establish a patent airway by intubation or to control seizures before securing more details of the history. All information pertinent to the poisoning episode, as well as the age, sex, breed, feeding schedule, and past illnesses and immunizations of the animal, are kept for future reference and need in possible legal action.

Once the veterinarian is reasonably confident poisoning is involved, efforts are made to *prevent further absorption of the toxicant.* Animals exposed dermally are thoroughly cleansed with water, and emesis may be considered to remove any toxic material still remaining in the stomach following ingestion. Apomorphine is the professional drug of choice (0.04 mg/kg IV or 0.08 mg/kg IM or SC)[7] for inducing vomiting, but syrup of ipecac, hydrogen peroxide, or table salt may be tried in its absence. (For contraindications, see "First Aid," No. 2.) The efficacy of emesis may be increased by prior administration of a slurry of activated charcoal, but in all cases induction of vomiting is with only minimal benefit if 2 hr or more has elapsed since the time of ingestion.[2]

Gastric lavage is helpful in removing any unabsorbed toxic material from the stomach of an unconscious or anesthetized patient. A cuffed endotracheal tube is inserted before passage of a large-bore stomach tube (e.g., 0.5 inch diameter for a 10- to 20-kg dog),[2] and the head of the animal is lowered slightly to prevent aspiration of stomach contents. Ten to 15 cycles of injecting and then aspirating 100–300 ml of tap water is usually sufficient, but the washings should continue until two consecutive washes are completely clear.[2] (*Remember*: the first few washings are kept for chemical analysis.) Following lavage, a thick slurry of activated charcoal (2–8 g/kg body weight in a concentration of 1 g charcoal/5–10 ml water)[7] is administered via the stomach tube and allowed to remain in the stomach. The passage of the black charcoal in feces is a practical indication that the digestive tract contents have been emptied since the time of poisoning.

Activated charcoal is an efficient adsorbent and is valuable when used in combination with emesis or gastric lavage. Although it has no effect on toxins already absorbed into the animal's bloodstream, it is effective in preventing absorption of most toxic materials remaining in the stomach after emesis or gastric lavage. It may also adsorb poisons that have passed into the intestine before stomach emptying. Suitable commercial preparations of activated charcoal include Norit (American Norit), Nuchar C (West Virginia Pulp and Paper), and Darco G-60 (Atlas Chemical).[7] A grape-flavored activated charcoal already in slurry form and compressed tablets are also available and avoid the untidiness associated with the powdered activated charcoal.

As an additional precaution to prevent absorption of toxins from the intestinal tract, a laxative is administered or colonic lavage performed approximately 1 hr after the activated charcoal treatment. Sodium sulfate (0.6–0.8 g/kg orally)[7] is preferable to magnesium sulfate as a cathartic. Mineral or vegetable oils, followed by a saline cathartic in 30–40 mins, may be suitable substitutes when lipid-soluble poisons are involved.[7] Colonic lavage is performed by administering approximately 1 L of warm water (to which a mild soap, salt, or activated charcoal may be added) rectally via an enema tube. The fluid is allowed to run in by gravity flow and is removed by placing the tube outlet below the level of the animal's body. Repeat this procedure several times, being sure to retain the colonic washings for further analysis.

The next step in any poisoning case is *detoxification and elimination of absorbed toxins* (specific chemical antidotes are dealt with under the appropriate subheadings). Most poisons are eliminated via the urinary tract, and careful manipulation by osmotic diuresis or alteration of urinary pH may be effective in removing a suspected poison. A properly hydrated animal with adequate kidney function is required before either of these methods is considered. Urine outflow is monitored by catheterizing the animal and frequently measuring urine flow; 0.1 ml/kg/min is the minimum adequate urinary outflow.[7] Mannitol (2 mg/kg/hr) or furosemide (4 mg/kg) are the most effective and frequently used diuretics.[7] Acidifying agents, e.g., ammonium chloride (200 mg/kg/day in divided doses),[7] may be used to help eliminate amphetamines, which remain in an ionized form in acidic urine. Sodium bicarbonate (5 mEq/kg/hr) is effective for alkalizing the urine for elimination of aspirin or barbiturates.[7]

The final aspect of successfully treating a poisoning victim is *adequate supportive care*. Maintenance of body temperature, respiration, cardiovascular function, acid-base balance, and control of central nervous system (CNS) activity is essential until the animal is recovered. Hypothermia may be controlled with the use of warm blankets, heat lamps, or hot water bottles under adequate supervision. Cold water baths or ice bags are effective in cases of hyperthermia. It may be necessary to provide mechanical respiration using a Bird Respirator or Ohio ventilator for anesthetized animals or those with severe respiratory distress. Proper hydration status is closely monitored along with the acid-base balance. Simple hypovolemia may be corrected by administering lactated Ringer's solution. The addition of sodium bicarbonate (2–4 mEq/kg every 15 min)[7] is recommended in cases of severe acidosis. When blood gas analysis is available, the guidelines described in Chapter 4 for sodium bicarbonate administration can be used. Although a base imbalance is rare in most small-animal toxicoses, when such a state (basic deficit) is clearly established the intravenous administration of physiological saline at 10 ml/kg is substituted for lactated Ringer's.[7] Phenobarbital is generally recommended to reduce CNS hyperactivity by maintaining the animal in a light plane of surgical anesthesia.[7] If the animal is already under some respiratory distress, it is best to utilize a muscle relaxant-sedative, e.g., Valium (5 mg IV) or Robaxin (110 mg/kg IV).[7] These techniques, plus frequently turning the animal, are usually adequate to maintain proper cardiovascular function. On occasions where a cardiac stimulant would seem beneficial, calcium gluconate can be given slowly intravenously, or inotropic drugs can be administered according to dosage regimens described in Chapter 2.[7]

Use of Poison Control Centers and Diagnostic Laboratories

Poison control centers and diagnostic laboratories are two important outside sources for aiding the veterinarian not only in making a diagnosis but also in prescribing a proper treatment regimen for small-animal toxicities. Most poison control centers have information on a wide variety of toxic materials, including those not commonly encountered. The centers are of particular value when labels or containers are presented with an acutely ill animal.

Because of the medicolegal ramifications frequently associated with poisoning cases, the use of good diagnostic services is often needed. However, their results are dependent upon proper tissue and sample collection by the veterinarian. Tissues are placed in wide-mouth plastic bottles or bags which have not been used before. The samples are then frozen to prevent putrefaction. If the patient dies, at least 1 lb (0.5 kg) each of liver, kidney, and brain is submitted in properly labeled, separate containers. In all cases, vomitus, gastric washings or contents, colonic lavage solutions, blood, and urine are also submitted.[8] However, a complete toxicologic screening is expensive and often impractical. A good history, including identification of possible or suspected poisons, can often point diagnostic personnel in the right direction.

SPECIFIC CLINICAL SYNDROMES

Strychnine

Source. Although the use of strychnine as a rodenticide has declined in recent years because of the development of more efficacious products, it remains a common agent of accidental and malicious poisoning in cats and dogs.

Strychnine is an indole alkaloid derived from seeds of the plants *Strychnos nux-vomica* and *Strychnos ignatti*. It is available in various formulations as baits, pellets, and powders. Products containing more than 0.5% strychnine are restricted by federal law to use by certified applicators, but baits containing lower quantities are still commercially available. These baits commonly consist of peanuts, wheat, milo, or barley colored with a red or green dye.[14]

The lethal oral dose of strychnine is reported to be 0.75 mg/kg body weight in the dog and 2.0 mg/kg in the cat.[33]

Clinical Signs.   Strychnine is rapidly absorbed from the small intestine. Clinical signs may develop within 10 min to 3 hr after ingestion. Onset is delayed by the presence of stomach ingesta or if the animal vomits.

Initial clinical signs include nervousness, apprehension, and increased muscular tone. Severe tetanic convulsions may occur spontaneously or be initiated by external stimuli, e.g., loud noises, a bright light, or a current of air. Convulsions are characterized by extensor rigidity, the animal commonly assuming a "sawhorse" stance, arching of the neck, and retraction of the lips. The pupils are dilated and the pulse weak and rapid; cyanosis is obvious, and respiration may temporarily cease. Convulsive episodes may vary from a few seconds to several minutes. Periods of relaxation follow, but these become less frequent and shorter in duration as the poisoning progresses. Death may occur less than 1–2 hr after strychnine ingestion and is usually attributable to anoxia or exhaustion during the convulsive period.[19,33]

Treatment.   Follow these guidelines:
1. If clinical signs are not yet evident, vomiting is induced with apomorphine or hydrogen peroxide, and activated charcoal is administered.
2. The primary objectives in animals already displaying characteristic seizures is maintenance of relaxation and control of respiratory depression by ensuring adequate ventilation.
   a. Intravenous administration of pentobarbital sufficient to control seizures and maintain muscle relaxation can be used for short-term therapy.
   b. Gastric lavage is performed and activated charcoal administered.
   c. Inhalation anesthesia or methocarbamol (150 mg/kg body weight) is utilized for maintenance of long-term muscle relaxation. It may be necessary to administer oxygen or provide artificial ventilation if respiratory depression is severe. Adequate respiration must be maintained.
   d. Frequent turning of the animal and prevention of hypothermia are essential for efficient recovery.
   e. Forced diuresis with 5% mannitol in 0.9% sodium chloride (7 ml/kg/hr) intravenously and oral administration of ammonium chloride (150 mg/kg) after establishment of adequate urine flow aids in strychnine elimination.
   f. Therapy continues for 12–48 hr.[19,33]

Sodium Fluoroacetate (Compound 1080)

Source.   Sodium fluoroacetate (compound 1080) and related compounds, e.g., fluoroacetamide and fluoroacetic acid, were developed for use as insecticides and rodenticides. Current United States law restricts their use to licensed exterminators. Compound 1080 is commonly mixed with a black dye and combined with bread, bran, cereals, or other baits at a concentration of 0.6%. These products are particularly popular in control of rodents around sewers, grain elevators, and mills. All fluoroacetate derivatives are extremely toxic and nonselective in their effects. Dogs are quite susceptible, 0.05 mg/kg being a large enough dose to produce death in some instances. Small animals may be poisoned by ingestion of birds or rodents killed by compound 1080.[13]

Clinical Signs. The primary route of exposure to sodium fluoroacetate is oral, but the compound can be readily absorbed through the gastrointestinal tract, respiratory tract, or abraded skin. Its toxic effect is the result of biotransformation of fluoroacetate to fluorocitric acid, which inhibits aconitase in the Kreb's cycle. The time required for biotransformation accounts for the 0.5- to 2-hr lag period between exposure and onset of clinical signs.[13]

Dogs. Initial signs are vomiting, urination, and repeated defecation. The animal may appear restless, wander aimlessly, and become hyperirritable. Aimless wandering progresses to wild, frenzied running and barking. The animal may be completely oblivious to its surroundings, colliding with walls and other obstacles. Tonic-clonic seizures with opisthotonus and paddling followed by prostration interrupt the frenzied cycle. Convulsions become weaker and more frequent, with death attributable to respiratory failure within 2–12 hr after clinical onset.

Cats. Generally, marked excitement as exhibited by dogs is not encountered. Cardiac arrhythmia, hyperesthesia, and vocalization are more usual.

Treatment. General emergency procedures must be applied, as no specific antidote for sodium fluoroacetate is available.

1. If no clinical signs are evident and known exposure has occurred, vomiting is induced with apomorphine or gastric lavage is performed.
2. Convulsions are controlled with a short-acting barbiturate. The plane of anesthesia should be deep enough to inhibit the more violent seizures without causing further respiratory depression.
3. Glyceryl monoacetate is administered at 0.125 g/kg IM. This compound may inhibit the biotransformation of fluoroacetate to fluorocitric acid. If glyceryl monoacetate is not available, 2 ml/kg each of 50% ethanol and 5% acetic acid can be given orally.[13]
4. Necessary supportive care is provided.

Anticoagulant Rodenticides

Source. Two commercial types of anticoagulant rodenticides are currently available: (1) coumarin derivatives, represented by warfarin, D-Con, fumarin, bromadiolone, and brodifacoum; and (2) indandione derivatives, e.g., pindone and diphacinone.[27] Bromadiolone and brodifacoum are relatively recent additions to the coumarin family; they were developed to be effective against warfarin-resistant rodents and have 10–20 times more activity than warfarin.[40] All animals are susceptible to the anticoagulant rodenticides, but dogs seem to be the species most frequently affected. Poisoning may result either from ingestion of the rodenticide itself or consumption of dead vermin.[16]

The single oral lethal dose of warfarin is 5–50 mg/kg in the dog. Repeated ingestion may also result in toxicity. Warfarin at doses of 5 mg/kg for 5–10 days in dogs and 1 mg/kg in cats is considered enough to produce clinical signs of the toxicity.[9]

Clinical Signs and Diagnosis.   Clinical signs resulting from ingestion of an anticoagulant rodenticide are attributable to their antagonistic effect on the vitamin K–enzyme complex. Presenting complaints may be highly variable depending on the amount of poison consumed and the degree of organ dysfunction induced by hemorrhage or hypovolemic shock. The most common indications of vitamin K antagonism are: (1) subchronic cases of anemia, weakness, dyspnea, multiple internal and external hemorrhages, blood-stained feces, epistaxis, and hematemesis. Extensive hemorrhage into the brain, spinal cord, or subdural space produces CNS signs, including ataxia, convulsions, paralysis, or severe depression; (2) animals may be simply found dead due to extensive hemorrhage into the brain, pericardial sac, or thorax.

Diagnosis is based on clinical signs and clinicopathologic findings (prolonged prothrombin time, activated thromboplastin time, and activated coagulation time).[18]

Treatment.   Therapy is aimed at correction of hypovolemia and replenishment of depleted vitamin K.

1.   When signs of hypovolemia are severe, whole blood is administered intravenously at a dose of 20 ml/kg. Approximately 50% of this quantity is given rapidly, with the remainder administered slowly by intravenous drip.[27]

2.   Vitamin K_1 is given intravenously every 12 hr for the first 1–3 days of therapy. In less acute cases, vitamin K_1 can be administered subcutaneously to avoid possible anaphylactoid reactions, which may result when it is given intravenously.[27]

3.   As blood coagulation tests approach normal limits, vitamin K_3 or K_1 may be utilized orally. Oral treatment is continued for an additional 5 days in the case of coumarin-derivative toxicities and for at least 3 weeks with indandione-related poisonings.[27]

Metaldehyde

Source.   Metaldehyde, a polymer of acetaldehyde, is commonly used as an ingredient in snail and slug baits. Older formulations, which contained as much as 6% metaldehyde, were highly attractive to small animals, and at one time metaldehyde intoxication ranked second only to strychnine as the principle cause of canine poisonings in the Puget Sound area in the United States. Through research efforts at the University of California at Davis, new metaldehyde-containing molluscicides have been developed which have largely lost their appeal for the canine appetite. With the decline in supplies of older preparations, the incidence of metaldehyde toxicity is expected to drop dramatically.[28]

The oral LD_{50} for metaldehyde is in the range of 100–500 mg/kg in the dog.[28,37] Although cats are highly susceptible to metaldehyde, poisoning cases have been largely restricted to the canine species.

Clinical Signs.   Onset of clinical signs is largely dependent on the amount of bait consumed and the condition of the digestive tract at the time of ingestion. Early signs may include ataxia, muscle fasciculations, apprehension, nervousness, and salivation. Progression of intoxication results in continuous muscle spasms and prostration that is easily confused with strychnine poisoning. However, convulsive episodes are not elicited by external stimuli. Hyperthermia, with temperatures as high as 108°F, and severe acidosis are also common features.[28,37]

Treatment.   Therapy is aimed at eliminating any unabsorbed toxicant, controlling muscular tremors, and restoring proper acid-base balance.

1.   Emesis is induced with apomorphine or hydrogen peroxide. If muscular tremors are severe, the animal is lightly sedated with a short-acting barbiturate and gastric lavage is performed.

2.   Diazepam 2–5 mg/kg IV or triflupromazine 0.2–2.0 mg/kg IV is usually sufficient to control muscular tremors.

3.   The use of lactated Ringer's solution to control acidosis is recommended.[28,37]

Phosphorus

Source.   White or yellow phosphorus is occasionally found as a component of rodent baits. Dogs are highly susceptible to phosphorus intoxication; as little as 50–100 mg produces death following ingestion, but clinical reports of poisoning are rare. Red phosphorus is nontoxic.[9]

Clinical Signs.   Acute indications of severe gastrointestinal irritation may occur immediately or several hours after initial exposure. Intense vomiting and abdominal pain are typical. An important diagnostic feature is the garlic odor of the vomitus and its ability to glow in the dark due to the phosphorus content. After the acute episode, the animal enters a period of apparent recovery which may last a few hours to several days. However, a relapse characterized by vomiting, abdominal pain, icterus, convulsions, and coma follows the quiescent stage in the majority of cases of toxic ingestion.[9]

Treatment.   Emergency measures must be initiated almost immediately after exposure for treatment to be successful.

1.   Vomiting is induced with apomorphine, or gastric lavage is performed.

2.   The stomach is rinsed with a 0.2% copper sulfate solution, or 0.1–0.2% potassium permanganate is administered orally.[9]

3.   Mineral oil (100–200 ml) is given to flush any remaining phosphorus from the intestinal tract.[9]

Thallium

Source. The heavy metal thallium was commonly used as a rodenticide, pesticide, and fungicide during the 1950s and 1960s. It is a highly toxic element which persists in the environment almost indefinitely. The general distribution of thallium was banned in 1965 by the U.S. Department of Agriculture, and manufacture was halted in 1972. Unfortunately, occasional cases of thallium intoxication are still reported, largely from urban areas where thallium was extensively employed as a rodenticide in condemned buildings and warehouses. The oral LD_{50} for thallium is in the range of 10–15 mg/kg for all species.[4]

Clinical Signs. The signs of thallium poisoning are dependent on the amount ingested and can be broadly divided into three categories: acute, subchronic, and chronic. It is possible for a single case to progress through all three stages and involve several body systems.

The clinical signs of an acute intoxication result from consumption of a large amount of thallium. The first indication of toxicosis is severe gastrointestinal distress developing 1–4 days after exposure. Hemorrhagic diarrhea, abdominal pain, anorexia, and vomiting are common. Trembling, paralysis, dyspnea, indications of renal damage [casts in the urine, proteinuria, and elevated blood urea nitrogen (BUN)], and death may follow within 24–40 hr.

Clinical signs of subchronic thallium intoxication develop 3–7 days after ingestion. Gastrointestinal signs and motor disturbances are encountered, but they are milder and of longer duration than those of acute cases. Skin lesions appear 4–7 days after exposure and are the predominant form of expression in subchronic thallium toxicities. Reddening of the skin and pustule formation beginning on the ears and nose and spreading to the axillary area and ventral abdomen are typical. A particularly striking lesion is the deep reddening of the oral mucosa.

The chronic form of thallium toxicity follows a course very similar to that of the subchronic case, but there is a further downplay of the gastrointestinal and nervous signs. Indication of thallium involvement may not be evident until 7–10 days after ingestion. Skin lesions are severe, with almost complete loss of body hair and crust development within 1–3 weeks. Death is usually attributable to secondary complications, including dehydration and malnutrition.

Diagnosis is based on clinical signs and detection of thallium in the urine.[4,45,48]

Treatment. Therapy has two main thrusts: removal of thallium from body tissues and good supportive care.

1. If a known thallium ingestion has occurred, every effort is made to remove what remains in the gastrointestinal tract. Induction of emesis, gastric lavage, or a through-and-through enema are beneficial if performed within 3–4 hr after exposure.

2. The chelating agent diphenylthiocarbazone (dithizone) has proved to be the most efficacious for detoxifying thallium and promoting its excretion during the first 24–36 hr after exposure. For dogs—administer at a rate of 50–

70 mg/kg PO three times daily for 2–3 days in acute and early subchronic cases. (Monitor the patient closely, as dithizone may cause cataracts or blindness.) There are questions about the safety of the use of diphenylthiocarbazone in the feline species; thus, if employed, it is administered at much lower dosages than those recommended for the dog.

3. Prussian blue (100 mg/kg) is substituted for diphenylthiocarbazone after the initial 24-hr treatment. This dose is repeated orally twice daily for at least 5 days. The remainder of the clinical signs are dealt with symptomatically.[4]

Organophosphate and Carbamate Insecticides

Source.   Since the introduction of organophosphate insecticides during the mid-1940s and the carbamates during the late 1950s, these compounds have grown in popularity for control of ectoparasites on companion animals and livestock, as agricultural pesticides for crop protection, and in homes and gardens for elimination of insect pests. Although, in general, they are more toxic than chlorinated hydrocarbons, their lack of persistence in the environment and lack of residual effects in animals have made the organophosphate and carbamate insecticides more acceptable to the public and government regulatory agencies. Poisoning of companion animals has resulted from ingestion of improperly stored or discarded insecticides, miscalculation of insecticide concentration in solutions used for spraying or dipping, retreatment of animals with organophosphate or carbamate preparations within a short time span, or following drug interactions with some anthelmintics or tranquilizers.[11]

Clinical Signs.   The organophosphate insecticides inhibit the action of acetylcholinesterase, which functions at nerve synapses to remove acetylcholine, the neurotransmitter of the parasympathetic system and myoneural junctions. Early signs are mild salivation, defecation, urination, emesis, and a "sawhorse" gait. Progression of intoxication produces profuse salivation, severe abdominal cramps, diarrhea, miosis, muscular tremors, cyanosis, dyspnea, and death due to respiratory paralysis.

Although the mode of action of organophosphate and carbamate insecticides is identical, there are some important differences between the two compounds. Compared to the organophosphates, carbamates are relatively rapidly reversible inhibitors of cholinesterase. Carbamates are not as easily absorbed through the skin, and toxicity usually results only from oral ingestion. Finally, oximes (2-PAM, protopam chloride), essential components in the treatment of organophosphate intoxication, seem to be contraindicated in carbamate poisoning cases.[11]

Treatment.

1. Atropine sulfate is given at an initial dose of 0.2 mg/kg, one-fourth intravenously and the remainder subcutaneously. The dose of atropine is given until effective atropinization occurs. The actual dosage is "to effect" and may exceed the calculated 0.2 mg/kg dosage, especially in severely poisoned animals. Relief of parasympathetic signs occurs almost immediately upon atropine

administration, but muscular tremors are not controlled. Atropine may be repeated at one-half the initial dose subcutaneously if parasympathetic signs are again exhibited.

2. Animals which have been dermally exposed are washed with water. Activated charcoal is given orally in cases of ingestion.

3. In general, one or two administrations of atropine sulfate are sufficient for reversal of carbamate poisonings. If cholinergic signs continue, organophosphate intoxication is probable. As atropine sulfate blocks only the effect on the organophosphate-acetylcholinesterase bond, oximes (2-PAM, protopam chloride) are administered at a rate of 20 mg/kg. Protopam chloride is an oxime which acts specifically on this bond.[11]

Chlorinated Hydrocarbon Insecticides

Source. With the increasing use of organophosphate and carbamate insecticides, toxicities attributable to chlorinated hydrocarbons have decreased dramatically in recent years. The majority of poisonings in companion animals result from bathing and dipping the animal in excessive amounts of the compound. Cats seem to be more commonly involved as a result of owners utilizing formulations intended for dogs. Of those chlorinated hydrocarbons remaining for public use, toxicities involving lindane, chlordane, and toxaphene are most frequently reported.[43]

Clinical Signs. Initial signs of hyperexcitability and hyperesthesia are followed rapidly by observable spontaneous muscle twitching. Muscle fasciculations usually begin in the facial area, proceed caudally to involve the entire body, and may result in a convulsive seizure reminiscent of those encountered with strychnine toxicity. Hyperthermia, respiratory depression, and excessive salivation can be expected during the convulsive period. Animals may die during a seizure or undergo several convulsive episodes with complete recovery over several days.[43]

Treatment. No specific antidote is available for poisonings involving chlorinated hydrocarbons. Treatment is aimed at alleviating clinical signs and enhancing elimination of the compound.

1. Seizures are controlled with a barbiturate anesthetic.

2. If dermal exposure has occurred, the animal is bathed in warm, soapy water.

3. In cases of ingestion, gastric lavage may be beneficial if initiated within 2 hr after exposure. Emetics are used with caution, as they may initiate a seizure and result in inhalation pneumonia. Activated charcoal may be administered orally to prevent further absorption of compound remaining in the gastrointestinal tract.

4. Intravenous administration of lactated Ringer's solution may be helpful in enhancing elimination of the insecticide.

5. The animal should be kept in quiet, dark surroundings.[43]

Ethylene Glycol

Source.   Ethylene glycol is an industrial solvent utilized in the manufacture of dyes, lacquers, de-icer solutions, and automobile coolants. The majority of small animal poisonings result from ingestion of antifreeze in which ethylene glycol constitutes 95% or more of most commercial preparations. Antifreeze poisoning is most likely to be encountered in the autumn when radiators are commonly drained for addition of new coolant. The minimum lethal dose of antifreeze is reported to be 4.2–6.6 ml ethylene glycol/kg in the dog and 1.5 ml/kg in the cat.[30]

Clinical Signs and Diagnosis.   Presenting clinical signs may be highly variable. Acute toxicity results from ingestion of a large dose of ethylene glycol, usually in excess of 6 ml/kg, with death attributable to acidosis 12–36 hr after ingestion. Animals consuming smaller quantities and surviving more than 24 hr display milder clinical signs but are prone to develop uremia and acute renal failure due to the nephrotoxicity of ethylene glycol metabolites and the formation of calcium oxalate crystals in the renal tubules. The additional time associated with chronic toxicities allows metabolism of ethylene glycol to oxalic acid, which combines with calcium to produce these crystals.

Acute toxicity.   At 30–60 min after ingestion there is apprehension, moderate depression, ataxia, and frequent vomiting. This is followed by progressive depression, paresis, coma, and possible convulsions. Coma usually appears 6–12 hr after ingestion, with death intervening within 8–40 hr.

Chronic toxicity.   Signs similar to those of acute toxicities are encountered but are of a milder degree. Ataxia, vomiting, depression, and paresis may develop 3–10 days after the initial exposure. A rise in BUN, to as high as 200 mg/dl when coma develops, plus anuria or oliguria and dehydration signal the onset of renal failure.

Although diagnosis is difficult, these clinical signs in combination with a rising BUN and the presence of numerous oxalate and hippuric acid crystals in urinary sediment or the absence of urine production aid in the differentiation of ethylene glycol toxicity from other toxemic and renal disorders.[30]

Treatment.   Initiation of emergency procedures as soon as possible after antifreeze exposure is necessary for successful treatment. Therapy is based on three critical factors: (1) prevention of further absorption of ethylene glycol from the digestive tract; (2) control of acidosis; and (3) halting the conversion of ethylene glycol to its more toxic metabolites.

Further absorption is prevented by inducing vomiting with apomorphine or hydrogen peroxide. Gastric lavage and administration of activated charcoal may also be used. To control acidosis and stop metabolism of ethylene glycol, 20% ethanol and 5% sodium bicarbonate are employed. Dogs are given 5.5 ml of 20% ethanol/kg IV and 8 ml of 5% sodium bicarbonate/kg intraperitoneally every 4 hr for a total of five treatments. Four additional treatments are then needed at 6-hr intervals.[30,38] Cats are given 5 ml of 20% ethanol/kg and 6 ml of 5% sodium bicarbonate/kg, both administered intraperitoneally, every 6 hr for a total of five treatments. Four additional treatments are then needed at 8-hr intervals.[30,34]

Lead

Source. Although it may be difficult or nearly impossible to determine the definitive source of a lead toxicity case, the potential origins of this poisoning are widespread and diverse. Lead-based paints are probably still the most common source of exposure, and a history of an animal from an environment in which remodeling of an older home is occurring is frequent. Lead contained within linoleum, batteries, drinking water from improperly glazed ceramic bowls, golf balls, and fishing weights also serve as likely sources.[25]

Clinical Signs and Diagnosis. Young animals, between the age of 2 and 8 months, are much more likely to be affected by lead toxicity because of their inquisitive nature and low tolerance for the metal. Cases are most often encountered during the summer months, as vitamin D produced by the skin with sun exposure increases intestinal absorption of ingested lead. Lead toxicosis has been infrequently reported in the cat.

The physical signs of lead toxicity usually involve the gastrointestinal tract, the nervous system, or both. The usual sequence of events is development of a gastrointestinal upset several days before the onset of clinical signs of nervous involvement. Kowalezyk surveyed 27 dogs affected with lead toxicosis and found that the gastrointestinal signs, in order of frequency, were vomiting, anorexia, tender abdomen, diarrhea, and constipation. The neurologic signs included hysteria, convulsions, ataxia, blindness, and mydriasis.[24]

Because clinical findings of lead toxicity closely mimic those of canine distemper, clinicopathologic results are essential for establishing a diagnosis. The presence of a large number of nucleated red blood cells (5–40/100 white blood cells) without evidence of a concomitant severe anemia is considered nearly pathognomonic for lead toxicity. The identification of basophilic stippling of erythrocytes is also indicative. For definitive diagnosis, a whole blood sample (use citrate or heparin, not EDTA, as an anticoagulant) is submitted to an appropriate laboratory for lead analysis. A lead level of 0.6 ppm or more is considered diagnostic in the dog and cat. Slightly lower blood lead levels indicate recent exposure and absorption of moderate amounts of lead.[20,23–25,28,46]

Treatment. Therapy is aimed at removing any unabsorbed lead from the gastrointestinal tract, reducing the body lead burden, and alleviating clinical signs.

1. Vomiting is induced with apomorphine or hydrogen peroxide. In more severe cases, gastric lavage and/or a through-and-through enema may be of more benefit. Laxatives may be used in chronic exposure circumstances.

2. CaEDTA (calcium ethylenediaminetetraacetate) is administered at a rate of 100 mg/kg for 2–5 days. The daily dose is divided into four equal portions, diluted to a concentration of 10 mg CaEDTA/ml 5% dextrose solution, and given subcutaneously. In moderate cases with no life-threatening clinical effects, removal from the lead sources may be all that is necessary.

3. Gastrointestinal and nervous signs are treated symptomatically.

4. The source of the lead must be identified and removed from the pet's environment.[25]

Arsenic

Source. Although government regulations have restricted the use of inorganic arsenicals, accidental ingestion of such compounds as lead arsenate and Paris green (commonly used agricultural insecticides) and lead arsenate (a cutaneous parasiticide for ticks and mites) still results in occasional reports of poisoning in farm pets. Arsenicals are also found as constituents of crabgrass control preparations, other defoliants, and ant baits, and these may serve as sources of intoxication. Finally, iatrogenic cases of arsenical poisoning have resulted from improper use of Sodium Caparsolate and Filcide, employed for treatment of heartworms in dogs.[9,17]

Clinical Signs. Inorganic arsenicals and trivalent organic arsenicals, e.g., thiacetarsamide and arsphenamine, exert their toxic effect by inhibiting sulfhydryl-enzyme systems, which are essential for cellular metabolism. Although a chronic form of arsenic poisoning exists, the primary syndrome in companion animals is acute, the onset of clinical signs occurring 30 min to several hours after ingestion. Gastroenteritis is the outstanding feature. Initial signs are restlessness, nausea, repeated vomiting, and severe abdominal pain. Progression of intoxication results in diarrhea (usually hemorrhagic), extreme weakness, subnormal temperature, a weak rapid pulse, and death due to shock resulting from fluid loss.[9,17]

Treatment. Therapeutic measures are aimed at inactivating any unabsorbed material remaining in the intestine, restoring fluid balance, protecting the digestive tract, and reversing toxic manifestations.

1. If ingestion of an arsenical is suspected but no clinical signs are yet evident, vomiting is induced with apomorphine or gastric lavage is performed. Vomiting should not be induced in clinically ill animals.

2. BAL (dimercaprol) is administered at 5 mg/kg IM three times daily until recovery. BAL may be used as a preventative in animals not showing evidence of intoxication. One administration of BAL at 5 mg/kg is recommended, repeated in 3–4 hours at a dose of 2 mg/kg if necessary. Because BAL itself is toxic, it must not be used for longer than 5 days. If longer therapy is required, administer BAL in 3-day cycles.

3. A 10% solution of sodium thiosulfate is administered at doses up to 1 g daily, divided into four doses. The use of 1 g of ascorbic acid daily is also beneficial.

4. Fluid balance may be restored with intravenous administration of lactated Ringer's solution.

5. A broad-spectrum antibiotic may be given to prevent secondary infections.

6. Good nursing care is essential for successful treatment.[17]

Although BAL is an effective antidote if administered within 24 hr after arsenic ingestion, animals presented with advanced clinical signs have a grave prognosis.

Garbage- and Food-Borne Intoxications

Source. Clinical signs of enterotoxemia may result from ingestion of garbage, infected viscera, bones, decaying organic matter, manure, sewage, or highly fermentable foods. The primary offenders are *Salmonella* spp., *Clostridium* spp., *Escherichia coli*, and *Staphylococcus* spp. Toxins may be preformed as in the case of *C. perfringens*, *C. botulinum*, and the enterotoxin of *Staphylococcus* spp., or they may arise from multiplication of toxin-producing bacteria within the intestine. Because of their nondiscriminatory eating habits, dogs are the species most frequently affected.[9,12]

Clinical Signs. There are two primary clinical syndromes associated with garbage- or food-borne intoxications: gastroenteritis and shock. The former is the more common and results from ingestion of dead carrion, spoiled foods, or material unusually high in carbohydrates. In the acute syndrome, vomiting, abdominal pain, and depression develop 2–6 hr after ingestion of the offending agent. Progression of the poisoning may result in a mucoid to watery diarrhea, weakness, ataxia, dehydration, and on occasion death. Less severe cases of enterotoxemia pursue a more chronic course characterized by anorexia, dull hair coat, mucoid feces, increased flatulence, halitosis, and lethargy. Signs identifiable with clinical shock—dyspnea, depression, weakness, rapid pulse, mucosal pallor, and circulatory collapse—may follow consumption of a clostridial exotoxin or release of *E. coli* endotoxin.

Mention should be made of the neurotoxic syndrome associated with *Clostridium botulinum*. Although dogs as a species are quite resistant to botulinum toxin, clinical cases have been reported. Typical signs included a flaccid ascending paralysis, dyspnea, and excessive salivation.[12]

Treatment. Use the following guidelines.

1. With acute or peracute intoxications, ingesta may remain in the stomach. Vomiting is induced with apomorphine, or a through-and-through enema may be given.

2. Dehydration, acid-base balance, and shock are corrected with appropriate intravenous fluid therapy; 5% dextrose in lactated Ringer's solution is recommended.

3. A broad-spectrum antibiotic and vitamin B complex are given. Antibiotic therapy is continued for a minimum of 5 days.

4. Food and water are withheld for 24 hr, and then the animal is returned to oral food gradually. A bland diet (rice and cottage cheese) or a prescription diet (e.g., i/d or k/d) is utilized for 3–5 days. After this period, the animal may be returned to its usual commercial preparation in one-fourth increments every 2 days.[12]

Acids and Alkalis

Source. Caustic agents, e.g., strong acids and bases, are frequent constituents of household cleaning products, disinfectants, and sanitizers. Improper storage or inadequate cleanup of spills are the usual methods of exposure to companion animals.

Clinical Signs. The primary effect of strong acids and bases is corrosion. Ingestion results in severe abdominal pain; burning of the mouth, pharynx, and esophagus; vomiting; and excessive thirst. The oral mucosa may be intensely hyperemic or frankly necrotic, assuming a grayish white to black, wrinkled appearance. Skin exposure may produce lesions varying from a mild dermatitis to severe loss of surface epithelium. Development of clinical shock and systemic infections must always be considered as possible sequelae in extensive cases.

Treatment. The treatment for external exposure is: (1) for acids—flushing with large quantities of warm soapy water; and (2) for alkalis—flushing with vinegar or acetic acid. An emollient cream, topical antibiotic, or sodium bicarbonate paste (alkalis only) is applied. A broad-spectrum antibiotic is given for 3–5 days. The treatment for internal exposure includes: (1) for acids—administration of magnesium hydroxide, egg whites, or milk; and (2) for alkalis—administration of large quantities of water, but not acids because of possible heat generation. DO NOT INDUCE VOMITING when strong acids or bases are involved. It may be necessary to perform a tracheotomy if pharyngeal or laryngeal edema is severe. A broad-spectrum antibiotic is also used for 3–5 days. The animal is reintroduced slowly to a bland, easily digestible diet (rice and cheese).[9]

Phenols

Source. Phenolic compounds are commonly used as wood preservatives, fungicides, herbicides, disinfectants, and photographic developers. Their frequent commercial and home use make exposure, either accidentally or through overzealous owner application of disinfectant products, a very real possibility.

Because of their inherent deficiency of the enzymes required to metabolize and excrete phenolic compounds, cats are more susceptible to phenolic intoxication than are other species. For example, dogs can adequately handle three times the quantity of phenol as cats. A similar argument is applicable to the neonate whose enzyme systems are incompletely developed for several weeks after birth.[15,32]

Clinical Signs. Phenolic compounds are rapidly absorbed through intact skin or from the gastrointestinal tract. Resultant clinical signs are largely dependent on the amount and type of phenol absorbed. Large concentrations produce acute signs as soon as 30 min after exposure, with death occurring within 12–24 hr. Smaller amounts result in only mild depression and occasional vomiting for several hours before progressing to the typical neurologic and respiratory manifestations. Early signs may include ataxia, mild muscular fasciculations, and depression. Coma and respiratory failure are the end result. Additional clinical signs which may be noted in cases of dermal exposure include intravascular hemolysis and terminal icterus or burning of the skin following exposure to concentrated solutions.[32]

Treatment. There is no specific antidote for phenol poisoning. General emergency procedures, i.e., washing the skin with soap in cases of dermal exposure or induction of emesis and administration of activated charcoal following ingestion, are the only recourse. Good supportive care is critical to allow the animal time to detoxify and eliminate the compound.[32]

Mycotoxicoses

Mycotoxins, metabolities of toxigenic fungi, may form on animal feeds under appropriate moisture and temperature conditions. Although over 30 mycotoxins have been identified as causative agents in animal disease, only two—aflatoxin, produced by *Aspergillus flavus*, and penitrem A, a metabolite of *Penicillium crustosum*—have been associated with problems in dogs.

Aflatoxin has a specific affinity for the liver, producing clinical signs of anorexia, icterus, melena, polyuria, polydipsia, and bleeding diathesis. In the past, aflatoxin-contaminated peanut meal occasionally was used in commercial dog food preparations, resulting in typical signs of aflatoxicosis. *Penicillin crustosum* is a common contaminant of refrigerated foodstuffs but also has been isolated from cereal grains and thus may contaminate commercial preparations. Its metabolite, penitrem A, causes acute muscle tremors, seizures, ataxia, and prostration.

No specific antidote is available for either mycotoxin, and clinical signs must be treated symptomatically.[6,29,35]

Algae

Source. Only blue-green algae (cyanophyta) are considered to be directly toxic and then only under certain environmental conditions. They are frequently found on surfaces of ponds and lakes, particularly in shallow areas. Poisonings are usually reported during late spring and early summer when increased temperature and warm, gentle breezes result in rapid growth and accumulation of blue-green algae in large quantities. Dogs are usually poisoned through ingestion of contaminated waters.[22]

Clinical Signs. The toxic principle seems to be several varieties of endotoxin. In most reports of algal poisoning, signs occur within 15–45 min after ingestion of a toxic dose. Nausea, vomiting, abdominal pain, diarrhea, prostration, muscular tremors, dyspnea, convulsions, and death within 24 hr is the usual progression of clinical signs. Those rare animals who do recover from acute toxicity commonly develop photosensitization 3–4 days after the initial exposure due to the hepatotoxic effect of the algae.[22]

Treatment. No truly effective treatment is available. Signs are dealt with symptomatically.[22]

Mushrooms

Source. Although there are a number of toxic genera of mushrooms a veterinary practitioner may encounter, the majority of small-animal poisonings arise from ingestion of members of the genus *Amanita*. These grow quite abundantly in pastures and wooded areas in warm, humid climates. Dogs are usually the species involved. Cases are seen in animals allowed to roam freely or after family outings.[22]

Clinical Signs.   Acute signs referable to the gastrointestinal and neuromuscular systems develop 6–10 hr after ingestion of a toxic dose. Severe abdominal pain, salivation, vomiting, diarrhea which may be blood-tinged, and incoordination may be seen. Affected animals may recover from this syndrome in several days, but approximately 20% of the dogs relapse within a week due to toxic hepatitis and nephritis. Animals become depressed, anorectic, lose weight, and develop jaundice 2 days into this secondary phase. Ten to 14 days may be required for complete recovery when liver involvement is severe, and a number of dogs and cats may succumb no matter how intensive the therapy.[22]

Treatment.   No specific antidote is available. Vigorous symptomatic therapy for animals in the early stages of the digestive-neuromuscular syndrome may help prevent later development of severe toxic hepatitis and nephritis. Once signs of liver degeneration develop, a high-carbohydrate/low-protein diet is recommended if the animal is still eating. Aggressive intravenous and subcutaneous use of fluids, electrolytes, amino acids, and glucose is required in animals who are completely anorectic.[22]

Ricinus (Castor Bean)

Source.   Ricinus is commonly planted as a hedge or screen along driveways or fences. The toxic principle, ricin (a phytotoxin), is present in all parts of the plant. Small-animal poisonings usually result from ingestion of the seed, in which the concentration of ricin is particularly high.[1,22]

Clinical Signs.   A latent period of several hours to a few days is usually required after ingestion before signs develop. However, because of the protein nature of phytotoxin, acute anaphylactic reactions have been encountered. Commonly, there is a high fever, gastroenteritis, muscular twitching, convulsions, coma, and death as early as 24 hr after the onset of signs.[1,22]

Treatment.   If a known ingestion has occurred and clinical signs are not yet evident, apomorphine and a laxative are given or a through-and-through enema performed. Clinical signs are treated symptomatically.[1,22]

Common House Plants

Many common household plants are potential sources of poisoning to small animals. Cats are especially prone to this type of toxicity because of their curious nature. The majority of clinical cases attributable to plant poisonings result from ingestion and are followed by classic signs of gastroenteritis. However, a few may cause allergic reactions, dermatitis, or mechanical injury. The following information is only a partial compilation of the most frequently encountered plant toxicities. For a more complete review, consultation of Kingsbury's work[22] is recommended.

Dumb Cane (*Dieffenbachia* spp.) and Philodendron. The toxic principle of dumb cane includes calcium oxalate crystals, which are present in all parts of the plant. At least one other unidentifiable principle is also present. Clinical signs result from the burning and irritative effect produced by these crystals when the plant is chewed. Excessive salivation and edema of the oral and pharyngeal mucosa are the signs most frequently observed. Treatment consists of immediate flushing of the oral cavity with large quantities of water. If burns are severe, hyperalimentation may be required, and the use of an antibiotic to prevent secondary infection is recommended.[1,22]

Laurel (*Kalmia* spp.). Laurels are indigenous in the United States, where they are commonly found in wooded areas. Because of their decorative nature, they are frequently used in floral arrangements. The toxic principle, andromedotoxin, is found in all parts of the plant. Clinical signs may include a serous ocular and nasal discharge, salivation, emesis, convulsions, and paralysis after ingestion. Treatment is aimed at removing any unabsorbed toxin via gastric lavage or production of emesis with apomorphine. Subsequent administration of activated charcoal is also considered beneficial. The remainder of the clinical signs are treated symptomatically.[1,22]

Mistletoe (*Phoradendron serotinum*). The berries of the mistletoe plant contain two toxic substances, β-phenylethylamine and tyramine, which result in a combination of gastrointestinal signs and bradycardia. Treatment consists of gastric lavage or induction of emesis, control of the bradycardia (Ch. 2), and good supportive care.[1,22]

English Ivy (*Hedera helix*). This is a commonly cultivated vine in the United States. Cases of poisoning attributable to this plant have been reported in children. Clinical signs are of a purgative nature, including salivation, emesis, abdominal pain, and diarrhea. Treatment is symptomatic.[1,22]

Poinsettia (*Euphorbia pulcherrima*). In most cases, poisoning is caused by an acrid principle which produces signs of severe gastrointestinal involvement and burning of the oral and pharyngeal mucosa. Ingestion of a single leaf may cause death of a small child. Treatment is symptomatic after removal of any undigested toxin from the intestinal tract by gastric lavage or induction of emesis. Administration of activated charcoal may also be beneficial.[1,22]

ADVERSE DRUG REACTIONS AND INTERACTIONS

Today's veterinarian has at his disposal a wide range of therapeutic agents of unquestioned value and benefit. However, any foreign substance, including pharmaceuticals intended to aid in treatment of a disease process, can affect an animal adversely. Recognition of an adverse drug reaction requires astute observation, as the clinical signs manifested are difficult to separate from those of the concurrent disease. However, realization that such reactions usually occur at the time of drug administration and that the clinical syndrome improves when treatment is discontinued aids the diagnostician in evaluating adverse drug reactions (ADRs) and effects.[3]

Classification of ADRs

In general, ADRs can be divided into six broad categories: side effects, disruption of control mechanisms, allergic reactions, drug interactions, predisposition due to patient status, and human error.[3]

Side Effects. Briefly defined, these are reactions which are expected but not necessarily considered to be desirable. Common examples include renal dysfunction produced by the antifungal agent amphotericin B, mydriasis produced by atropine, or bronchoconstriction and gastrointestinal side effects produced by dinoprost (Lutalyse).[3]

Disruption of Control Mechanisms. Drugs may interfere with normal metabolic pathways, particularly after prolonged administration. Adrenocorticosteroids may reduce the animal's resistance to infection, and intensive antimicrobial therapy has been known to produce overgrowth of normal intestinal flora.[3]

Allergic Reactions. Allergic reactions may result when prior exposure to the drug has produced sensitization, or they may occur because of a preexisting genetic basis. Although not well documented in animals, allergic reactions have been reported with tetracycline and penicillin.[3]

Drug Interactions. Drugs administered concurrently may be additive, react unfavorably, have no effect on each other, or actually potentiate one another. Examples include enhancement of biotransformation of digoxin in dogs by phenobarbital, precipitation of phenytoin toxicity by chloramphenicol, and decreased absorption of tetracycline with comcomitant administration of Kaopectate, milk, or iron formulations.[3]

Predisposition Due to Patient Status. Age, species, and current health status have a profound effect on the results obtained with drug therapy. The neonate and aged animal do not have the biotransformation capabilities of the young adult. Animals with liver disease also have an impaired ability to metabolize many compounds, and those with kidney disease may be unable to properly eliminate drugs which normally undergo renal excretion. Corticosteroids may exacerbate diabetes mellitus. Cats are inherently more sensitive to aspirin, acetaminophen, and phenolic compounds; greyhounds have prolonged sleeping times with barbiturates, and brachycephalic breeds may develop a sinoatrial block upon administration of acepromazine.[3]

Human error. Incorrect dosage or an inappropriate method of administration may result in adverse reactions.[3]

Treatment

Treatment is aimed at relieving the drug-induced signs and enhancing drug excretion if possible. Frequently simple discontinuance of therapy is adequate. Administration of activated charcoal may be beneficial as a nonspecific antidote if the adverse reaction is severe and the drug involved undergoes an enterohepatic cycle. Allergic reactions are dealt with by either intravenous administration of epinephrine (1:10,000) if anaphylaxis is acute or antihistamines and corticosteroids for subacute reactions.[3]

Following is a summary of some of the more common adverse drug reactions which may be encountered by the practitioner. It is not our purpose to provide a complete listing. For further information, a standard text in veterinary pharmacology should be consulted.

Analgesics. *Aspirin.* Aspirin may produce depression, ataxia, anorexia, blood dyscrasias, gastric ulceration, and death. The reaction encountered is of greatest severity in cats, which have a limited ability to metabolize the drug (25 mg/kg every 24 hr is adequate to maintain therapeutic blood levels in the cat).[3,10]

Acetaminophen. Acetaminophen can cause depression, facial edema, cyanosis, vomiting, and death. Because of an inherent deficiency of glucuronyl transferase, cats have a lower tolerance for acetaminophen than dogs. (One extra-strength acetaminophen tablet, 500 mg, is sufficient to cause death in cats.) Administration of acetylcysteine at 140 mg/kg orally at 4-hr intervals for four treatments is recommended for dealing with an overdose.[3,21,26,39]

Anthelmintics. *Arsenamide (Caparsolate, Thiacetaraside).* Gastroenteritis, depression, anorexia, icterus, proteinuria, and elevation of liver enzymes are sometimes seen after arsenamide ingestion. Accidental administration of this drug perivenously can result in severe local swelling and dermal necrosis.[3,5,21]

Bunamidine (Scolaban). Bunamidine can cause emesis, diarrhea, dyspnea, ventricular fibrillation, and death. It should be administered only to a fasted animal, and exercise is to be avoided for 24 hr after treatment.[3,5]

Dichlorophen (Dicestal). Dichlorophen may produce emesis, diarrhea, abdominal pain, ataxia, hyperthermia, tachycardia, and death.[3,5] Hyperthermic reactions are controlled with ice baths. The use of atropine and phenothiazine derivative tranquilizers in therapy is to be avoided.

Dichlorvos (DDVP, Task). Dichlorvos may cause gastroenteritis, profuse salivation, abdominal pain, and death. Dichlorvos is an organophosphate parasiticide. It is cumulative in action and produces toxic effects with carbamates and other organophosphorus-induced toxicities. (Administration of an organophosphate to a dog infested with adult heartworms can produce terminal prostration and rapid death.)[3,5,21]

Diethylcarbamazine (DEC, Caricide). Gastroenteritis, anaphylactoid reactions, and rapid death may occur if diethylcarbamazine is administered to microfilaria-infected dogs.[3,5,21]

Disophenol (DNP). Disophenol can cause emesis, diarrhea, abdominal pain, ataxia, hyperthermia, tachycardia, and death. Hyperthermic reactions are controlled with ice baths. The use of atropine and phenothiazine derivative tranquilizers in therapy should be avoided.[3,5,21]

Mebendazole (Telmintic). Idiosyncratic reactions have been encountered in dogs after administration of mebendazole. Resultant signs are attributable to rapidly developing liver necrosis.[3,5,41,42]

Antimicrobials. *Amphotericin B.* Nephrotoxicity, convulsions, phlebitis, anemia, and hypokalemia are sometimes seen. Amphotericin B may precipitate digitalis toxicity. The BUN should be carefully monitored during therapy with this compound.[36]

Aminoglycosides (Dihydrostreptomycin, Neomycin, Kanamycin, Gentamicin). Nephrotoxicity and ototoxicity may be seen. Simultaneous administration of furosemide (Lasix) may potentiate ototoxicity. These drugs may enhance the muscle relaxation induced by ether, halothane, and methoxyflurane, leading to respiratory failure when administered parenterally. Aminoglycosides must be used with extreme caution in pregnant animals or in those with preexisting renal dysfunction.[4,6,10,21]

Chloramphenicol. Anorexia, depression, vomiting, diarrhea, and bone marrow depression may result. Chloramphenicol doubles the sleeping time of phenobarbital anesthesia if administered 2 hr before or at the time of induction. Chloramphenicol can potentiate phenytoin toxicity.[3,5,10,21]

Penicillin. Facial edema, prostration, and death are sometimes produced.

Tetracycline. Emesis, hyperthermia, and anaphylactic reactions may be seen.[3,5,44] Tetracycline may cause staining and pitting of the enamel if administered to young animals.

Central Nervous System Depressants (Anesthetics, Muscle Relaxants, Tranquilizers). *Fentanyl (Sublimaze).* Defecation, salivation, bradycardia, respiratory depression, and death may occur. Fentanyl is additive with sodium pentobarbital anesthesia. It should not be utilized in conjunction with, or at least 8 hr before, the administration of tranquilizers, analgesics, or antitussives.[3,5]

Halothane (Fluothane). Hepatic dysfunction, cardiac arrhythmias, hypotension, hypothermia, or malignant hyperthermia may occur. Ganglionic blocking agents may augment halothane's hypotensive effect. Epinephrine and norephinephrine may precipitate cardiac arrhythmias. Aminoglycoside antibiotics may contribute to circulatory depression.[3,5]

Ketamine (Ketaset). Respiratory depression, emesis, excessive salivation, prolonged recovery, convulsions, and cardiac arrest may occur.[3,5]

Lidocaine. Hyperexcitability, depression, convulsions, unconsciousness, urticaria, edema, and respiratory arrest may be seen.[3,5] Lidocaine in conjunction with diphenylhydantoin can cause depression.

Methocarbamol (Robaxin). Emesis, muscular weakness, and ataxia may occur.[3,5]

Methoxyflurane (Metofane). Emesis, cardiac arrest, delayed hepatopathy, and death may occur. Epinephrine and norepinephrine may precipate cardiac arrhythmias. Methoxyflurane may potentiate the nephrotic effects of the aminoglycosides.[3,5]

Phenothiazine Derivative Tranquilizers (Acepromazine, Propriopromazine Hydrochloride, Trimeprazine). Hypotension, prolonged depression, blood dyscrasia with prolonged administration, and decreased threshold for convulsions may be apparent. These drugs may potentiate the toxicity of organophosphates. Epinephrine should not be utilized in conjunction with these products. They are additive in action with other depressants and general anesthesia.[3,5]

NECESSARY EMERGENCY EQUIPMENT AND MEDICATION

Because of the acute nature of most toxicities occurring in companion animals, it is wise to have certain therapeutic medications and equipment readily available. Parenteral solutions—including apomorphine, atropine sulfate, calcium disodium EDTA, 5% dextrose, dimercaprol (BAL), 20% ethanol, lactated Ringer's, normal saline, 5% sodium bicarbonate, vitamin K_1, pentobarbital, and 10% methocarbamol (Robaxin)—should be placed in a small kit or empty drawer. Designation of one shelf in the pharmacy for oral medications— e.g., activated charcoal, diphenylthiocarbazone, hydrogen peroxide, ipecac syrup, milk of magnesia, mineral oil, D-penicillamine, sodium chloride, prussian blue, and tannic acid—may well save valuable time when a toxic emergency arises. Quick availability of blankets, endotracheal tubes, an enema kit, intravenous catheters, a mechanical respirator or compression bag, syringes, and stomach tube may be the difference between life and death for an animal acutely poisoned.[31]

REFERENCES

1. Arena JM: Pretty poisonous plants. Vet Hum Toxicol 21:108, 1979
2. Aronson AL: Chemical poisonings in small animal practice. Vet Clin North Am 2:379, 1972
3. Aronson AL, Riviere JE: Adverse drug reactions. In Kirk RW (ed): Current Veterinary Therapy VIII. p. 122. Saunders, Philadelphia, 1983
4. Aronson CE: Thallium intoxication. In Kirk RW (ed): Current Veterinary Therapy VI. p. 124. Saunders, Philadelphia, 1977
5. Aronson CE: Veterinary Pharmaceuticals & Biologicals 1982/1983. Veterinary Medicine Publishing Co., Edwardsville, KS, 1983
6. Arp LH, Richard JL: Intoxication of dogs with the mycotoxin penitrem A. J Am Vet Med Assoc 175:565, 1979
7. Bailey EM: Emergency and general treatment of poisonings. In Kirk RW (ed): Current Veterinary Therapy VII. p. 105. Saunders, Philadelphia, 1980
8. Buck WB: Use of laboratories for the chemical analysis of tissues. In Kirk RW (ed): Current Veterinary Therapy VII. p. 115. Saunders, Philadelphia, 1980
9. Buck WB, Osweiler GS, VanGelder GA: Clinical and Diagnostic Veterinary Toxicology. 2nd Ed. Kendall-Hunt Publishing Co., Dubuque, IA, 1976
10. Burrows GE: Selected drug toxicities. In Kirk RW (ed): Current Veterinary Therapy VIII. p. 118. Saunders, Philadelphia, 1983
11. Carson TL: Organophosphate and carbamate insecticide poisoning. In Kirk RW (ed): Current Veterinary Therapy VII. p. 147. Saunders, Philadelphia, 1980
12. Eberhart GW: Garbage- and food-borne intoxications (enterotoxemias). In Kirk RW (ed): Current Veterinary Therapy VI. p. 176. Saunders, Philadelphia, 1977
13. Edwards WC: Sodium fluoroacetate (compound 1080) poisoning. In Kirk RW (ed): Current Veterinary Therapy VI. p. 119. Saunders, Philadelphia, 1977
14. Edwards WC, Kerr LA, Whaley MW: Strychnine poisoning in dogs—sources and availability. Vet Med. Small Animl Clinician 76:823, 1981

15. Ernst MR: Susceptibility of cats to phenol. J Am Vet Med Assoc 138:197, 1961
16. Evans J, Ward AL: Secondary poisoning associated with anticoagulant-killed nutria. J Am Vet Med Assoc 151:856, 1967
17. Furr A: Arsenic poisoning. In Kirk RW (ed): Current Veterinary Therapy VI. p. 134. Saunders, Philadelphia, 1977
18. Green RA, Buck WB: Warfarin and other anticoagulant poisonings. In Kirk RW (ed): Current Veterinary Therapy VII. p. 131. Saunders, Philadelphia, 1980
19. Harris WF: Clinical toxicities of dogs. Vet Clin North Am 5:605, 1975
20. Jacobs G: Lead poisoning in a cat. J Am Vet Med Assoc 179:1396, 1981
21. Keen P, Livingston A: Adverse reactions to drugs. In Pract 5:174, 1983
22. Kingsbury JM: Poisonous Plants of the United States and Canada. Prentice-Hall, Englewood Cliffs, NJ, 1964
23. Knecht DC, Crabtree J, Katcherma A: Clinical pathologic and electroencephalographic features of lead poisoning in dogs. J Am Vet Med Assoc 175:196, 1979
24. Kowalezyk DV: Lead poisoning in dogs at the University of Pennsylvania Veterinary Hospital. J Am Vet Med Assoc 168:428, 1976
25. Kowalezyk DF: Lead poisoning. In Kirk RW (ed): Current Veterinary Therapy VII. p. 136. Saunders, Philadelphia, 1980
26. Kujala C, Randall JW: Iatrogenic acetaminophen poisoning. Fel Pract 11:12, 1981
27. Mount ME, Feldman BF: Topics in drug therapy: vitamin K and its therapeutic importance. J Am Vet Med Assoc 180:1354, 1982
28. Mull RL: Metaldehyde poisoning. In Kirk RW (ed): Current Veterinary Therapy VII. p. 135. Saunders, Philadelphia, 1980
29. Nicholson SS: Mycotoxicosis. In Kirk RW (ed): Current Veterinary Therapy VIII. p. 167. Saunders, Philadelphia, 1983
30. Oehme FW: Antifreeze (ethylene glycol) poisoning. In Kirk RW (ed): Current Veterinary Therapy VI. p. 135. Saunders, Philadelphia, 1977
31. Oehme FW: Emergency kit for treatment of small animal poisoning. In Kirk, RW (ed): Current Veterinary Therapy VIII. p. 201. Saunders, Philadelphia, 1983
32. Oehme FW: Poisonings from phenolic chemicals. In Kirk RW (ed): Current Veterinary Therapy VI. p. 145. Saunders, Philadelphia, 1977
33. Osweiler GD: Strychnine poisoning. In Kirk RW (ed): Current Veterinary Therapy VII. p. 129. Saunders, Philadelphia, 1980
34. Penumarthy L, Oehme FW: Treatment of ethylene glycol toxicosis in cats. Am J Vet Res 36:209, 1975
35. Pier AC, Richard JL, Cysweski SJ: Implications of mycotoxins in animal disease. J Am Vet Med Assoc 176:719, 1980
36. Pyle RL: Clinical pharmacology of amphotericin B. J Am Vet Med Assoc 179:83, 1981
37. Samuelson ML: Metaldehyde poisoning. In Kirk RW (ed): Current Veterinary Therapy VI. p. 123. Saunders, Philadelphia, 1977
38. Sanyer JL, Oehme FW, McGavin MD: Systematic treatment of ethylene glycol toxicosis in dogs. Am J Vet Res 34:527, 1973
39. Savides MC, Oehme FW: Acetaminophen and its toxicity. J Appl Toxicol 3:96, 1983
40. Stowe CM, Metz AL, Arendt TD, Schulman J: Apparent brodifacoum poisoning in a dog. J Am Vet Med Assoc 182:817, 1983
41. Thornburg LP, Rottinghause GB: Drug-induced hapatic necrosis in a dog. J Am Vet Med Assoc 183:327, 1983

42. VanCauteren H, Marsboom R, Vandenberghe J, Well JA: Safety studies evaluating the effect of mebendazole on liver function in dogs. J Am Vet Med Assoc 183:93, 1983
43. VanGelder GA: Chlorinated hydrocarbon insecticide toxicoses. In Kirk RW (ed): Current Veterinary Therapy VI. p. 141. Saunders, Philadelphia, 1977
44. Ward GS, Guiry CC, Alexander LL: Tetracycline-induced anaphylactic shock in a dog. J Am Vet Med Assoc 180:770, 1982
45. Wilson JE: Thalltoxicosis. J Am Vet Med Assoc 189:1116, 1961
46. Zook BC, Carpenter JL, Leeds, EB: Lead poisoning in dogs. J Am Vet Med Assoc 155:1329, 1969
47. Zook BC, Gilmore CE: Thallium poisoning in dogs. J Am Vet Med Assoc 151:206, 1967
48. Zook BC, Holzwoth J, Thornton GW: Thallium poisoning in cats. J Am Vet Med Assoc 153:285, 1968

12 | Environmental Injury

Todd R. Tams

There are several environmentally induced injuries with which the veterinarian must deal. These include smoke inhalation injuries, thermal injuries, chemical injuries, hypothermia, frostbite, heatstroke, snake bites, and insect and arachnid stings and bites.

SMOKE INHALATION INJURY

Each year, many animals die as a result of fire-related injury. The majority of these deaths occur in the fire, and most are due to carbon monoxide (CO) poisoning. Those animals who survive and are presented to veterinarians may have sustained appreciable smoke or thermal damage to the respiratory tract as well as CO intoxication. Because the survival of fire victims often depends on proper emergency treatment, an understanding of the pathophysiology of smoke inhalation injury is essential.

Pathophysiology

Two distinct mechanisms of bronchopulmonary injury that follow smoke inhalation have been identified: carbon monoxide intoxication and smoke toxicity.[8,15] Smoke toxicity is further divided into direct injury from smoke and smoke poisoning from noxious chemicals formed by the incomplete combustion of various natural and synthetic products. Although these conditions may coexist and overlap, each has distinct characteristics.

Carbon monoxide is an environmental poisonous gas that is produced by the incomplete combustion of materials that contain carbon. It has an affinity for hemoglobin 240 times greater than oxygen, and the resulting carboxyhemoglobin (COHb) is unable to function in O_2 transport. The toxicity of COHb

355

depends on the concentration of CO in the inspired air and the duration of the exposure, although very small concentrations of CO cause high COHb levels.

The resulting physiological abnormality of CO intoxication is that of inadequate tissue oxygenation. All organs show the effects of this failure of O_2 delivery, but the brain is most sensitive to the O_2 deprivation. COHb levels below 10% do not cause clinical signs, whereas at levels of 20% shortness of breath on moderate exertion, mild dyspnea, and confusion may result. At 30% there is increasing irritability, dizziness, nausea, vomiting, and loss of coordination. Levels beyond 40% result in confusion, collapse, and even unconsciousness. Convulsions, respiratory failure, and death may occur at levels greater than 50–60%. Decreased O_2 content in the burning room and the additional pulmonary effects of smoke poisoning potentiate the effects of CO in a fire.[14] As COHb levels increase, the victim often loses both the interest and the ability to flee the smoke.

Excessive heat may directly injure the upper respiratory mucosa, producing airway obstruction from laryngeal spasm, erosions, and edema. True thermal damage to the lower respiratory tract and lung parenchyma is extremely rare unless live steam or explosive gases are inhaled. In dogs, the lungs are especially protected from substantial inhalation of smoke because of elongated nasal passages, epiglottic closure, or early bronchospasm. Mucosal burns of the mouth, nasopharynx, pharynx, and larynx may lead to upper airway obstruction at any time during the first 24 hr after the burn.

Direct airway damage may also be caused by inhalation of soot and other superheated particles that result from incomplete combustion. Moreover, these particles may carry noxious gases and other contaminants into the lungs which, on contact with water in the lungs, may form corrosive acids and alkalis.[8]

Smoke poisoning results from toxic by-products produced during burning of various materials. Some important by-products include oxides of sulfur and nitrogen, and an aldehyde, acrolein, which causes irritation and pulmonary edema at levels as low as 10 ppm. Some plastics also produce large amounts of benzene, whose anesthetic action may promote easier passage of acids and alkalis into the respiratory tract and their subsequent absorption by the alveoli.[15]

Pulmonary alveolar macrophages are also poisoned by smoke. This severely impairs macrophage function, contributing in part to the high incidence of late bacterial pneumonia.[14]

Diagnosis

The diagnosis of smoke inhalation injury is usually apparent from a history of exposure to fire or smoke in an enclosed space. Any animal with a flame burn or the acrid smell of smoke on its coat is assumed to have sustained smoke inhalation until it is proven otherwise. The rescuers are questioned carefully regarding where the animal was found, whether it was able to move away from the fire under its own power, and the duration of exposure.

Careful examination of facial burns, a search for oral burns, and laryngeal examination to check for laryngospasm are performed immediately. Hoarseness, expiratory wheeze, and carbonaceous sputum are indicators of potentially serious involvement. Inhalation injury may cause auscultable rales or rhonchi which may be evident on presentation or delayed until hours later. Cough, stridor, tachypnea (early), and bradypnea (later) may also be evident.[3] A cherry red color of the skin and mucous membranes, which may result from CO toxicity, burns, or heat from the fire, may mask cyanosis and poor perfusion from shock. The eyes are examined for evidence of conjunctivitis or corneal abrasions.

The presence of soot in the sputum or history of exposure confirms the diagnosis of smoke inhalation, and treatment is started at once. No further immediate diagnostic studies are required. However, several diagnostic aids are especially useful for better defining the initial condition of the patient and monitoring progress: carboxyhemoglobin determination, blood gas analysis, and thoracic radiographs. Iced venous blood samples for COHb determination are transported as soon as possible to a human hospital. High COHb levels alert the clinician to the possibility of ensuing serious neurologic complications from CO-induced hypoxia. Serial arterial blood gas analyses are of value in monitoring respiratory function. Thoracic radiographs are often normal initially, but after 16–24 hr pulmonary atelectasis, edema, hemorrhage, and infection may be found. The radiographic abnormalities in smoke inhalation cases do not always correlate with the degree of existing pulmonary injury.[3]

Treatment

The initial treatment priority in the smoke inhalation patient is establishment of an adequate airway. This may involve simply oropharyngeal suction, removing debris, and maintaining an unobstructed flow of air. If laryngeal examination reveals significant laryngospasm or swelling, nasotracheal or endotracheal intubation is performed. Alternatively, a tracheostomy can be performed before it is required as a last-minute emergency effort, using the technique described in Chapter 1.

Definitive therapy for CO poisoning is the administration of 100% O_2.[15,17] Reaching this concentration is impossible at the scene of the fire where inspired O_2 concentrations of only 30–35% can be achieved by the O_2 mask commonly used by firemen. The immediate goals are to reverse cerebral and myocardial hypoxia, and to accelerate CO elimination, all of which can be accomplished by a high concentration of inspired O_2. The half-life of COHb is 4 hr when breathing room air compared to 30 min when 100% O_2 is administered.

Patients that are fairly alert at presentation are usually placed in a conventional O_2 cage with a delivered O_2 concentration capacity of up to 40%. If an O_2 cage is not available, O_2 can be administered by mask, although alert animals often resist. If clinical signs of hypoxia develop despite these measures (irritable or aggressive behavior, incoordination, somnolence, collapse, or convulsions), the patient is intubated so that 100% O_2 can be administered.[14] Pentobarbital, diazepam (Valium), and, in dogs, narcotics such as morphine or oxymorphone (Numorphan) can be used as sedatives. Once sedated, the animal is intubated with a sterile, cuffed endotracheal tube and ventilated with positive pressure at a rate of 8–12 respirations/min for 30–40 min using the rebreathing bag of an anesthetic machine, a mechanical ventilator, or for short-term use a positive-pressure breathing bag (Ambu bag).[14] Oxygen therapy is also beneficial for the pulmonary edema which may occur after smoke inhalation injury resulting from altered alveolocapillary permeability.

Intravenous fluids are indicated in hypoxic states and shock to help maintain cardiac output, as reduced perfusion aggravates tissue hypoxia. Lactated Ringer's solution is the fluid of choice, and fluid administration is monitored carefully to avoid overhydration which could potentiate interstitial pulmonary edema.

The use of corticosteroids in inhalation injury is controversial. These agents have been used in the past for the early treatment of smoke inhalation injury on the assumption that they would help prevent or decrease the tracheobronchial inflammatory response associated with smoke inhalation. Steroids have also been used to treat cerebral edema and increased intracranial pressure associated with CO-induced brain hypoxia. However, studies using animal models have shown significant immunosuppression and decreased tracheobronchial clearance mechanisms when steroids are used. Steroid use in patients which have sustained both smoke inhalation injury and thermal injury results in increased mortality, and recent human studies involving isolated smoke inhalation injury strongly suggest that there is no difference in morbidity and mortality when comparing steroid- and nonsteroid-treated groups.[9] Because the risks of steroid use may outweigh the benefits, the author does not recommend the use of steroids in smoke inhalation patients.

Studies have also failed to document the efficacy of antibiotics for prophylaxis against late-developing pneumonia. Antibiotics given early may even be detrimental by selecting for resistant bacteria. Antibiotics, however, are used whenever a bacterial complication is suspected, and the choice of an antibiotic is preferably based on an airway culture and sensitivity test. In animals, pulmonary infections are most often caused by gram-negative bacteria; thus the initial choice of an antibiotic is made with this in mind.

Bronchodilator therapy is often used to help alleviate the reflex bronchospasm caused by inhalation of soot particles. Some useful bronchodilators include: aminophylline 6–10 mg/kg IM, IV, or PO tid; theophylline (Elixophyllin Elixir) 0.4 ml/kg PO tid; or a combination bronchodilator and expectorant (Quibron) at 0.6 ml/kg PO tid.

Complicating Factors

Inhalation injury in conjunction with body surface burns has a poorer prognosis for survival than that of inhalation injury alone. The incidence of postinhalation bronchopneumonia is increased if there are complicating factors, including surface burns or the use of tracheostomy tubes. Improper handling of tracheal tubes and poor management of tracheostomies may significantly increase the incidence of bronchopneumonia.

THERMAL INJURY

Thermal burns in animals may be due to a variety of causes. Flame burns are sustained in house, apartment, or brush fires; furnace or stove blasts; or malicious assault (e.g., gasoline dousing, firecrackers). Scald injuries result from spilled or spattered boiling water or cooking oil. Chemical burns are caused·by hot tar, corrosive acid, or alkalis.

Classification

The burn classification scheme of first, second, and third degree burns in humans, based on the severity and type of lesion produced, is not closely applicable to animals because of differences from humans in skin thickness and skin blistering characteristics.[6] A more practical classification scheme for animals categorizes burns into partial thickness and full thickness. Partial-thickness burns involve incomplete destruction of the skin and clinically are characterized by erythema, local edema, evidence of persistent capillary circulation, and partial sensation to touch.[6] In contrast, full-thickness burns involve complete destruction of all skin elements. There is a lack of superficial blood flow, insensitivity of the skin to touch, and easy epilation of hair.[6] These lesions often become leather-like.

The extent of surface injury may be estimated by measuring the burned area and comparing it to the total body surface area of the animal. Early assessment of depth and extent of burn injuries is important in determining a comprehensive treatment plan for specific burn and systemic therapy.

Pathophysiology

The emergency clinician must be acutely aware of the various systemic disorders that can occur in conjunction with thermal injuries, especially those which can be life-threatening. Hypovolemic shock begins very soon after infliction of major burns, and unless treated rapidly serious decreases in blood flow to the heart, brain, lungs, kidneys, and liver occur. Burns involving greater than 15% of the body surface area can result in serious hypovolemic shock in dogs and cats.[6]

Pulmonary complications are common in burned patients. Early problems include ventilation-perfusion abnormalities complicated in some cases by increased pulmonary resistance. If there is concurrent inhalation injury, there may be severe laryngeal edema and toxic damage to both upper and lower airways. Pulmonary edema may occur secondary to the injury and be worsened by overzealous fluid therapy. Late complications in burn patients include pulmonary infection, atelectasis, and embolism.

Acute renal failure may result from the effects of hypovolemia or, later, from burn-related sepsis. Hypoxic hepatic parenchymal damage may also result from hypovolemia. A significant anemia may occur early (first several days) in the syndrome due to the effects of the burn on blood cells traversing the vessels in injured areas or to a consumptive effect within the burn itself. Transfusions may become necessary.

Duodenal ulceration can be a complication of severe thermal trauma, and hemoconcentration may be a predisposing factor. Perforation and peritonitis may result.

Immunologic capabilities in burn patients are often decreased, causing impaired polymorphonuclear leukocyte migration and phagocytosis. Thus sepsis is a common cause of death in both human and animal burn cases.

Finally, thermal injury initiates more rapid erosion of lean body mass than does any other disease process.[16] Consequences of increased metabolic activity in burn patients include a negative nitrogen balance and a rapid decrease in body weight. Energy and protein stores essential to wound healing may become severely depleted.

Emergency Management of Major Burns

Initially, the treatment of major burns is the same as for all forms of trauma; quickly assess vital signs and ensure that the patient is able to breathe. Adequate ventilation and oxygenation may be possible in room air; however, if any concurrent inhalation injury has occurred, the patient is placed in an oxygen-enriched environment or sedated and administered 100% O_2, as discussed earlier for smoke inhalation.

Placing an intravenous line for fluid administration is the next priority. Support of the circulation is critical in treating hypovolemic shock and the fluid losses which occur into large burn spaces. It is extremely important that catheter sites be prepared aseptically to prevent infection. Large dogs may require two intravenous lines to meet initial fluid requirements. The initial fluid used is lactated Ringer's given in shock doses using the guidelines described in Chapter 2. After fluid therapy has been started, the patient is sedated for pain relief. This helps to relieve some of the anxiety, fear, and stress associated with major burn injuries and which is responsible for excessive energy utilization. Morphine or meperidine (Demerol) is useful for this purpose. The duration of action of morphine in dogs and cats is 6 hr, whereas meperidine is active for only approximately 45 min in dogs and 2 hr in cats. Pain relief is provided at a morphine dosage of 0.25–0.5 mg/kg in dogs. To avoid excitement in cats the dosage should not exceed 0.1 mg/kg. Meperidine is dosed at 10 mg/kg in dogs and 3 mg/kg in cats. Intramuscular administration is preferred because subcutaneous doses may be absorbed less reliably in shock states.

Local management of the burn wounds is begun only after the above treatments have been instituted. The hair is gently clipped from all wounds, being careful to avoid further damage from the clippers. Contamination and debris may be removed by flushing with saline or cleansing with dilute povidone-iodine solution (not scrub). If referral of the patient to an institution with intensive care facilities is planned, it can be done at this point. The patient is wrapped in clean sheets and blankets for warmth and comfort during transport. Hypothermic stress must be avoided in an already critical patient.

After cleansing, the burn wounds are covered with a topical antimicrobial cream to aid in prevention of wound sepsis. Ointments such as 1% silver sulfadiazine (Silvadene cream) and mafenide acetate (Sulfamylon) are the most effective. Because significant quantities of topical medications may be absorbed systemically in patients with major burns, adverse reactions attributable to sulfonamides are watched for carefully. Oils and greasy topical agents should not be applied to burns because they macerate tissue and delay healing.[2]

Large wounds are then covered with saline-moistened gauze sponges to keep the wounds moist and clean. A cast stockinette can be used as a loose body wrap to keep the sponges in place and to aid in keeping the wounds clean. Blankets and sheets are used as needed to maintain warmth.

Further care then consists of hourly monitoring of the temperature, quality of respiration, and urine output. An apparent reset in central temperature regulation occurs in the thermal-injured patient, such that animals with large burns frequently maintain a body temperature of 103.5–105°F. Monitoring the stable core temperature is important because infection is most often recognized initially by marked deviation from the baseline level.[16] Pulmonary function is monitored for signs of pulmonary edema or pneumonia; serial packed cell volumes are monitored for anemia and the possible need for blood transfusion; total plasma protein is monitored for hypoproteinemia; and clinical status is monitored for signs of septic shock. Urine output is a good indicator of the adequacy of fluid therapy. All intravenous catheters are changed every 72 hr or, if placed through burn tissue, every 48 hr.

Maintenance Burn Care

Maintenance care in patients with major burns consists primarily of local wound treatment and ensuring adequate nutritional intake. Because thermal injury initiates a rapid erosion of body mass, vigorous nutritional support must be instituted as soon as possible.[16] If the patient is not eating well on its own, tube feeding is used to meet caloric requirements (80–100 Kcal/kg/day).

Eschar excision of full-thickness burns usually begins on the second or third day to help prevent heavy bacterial colonization of the underlying tissues. Burned tissue acts as an excellent medium to support bacterial growth. Leather-like patches of skin are excised tangentially using a scalpel or sharp scissors. This is best done as soon as tissue surfaces are observed to be separating or cracking. After eschar excision, a 15- to 20-min full-body soak in a tub with water temperature of 106–110°F is beneficial. Povidone-iodine solution is added to the water, and infected tissue sites are gently massaged to further remove loose eschar. As soon as the soak is complete, the patient is dried quickly using sterile surgical towels. Heat lamps can be used to help minimize the tremendous tissue cooling which the patient experiences when removed from the tub. Topical antimicrobial preparations, moist gauze, and a stockinette body wrap are then applied as before. This procedure is followed twice daily. Although antibiotic use cannot be expected to sterilize a burn wound, topical antibacterial treatment has been shown to significantly reduce the number of microorganisms and minimize the spread of infection, or septicemia.

Use of systemic antibiotics is limited to confirmed cases of bacterial septicemia. Ideally, exudate obtained from a burn wound is submitted for culture and sensitivity testing as soon as it appears purulent. Gram stains are useful in selecting proper antibiotics while awaiting sensitivity test results. The most commonly isolated organisms from burn wounds are *Pseudomonas*, *Proteus*, *Escherichia coli*, and *Staphylococcus*. Life-threatening burn sepsis is best treated with cephalosporin and aminoglycoside antibiotics in combination.

A new synthetic skin substitute, comprised of a silicone-nylon composite with peptides derived from dermal collagen and bound to the nylon mesh, is now available as an alternative burn wound covering (Biobrane). It has excellent wound adherent properties and allows good penetrability of topical antibiotic preparations. These skin meshes need be changed only every 48 hr during maintenance treatment. Finally, after infection has been controlled and granulation tissue has developed (days to weeks), large remaining skin defects can be closed using grafting techniques.

SPECIAL CATEGORIES OF CHEMICAL INJURY

Skin injuries produced by chemicals can lead to special problems in management. Because of the diverse mechanisms of injury, treatment must be tailored to the specific etiologic agent. The possibility of wound progression after the chemical exposure must be anticipated.

Tar Burns

Burns caused by hot tar or asphalt are uncommon in veterinary medicine. More commonly, veterinarians are presented with patients who have contacted soft but not hot asphalt or tar. Nonetheless, if an animal has contacted or been splattered with hot tar, the treatment is immediate cooling of the burned areas with large volumes of cold water. Clients seeking telephone advice are instructed to avoid use of any irritating petroleum products (e.g., motor oil, gasoline) which may produce further tissue damage.

Once the tar has cooled off, the most effective way of removing it without injuring the skin is to dissolve it slowly in topical agents, e.g., antibiotic ointment (Polysporin, Neosporin), petrolatum, mineral oil, or lanolin.[4] An advantage of the antibiotic-containing ointments is that they may help to limit bacterial proliferation on the burn. The ointment base is a bland petroleum with the surface-active emulsifying agent polyoxyethylene sorbitan (Tween 80). Neosporin contains neomycin, which causes skin sensitivity in some dogs. The topical agent is applied liberally and gently rubbed over the tar until it begins to dissolve; it can then be washed away. Any tar not initially removed can be coated with a layer of ointment and covered with a dressing. Dressing changes two to three times daily aid in removal of the remaining asphalt. Tar burns are treated right away because of the risk of developing infection beneath adherent material.

Chemical Injury

Burn injury caused by a chemical often continues until the chemical has been remove or neutralized by an external agent or the skin itself. As a general rule, initial treatment for any chemical burn involves irrigation with large amounts of cool water for a sufficient length of time to achieve both dilution and removal. This may involve time periods of up to several hours. By decreasing the concentration, as well as physically removing the agent, water irrigation decreases the rate of reaction between the chemical and the tissue. In addition, the hygroscopic action of some concentrated acids and bases is reduced, and burn wound pH levels are returned toward normal. The hair in affected areas is clipped as soon as possible. Gloves are worn to help avoid contact with the chemical. It is recommended that alkaline burns be irrigated for at least several hours. For smaller burns this may involve simply holding the affected area under tap water.

Neutralizing agents are not indicated for most chemicals because many produce heat when they interact with the chemical. Special cases in which specific neutralization is important, however, include burns resulting from hydrofluoric acid and phenol compounds.[4] Upon contact with the skin, hydrogen gas and fluoride ions are released and the fluoride ions rapidly penetrate the skin, producing deep damage. Severe burn injury is caused by ongoing binding of fluoride ions with various salts in the skin. In addition to copious water irrigation, a 10% calcium gluconate solution is injected into the burn wound in quantities small enough to avoid tissue distention. Approximately 0.5 ml calcium gluconate per square centimeter of burn surface area is injected and is extended to include normal surrounding tissue.[4] If burn pain does not subside within 15 min the treatment is repeated.

Phenol, a widely used disinfectant in cleaning agents, can produce direct caustic skin injury as well as systemic toxicity after absorption through the skin. Diluted solutions are more rapidly absorbed, and therefore swabbing the skin with water is not advised. Rather, copious water irrigation is begun immediately. Following irrigation, the wound is swabbed with a solvent, e.g., propylene glycol, vegetable oil, or soap and water. Systemic side effects due to phenol injury include cardiac arrhythmias, hemolysis, and muscle irritability. Epidermal sloughs should be removed via vigorous scrubbing of the wound.

Maintenance wound care for chemical wounds involves application of topical antibiotic preparations, e.g., silver sulfadiazine (Silvadene), mafenide acetate (Sulfamylon), or povidone-iodine (Betadine), and grease-gauze (Adaptic Vaseline) wrappings, which are changed every 1–2 days. Systemic antibiotics are rarely indicated.

Gasoline Immersion Injury

Occasionally, veterinarians may be presented with patients suffering from gasoline immersion injury. These cases are usually the unfortunate result of malicious activities, e.g., spraying or dousing animals in gasoline. In addition, unknowing owners sometimes use gasoline or other petroleum products to treat external parasites. Gasoline vapor can cause severe intoxication in poorly ventilated areas. Gasoline immersion injury can be a benign cutaneous chemical burn or a life-threatening multisystem injury. The hydrocarbon content of gasoline is responsible for the major toxic effects, which include chemical cutaneous burns, neurologic disorders, pulmonary injuries, cardiovascular abnormalities, gastrointestinal disturbances, and renal and hepatic injuries.[12] The cutaneous burns result from the fat-solvent action of gasoline.

Treatment of the cutaneous wounds involves prolonged hydrotherapy (1–2 hr) followed by application of topical antibiotics. Intense fluid therapy and prevention of hypothermia are important in treating animals with systemic involvement.

Injuries involving leaded gasoline may also include lead poisoning. The organic lead compound, tetraethyl lead, easily penetrates the skin and has a high affinity for nervous tissue.[12] Significant absorption occurs through the respiratory tract. Treatment with Ca-EDTA (calcium versenate) as an injectable chelating agent is used to treat lead poisoning, as described in Chapter 11. Alternatively, an oral chelating agent (penicillamine) may be used.

HYPOTHERMIA

Hypothermia, a spontaneous decrease in core temperature as a result of environmental exposure, is most commonly seen in animals who are injured, debilitated, old, or unconscious; animals immobilized by leg-hold traps; animals immersed in cold water; and animals who become wet and exhausted and are unable to find shelter in a cold environment. Accidental hypothermia of anesthetized small animal surgical patients is a common and potentially dangerous problem.

Diagnosis

Hypothermia can be easily overlooked; standard thermometers read only as low as 94°F (34.4°C), and the signs and symptoms of hypothermia may be vague and misleading. Mental confusion, impaired gait, and lethargy are early signs. The pulse may be slow and shallow, or absent, and respirations infrequent. At temperatures less than 90°F (32°C), shivering is absent and considerable muscle stiffness may be apparent. As the temperature drops further, the pupils may be dilated and fixed, pulse and respirations may be difficult to detect, and the animal may even appear dead. Because of decreased oxygen requirements of cold organs, patients with severe bradycardia can recover without serious sequelae. A low-reading thermometer is necessary for accurate diagnosis. Glass thermometers that read down to 75°F (23.8°C) are available (Dynamed, Inc.).

Treatment

Severely hypothermic patients must be handled as gently as possible because the cold, bradycardic heart is extremely irritable and unnecessary movements can precipitate cardiac arrhythmias. A full minute or even longer may be required to detect the presence of vital signs in severely hypothermic patients. If the patient is in cardiac arrest, cardiopulmonary resuscitation efforts are begun, although the cold heart is relatively unresponsive to drugs or electrical stimulation. Injected drugs tend to accumulate in peripheral tissues and may cause serious toxicity when vasodilation occurs during rewarming.

Initial vigorous rewarming should be avoided because the resulting peripheral vasodilation may lead to shunting of cold acidotic blood to major core organs, which can precipitate cardiac arrhythmias. Rather, external rewarming is more safely accomplished by initially surrounding the patient with blankets. Hot water bottles and heating blankets must be used cautiously because of the increased risk of thermal burns to tissues that are underperfused. Passive external rewarming is often the only treatment necessary for mildly to moderately hypothermic patients with a stable cardiac status.

Prolonged hypothermia often causes depression of renal function, hypovolemia, and acidosis. Warmed intravenous fluids are administered to these patients and renal function carefully monitored. Fluids containing potassium are not used initially.

Core rewarming techniques, e.g., peritoneal dialysis, colonic irrigation, and intragastric lavage, are reserved for patients with severe [core temperature less than 90°F (32°C)] or prolonged (>12 hr) hypothermia or those with cardiovascular instability.[18] Peritoneal dialysis is an excellent and inexpensive means of rewarming. The dialysate is warmed to 109°F (43°C) and instilled into the peritoneal cavity as fast as gravity permits.[18] The fluid is removed immediately and the procedure repeated until normothermia is reached.

Hypothermia in surgical patients must not be overlooked. Any patient recovering more slowly from anesthesia than expected is monitored for hypothermia. Hypothermia can be minimized by avoiding excessive use of cold fluids (e.g., alcohol) for preparation of the skin and by avoiding direct patient contact with cold surgery table surfaces. Also, fluids for intravenous use and for lavage are warmed. If there is pronounced shivering during recovery from anesthesia, continued use of oxygen may help prevent tissue hypoxia.[11] Neonates less than 2 months of age are especially susceptible to hypothermia because they have a poorly developed thermoregulatory system and are unable to shiver to maintain body temperature.

FROSTBITE

The treatment of frostbite injury primarily involves prompt and thorough rewarming. Because refreezing results in increased tissue loss, frozen areas are not thawed if there is any possibility that thawing could be followed by refreezing. Rapid thawing is best accomplished by submerging the tissue in warm water (104–108°F) for 20–30 min. Thawed tissues are extremely sensitive and must not be rubbed.

Recent studies suggest that thromboxane and prostaglandins play a significant role in the pathogenesis of tissue damage from frostbite injury. Furthermore, treatment with a topical thromboxane inhibitor, *Aloe vera* (Dermaide Aloe), and aspirin as a systemic antiprostaglandin agent have shown promising results in humans with frostbite injury. Topical *Aloe vera* is applied to injured tissues every 6 hr, and aspirin is administered three times daily for 72 hr.[5]

Antibiotics are recommended to help prevent secondary infections. Amputation of injured limbs is done only as a last resort and not until at least 3 weeks have elapsed to allow sufficient time to determine tissue viability.

HEATSTROKE

Heatstroke is a true medical emergency associated with high mortality. It is characterized by hyperthermia with a rectal temperature of 105–111°F (41–44°C) or higher in conjunction with alteration in consciousness. In most cases the patient has been confined in a poorly ventilated enclosure on a hot, humid day, e.g., in a hot apartment or automobile. The condition can also occur in animals confined outdoors in direct sunlight on hot, humid days. Highly humid conditions impair evaporation of water from the oral and nasal cavities, which renders panting ineffective as a cooling mechanism. Studies have documented a tremendous level of heat buildup inside cars parked in direct sunlight.[13] It should be noted that leaving car windows partially or fully open does not prevent this heat buildup.[13] Thus a pet confined to an automobile under these conditions is subject to tremendous heat stress. Cats seem to tolerate higher temperatures better than dogs and are rarely presented for heatstroke. Among dogs, the brachycephalic breeds are most susceptible.

Pathophysiology

Successful therapy of heatstroke depends on understanding the pathophysiology of hyperthermic injury and anticipating the many complications that can occur. Excessive panting in response to temperature elevation may result in respiratory alkalosis. Later, excessive muscle activity associated with panting may contribute to combination of respiratory alkalosis and metabolic acidosis.[10] Electrolyte changes, including hyperkalemia and hypophosphatemia, have been documented in dogs with experimental hyperthermia.[10] Significant hemoconcentration may occur (packed cell volume greater than 70%). The important life-threatening complications which can result from heatstroke include cerebral edema, acute renal failure, and disseminated intravascular coagulation (DIC). Clinically, many patients are stuporous and exhibit involuntary tremors and paddling movements due to central nervous system (CNS) disturbances. With severe or prolonged hyperthermia animals may be presented in a coma, which often culminates in death from respiratory arrest. Renal dysfunction secondary to myoglobinuria from heat-induced rhabdomyolysis must be anticipated and treated aggressively if it becomes evident. Hemorrhagic diathesis may result from DIC.

Treatment

The key to treatment of heatstroke involves rapid, aggressive care and early anticipation of complicating factors. Rapid cooling using any method available to actively lower the patient's temperature is the first priority of treatment. This is best accomplished by lowering the trunk and limbs into a tub of cold or iced water or by hosing the animal with water. If the animal is comatose, it is intubated immediately and ventilated with oxygen, as hypoxia potentiates CNS edema. Additional emergency care includes administration of intravenous fluids in shock doses using lactated Ringer's solution or normal saline. Fluid administration helps alleviate hemoconcentration and peripheral circulatory failure and may be of benefit in preventing acute renal failure and DIC.

The rectal temperature is taken every 5–10 min, and cooling is discontinued when the temperature reaches approximately 103°F (39.5°C). Further cooling may result in hypothermia. When hyperthermia recurs, recooling may be necessary. Use of alcohol sponge baths should be avoided because they may induce shivering, which may raise rather than lower the core temperature.

Dexamethasone is administered intravenously to treat cerebral edema. An initial dosage of 1.0–2.0 mg/kg is followed by the same amount on a daily basis divided into two or three doses for several days depending on neurologic response. If recovery is rapid, only one or two doses may be necessary. If seizures occur they can be controlled with phenobarbital or intravenous diazepam (Valium). Initial baseline laboratory data should include a complete blood count, biochemistry profile, and urinalysis. Urine output and renal function are monitored closely for signs of inadequate volume replacement as well as for any indications of acute renal failure. Oliguria or azotemia are managed as discussed for acute renal failure in Chapter 6. Blood chemistries are followed daily for the first several days so that imbalances can be identified and managed as quickly as possible.

When DIC is associated with heatstroke, it may be indicated by excessive bleeding from venipuncture sites, hemorrhagic diarrhea, and development of petechiae or ecchymoses. Coagulation studies which help to verify the presence of DIC include the platelet count, one-stage prothrombin time (OSPT), activated partial thromplastin time (APTT), and fibrin degradation products (FDP) assay. If it is not possible to perform these tests and bleeding tendencies are recognized, treatment is initiated with the presumption that DIC is present. The treatment of DIC is described in Chapter 8.

Occasionally heatstroke episodes are followed by icterus or biochemical evidence of liver damage. In some cases liver failure ensues and may be complicated by DIC. If liver involvement becomes clinically evident, intravenous fluids should consist of half-strength saline with 2.5–5% dextrose.

SNAKEBITE

Approximately 20 species of poisonous snakes exist in the United States. Most are rattlesnakes, cottonmouths, and copperheads, all of which are called vipers because they have deep pits lined with heat receptors in the cheeks between the eyes and nostrils. Pit vipers are widely distributed throughout the United States, but the majority of poisonous snakebite cases occur in the southern and southwestern states. It has been estimated that 15,000 animals are bitten annually in the United States, and that rattlesnakes account for approximately 80% of snakebite deaths.

Snake venoms are highly complex mixtures of many proteins and peptides, including some enzymes. The venom of pit vipers is predominantly hemotoxic, affecting blood vessel wall integrity and the clotting mechanism. This results in severe local swelling after the bite injury. Coral snake venom is predominantly neurotoxic and may produce neuromuscular block. Coral snake envenomization has a grave prognosis; fortunately, animals are seldom bitten by these snakes.

Diagnosis

The initial step in snakebite injury is to identify the offending snake as poisonous or nonpoisonous, if possible. If the snake is caught, the head should not be damaged as it may be required for species identification. The recognition of clinical signs is the major guide to diagnosis, as some episodes of snakebite occur without envenomation. In most cases of envenomation, signs occur within 30–60 min and consist of local pain, swelling, and ecchymosis.[7] Dark, bloody fluid may ooze from the puncture wounds. Systemic effects, e.g., hypotension with tachycardia, pulmonary edema, salivation, and shock may occur within the first several hours. Hemolytic anemia, hemoglobinuria, and acute renal failure may follow. Snakebite injuries in the head or neck area may cause severe swelling around the upper airway resulting in respiratory distress.

Treatment

If an animal has been bitten by a harmless snake, or there is no evidence of envenomation from a venomous snake, cleaning and debriding the wound and administration of a broad-spectrum antibiotic should be sufficient treatment. Antibiotics are indicated because the oral cavity of the snake is grossly contaminated by a wide variety of bacteria. Aspirin or other suitable drug for relief of pain may also be necessary.

Emergency treatment of pit viper bites that show evidence of envenomation is administered immediately. Polyvalent antivenin compound (Antivenin) is given intravenously or intraarterially as soon as possible[7]; 10–20 ml (one to two vials) is given in most cases.[1] The sooner the venom is neutralized, the better is the therapeutic result. Clinicians experienced in treating snakebite cases have observed anaphylactic reactions in cats following intravenous antivenin administration. Thus antivenin is given to cats cautiously and only if absolutely necessary.

Intravenous fluids are administered to counteract the danger of shock. The use of corticosteroids, e.g., dexamethasone (Dexamethasone Sodium Phosphate) or prednisone sodium succinate (Solu-Delta-Cortef), has been advocated as an emergency measure to treat shock, relieve pain, and reduce swelling. Another potent antiinflammatory agent which seems to be useful in alleviating swelling and pain in injured tissues is DMSO. It may also potentiate the action of corticosteroids. DMSO is usually applied topically, but it has also been used intravenously in dogs with snakebite at a dose of 10 ml, regardless of the size of the dog.[1]

Broad-spectrum antimicrobial therapy is recommended because of the complex oral flora of snakes. The most common species isolated include *Pseudomonas aeruginosa*, *Proteus* spp., *Clostridium* spp., and staphylococci. Tetanus antitoxin is probably indicated in victims of snakebite.

Thoughtful attention must be given to pain relief in any case of snakebite. Severe pain may be a significant factor in the onset of shock. Demerol (10 mg/kg IM) is useful but short-acting. Flunixin meglumine (Banamine) affords pain relief as well as having an antiinflammatory effect at a dosage of 1–2 mg/kg IV.

BITES AND STINGS OF BEES, WASPS, HORNETS, AND SPIDERS

Insect stings involving bees, wasps, and hornets cause a painful local inflammatory reaction with a variable degree of swelling. Multiple stings may result in shock. The most important clinical consideration related to an insect bite is the possibility of a life-threatening anaphylactic reaction in a hypersensitized animal. Anaphylaxis can result from a single sting in a previously hypersensitized animal. Furthermore, bites in the pharyngeal or cervical area can result in severe local swelling surrounding the upper airway, leading to respiratory distress and even asphyxiation.

Emergency treatment of insect bites consists of epinephrine (1:10,000) at a dose of 1–5 ml subcutaneously when anaphylaxis is evident. The onset of anaphylaxis may be delayed so the bitten animal must remain under close observation. Corticosteroids can be given to reduce the inflammatory response and relieve pain. Antihistamines are also helpful. Emergency tracheostomy may be necessary if pharyngeal or cervical swelling causes tracheal compression. Minor bites usually require only cold packs, rest, and careful observation for complications.

Spider bites are difficult to diagnose because the incident is rarely observed and the bite marks are so small. The venom of *Lactrodectus* spp. is highly toxic to mammals.[7] Bites cause initial local swelling and pain, but envenomation may then lead to neurotoxic manifestations, including muscle spasms, ataxia, and salivation. Convulsions and paralysis may ensue within 6 hr in acute cases, or not until several days later when less severe envenomation has occurred.[7] Antivenin is given as soon as possible if it is available. Intravenous fluids and corticosteroids are also administered. Meperidine (Demerol) may be given for pain, and sedation may be necessary if there are severe muscle spasms. Supportive care may be necessary for at least several days.

Bites caused by spiders of the *Loxoceles* spp. result in longer-term manifestations, beginning with initial pruritus and swelling and leading to eventual blister formation and focal ulceration (1–2 weeks). These lesions do not heal quickly, and often self-trauma of the area complicates improvement. In some cases fever, convulsions, hemolysis, and thrombocytopenia occur.[7] Corticosteroids are given initially along with application of cold packs. Focal ulcerations are excised early to promote more rapid healing.

REFERENCES

1. Clark KA: Management of poisonous snakebites in dogs and cats. Mod Vet Pract 6:427, 1981
2. Davis LE: Thermal burns. In Swaim SF (ed): Surgery of Traumatized Skin. p. 214. Saunders, Philadelphia, 1980
3. Farrow CS: Inhalation injury. In Kirk RW (ed): Current Veterinary Therapy VIII. p. 173. Saunders, Philadelphia, 1983
4. Frank DH: Special categories of thermal injury: evaluation and management. Top Emerg Med 3:45, 1981
5. McCauley RL, Hing DN, Martin CR, et al: Frostbite injuries: a rational approach based on the pathophysiology. J Trauma 23:143, 1983
6. McKeever PJ: Thermal Injury. In Kirk RW (ed): Current Veterinary Therapy VIII. p. 180. Saunders, Philadelphia, 1983
7. Meerdink GL: Bites and stings of venomous animals. In Kirk RW (ed): Current Veterinary Therapy VIII. p. 155. Saunders, Philadelphia, 1983
8. Mellins RB, Park S: Respiratory complications of smoke inhalation in victims of fires. J Pediatr 87:1, 1975
9. Robinson NB, Hudson LD, Riem M, et al: Steroid therapy following isolated smoke inhalation injury. J Trauma 22:876, 1982
10. Schall WD: Heat Stroke. In Kirk RW (ed): Current Veterinary Therapy VIII. p. 183. Saunders, Philadelphia, 1983
11. Seeler DL: Hypothermia and the small surgical patient. Vet Prof Top 6:22, 1981
12. Simpson LA, Cruse CW: Gasoline immersion injury. Plast Reconstr Surg 67:54, 1981
13. Surpure JS: Heat-related illness and the automobile. Ann Emerg Med 11:263, 1982

14. Tams TR, Sherding RG: Smoke inhalation injury. Comp Contin Educ 3:986, 1981
15. Trunkey DD: Inhalation injury. Surg Clin North Am 58:1133, 1978
16. Wilmore DW: Metabolic changes in burns. In Arty CP, Moncrief JA, Pruitt BA (eds): Burns A Team Approach. p. 120. Saunders, Philadelphia, 1979
17. Winter PM, Mill JN: Carbon monoxide poisoning. JAMA 236:1502, 1976
18. Zenoble RD: Accidental hypothermia. In Kirk RW (ed): Current Veterinary Therapy VIII. p. 186. Saunders, Philadelphia, 1983

13 | Life-Threatening Sepsis

Richard B. Ford

Although the incidence of bacterial septicemia in companion animal practice is not precisely documented, septicemia must be regarded as one of the major infectious diseases of dogs and cats. The presence of bacteria in the blood of an animal may be transient and self-limited and therefore of little or no detectable significance clinically. On the other hand, the extension of localized infections, e.g., those involving the skin or oral cavity, can result in blood-borne bacterial infections that cause serious manifestations of systemic disease. The onset of clinical signs associated with bacterial septicemia may be acute or chronic, but in either case must be regarded as a true medical emergency that requires an organized diagnostic approach and aggressive implementation of specific therapeutic protocols directed at eliminating the infecting microbe as well as correcting secondary pathophysiological consequences of the infection.

The native microbial flora of companion animals is abundant and, in the healthy host, necessary to the well-being of the animal. It may seem paradoxical that the microorganisms involved in host defense mechanisms are the same organisms involved in life-threatening septicemic infections. There are, however, several explanations for this phenomenon. One principle factor seems to be that of microbial opportunism in the face of significant compromise of host defenses. The animal that presents with a true medical emergency requires specific intervention as discussed in the individual chapters of this text; yet it is this animal that, because of the potential for sustained suppression of normal defense mechanisms, deserves special attention with regard to risk of becoming septic. Hence it is the recognition of the patient that is at risk for developing life-threatening sepsis that is the key to sepsis management.

This chapter addresses the techniques available for diagnosing and managing ongoing sepsis and the physiological alterations that make sepsis life-threatening; the chapter also addresses the importance of recognizing and treat-ing those patients at risk of becoming septic.

SEPSIS DEFINED

The term bacteremia refers to invasion of the bloodstream by a microbial agent.[6] On the other hand, septicemia, or bacterial sepsis, refers not only to invasion of the bloodstream by bacteria but also to the production of clinical signs, e.g., fever and lethargy.[6,8] It is important to appreciate the fact that the presence of bacteria in blood and the colonization of bacteria in tissues does not suggest that a life-threatening condition exists or even that one will exist. Indeed, transient bacteremias are expected in virtually all animals undergoing routine dental prophylaxis; yet relatively few of these patients have serious complications. Sepsis does become life-threatening when the host animal is unable to mount an adequate defense response in the face of bacterial colo-nization and proliferation in tissue. Because bacterial sepsis is associated with hypotension, this term is often referred to as "septic shock."

Endotoxemia, on the other hand, implies the presence of a heat-stable bacterial toxin, found primarily in gram-negative organisms, circulating in the blood.[2] Endotoxin is a lipopolysaccharide complex that in human medicine has been the focus of attention in gram-negative rod septicemia. There is strong evidence that endotoxin can induce several circulatory and hemodynamic al-terations that result in shock, hence the term *endotoxin shock*. This term is frequently used interchangeably with "gram-negative sepsis with shock."[2,6,8]

Defined, bacterial endocarditis is a septic condition recognized in animals that is characterized by colonization of the endocardium by relatively avirulent bacteria, usually derived from normal flora of the oral cavity, gastrointestinal tract, or genitourinary tract. Bacterial endocarditis is a potentially debilitating, as well as life-threatening, condition which, unlike endotoxemia, produces sys-temic manifestations as a direct result of emboli that originate from endocardial and valvular vegetations of microbes.[1,7]

PATHOGENESIS OF SEPSIS

The mortality rates of septic patients, human and animal, are high and the prognosis of any patient with confirmed bacterial sepsis, whether caused by gram-negative or gram-positive organisms, must be regarded as grave. How-ever, the low survivability of sepsis cannot be primarily attributable to the inability of antimicrobial agents to control bacterial proliferation. There are, in fact, several complex physiological factors, the clinical aspects of which are reviewed below, that are the principle mediators of progressive deterioration, shock, and death.

The pathogenesis of shock in septic patients is best described in terms of host-endotoxin interactions. Endotoxin, which is actually a component of the cell walls of aerobic (and some anaerobic) gram-negative bacteria, elicits in-tense, widespread intravascular inflammation. The endotoxin-induced inflammation has been divided into three phases: (1) the mediator phase, the result of endotoxin activation of inflammation; (2) the phagocytosis phase, the intravascular phagocytosis of bacteria along the endothelium of tissue capillaries and venules; and (3) the shock phase, characterized by cellular hypoxia, lactic acidosis, and hypotension.[2]

During the mediator phase, endotoxin activates the complement system, generates kinin activity, activates coagulation, and increases prostaglandin activity. Clearly the patient is predisposed to disseminated intravascular coagulopathy as platelets release factor III, which in turn leads to thromboplastin generation. Endotoxin also activates Hageman factor (factor XII), which further potentiates coagulation. Recently it has been shown that endorphins, in response to endotoxin, can induce hypotension in experimental animals. Naloxone hydrochloride, a specific opiate antagonist, dramatically reverses endotoxin-induced hypotension and therefore may play an important role in the management of septic patients.

The phagocytic phase is characterized by the diffuse damage to the endothelium of capillaries and is likely associated with many of the clinical manifestations of septic shock, e.g., fever, reduced venous return (venipuncture may be difficult due to poor venous filling), and decreased cardiac output. Evidence of organ system failure may become apparent. Gastrointestinal hemorrhage and mucosal sloughing is well recognized in the dog and can be attributed to the development of villous hypoxia as blood pressure falls.[3] Splanchnic vascular pooling contributes to liver failure as manifested by increased levels of circulating hepatic enzymes, decreased clearance of indocyanine green, cholestasis, and icterus. Laboratory evidence of acute renal failure may also be seen in septic dogs. Renal infarction caused by microembolization, particularly in bacterial endocarditis, altered renal blood flow, and direct nephrotoxic injury caused by bacteria and endotoxin are the major causes of renal failure. Spontaneous bleeding and abnormal coagulation profiles are attributable to thrombocytopenia, decreased synthesis of clotting factors, and disseminated intravascular coagulation.[3]

The tissue anoxia phase is a terminal event that occurs after several hours of bacteremia/endotoxemia. It is characterized by profound reductions in blood flow within the microcirculation. Metabolic alterations associated with this phase include hypoglycemia, despite high levels of glucagon and epinephrine, decreased oxygen consumption with only slight differences in arteriovenous oxygen tension, lactic acidosis caused by anerobic carbohydrate metabolism, progressive intravascular coagulation, profound hypotension, and death.[2,3]

CLINICAL FEATURES OF SEPSIS

Clinical Signs

The variability of clinical signs associated with sepsis, the unpredictable clinical course, and the lack of a sensitive diagnostic test for septicemia or endotoxemia contributes substantially to the difficulty in confirming septicemia and to the poor prognosis associated with clinical sepsis.

Table 13-1. Conditions and Procedures Predisposing Patients to Sepsis and Septic Shock

Routine dentistry and extractions (particularly in older dogs)
Pyometra
Prostatic abscess
Pyothorax
Pneumonia
Peritonitis
Mitral insufficiency
Penetrating wounds
Compound fractures
Neoplasia
Intestinal obstruction/surgery
Placement of intravenous catheters (particularly long term)
Urinary catheterization; urinary tract infection
Malnutrition
Severe burns
Severe ectoparasitism
Immunosuppressive drugs

Persistent fever, lethargy, and leukocytosis are classic features of clinical sepsis. Although the diagnosis can be relatively straightforward in these patients, the onset of sepsis can be subtle and the patient's clinical features much less clear, particularly in the face of concurrent disease. A number of host factors, discussed below, must be taken into consideration when evaluating any patient at risk of becoming septic or presumed to have existing septicemia.

Host Risk Factors

Age. Although animals of any age may become septic, patients at greatest risk of developing septic shock and dying are the very young and the very old. The reasons for this are not completely understood, but it seems likely that defects in humoral and cell-mediated immunity are involved.

Underlying Disease. It is well known that bacterial sepsis is most often associated with some underlying defect in host defense mechanisms. Therefore it is not surprising that the single most significant factor favoring the development of sepsis is the presence of underlying disease. Table 13-1 lists those patients considered at greatest risk of developing septicemia or bacterial endocarditis.

Surgery. Surgery, particularly involving the urinary tract, oral cavity, or gastrointestinal tract, is a likely initiating factor in the development of sepsis. In addition, prolonged use of intravenous or urinary catheters can result in loss of normal anatomic barriers important in preventing bacteremia.

Drug Therapy. The increased use of immunosuppressive drugs in veterinary medicine, e.g., cyclophosphamide, plays an important role in the risk of clinical sepsis. These drugs have powerful suppressive effffects on host defense immune mechanisms, particularly bone marrow. Ironically, prior antibiotic therapy in humans, especially with broad-spectrum drugs such as chloramphenicol, predispose patients to gram-negative bacteremia. Presumably this occurs because of the ability of the antibiotic to alter normal microbial flora of the respiratory and gastrointestinal tracts with resultant colonization by antibiotic-resistant gram-negative bacteria.[6]

Miscellaneous. Trauma, widespread or severe burns, deep pyoderma, severe mite or flea infestations, and whelping are additional factors that may predispose a patient to the development of sepsis, as in each instance the integrity of normal anatomic barriers may be compromised.

Laboratory Findings

As with the physical examination, there are no consistent laboratory findings that confirm septicemia. If a discrete focus of infection is present, e.g., in the urinary tract, routine laboratory tests primarily support involvement of that organ system. Even when a focus is not present, leukocytosis and monocytosis support the presence of an infection but do not constitute a diagnosis.

The principle diagnostic test in patients suspected of having bacterial septicemia is the blood culture. Whole blood, usually 5–10 ml, is collected aseptically from a vein and inoculated into a liquid aerobic culture medium; when available, blood is also inoculated into anaerobic culture media. The skin over the vein from which the blood is collected must be clipped, cleansed with a surgical soap, and rinsed prior to venipuncture. Studies in humans indicate that collection of blood during febrile episodes in septic patients will likely yield a positive culture in bacteremic patients.[6] This probably applies equally in veterinary medicine. In addition, it has been shown that within a 24-hour period obtaining more than three blood cultures does not significantly improve the chances of obtaining a positive culture in a septic patient.[6] In severely ill patients, collecting one blood sample every 8 hr may be impractical. In these cases it is feasible to obtain three blood cultures over the span of only a few hours. Furthermore, there is no advantage to obtaining a single, large blood sample and inoculating serial blood culture vials.

Blood is inoculated into a liquid medium usually containing trypticase soy broth or thioglycollate broth. The media may also contain sodium polyanethole sulfonate, a compound that possess antiphagocytic, anticomplementary activity and inactivates some antibiotics. After inoculation, the blood culture medium is submitted to a laboratory where it is incubated at 37°C. The medium is then inspected for turbidity at least daily for the first 7 days. A sample of blood culture medium is gram-stained within 24 hr to detect the presence of small numbers of bacteria. Most laboratories do not keep blood cultures beyond 2 weeks. The usual time for detection of blood cultures is 3 days for both aerobes and anaerobes.

The fact that a patient has received prior antibiotic therapy does not preclude attempts to culture the blood. It is true that recovery of bacteria from a blood specimen is delayed or prevented in patients receiving antibiotics. However, it is possible to remove antimicrobial agents from blood specimens. A combined product containing polymeric adsorbent resin and a cation-exchange resin is commercially available (Antimicrobial Removal Device, Marion Scientific, Kansas, MO 64114). This procedure entails processing the blood specimen by mixing with the resins for approximately 15 min, after which the blood is aseptically transferred to an appropriate culture medium.

Gram-negative bacteremia is associated with circulating endotoxin. Efforts directed at developing a rapid, sensitive test that detects the presence of circulating endotoxin have centered around the *Limulus* gelation test.[6] *Limulus polyphemis*, the amebocyte of the horseshoe crab, is extracted and prepared as a lysate. Mixing minute quantities of endotoxin with *Limulus* lysate in vitro causes a gelation reaction. This test has proved somewhat disappointing in clinical trials in humans as false-positive as well as false-negative reactions are reported. Efficacy of the *Limulus* gelation test has not been reported in veterinary medicine.

TREATMENT

The treatment regimen for septic patients includes: (1) prompt recognition of bacteremia: (2) identification of the causative agent and its susceptibility to antimicrobial drugs; (3) use of appropriate dosages of antimicrobial agents; (4) use of the appropriate route for administering antimicrobial agents; (5) identification and elimination of the source of infection; and (6) prompt management of complications.

Antimicrobial Therapy

Ideally, the selection of an antibiotic is based on the bacterial species most likely to cause the septicemia. This is possible when time is available to obtain blood cultures and the culture results are positive. Table 13-2 summarizes primary and alternative treatment regimens for septic patients. When the specific causative organism has not been determined but it is deemed necessary to initiate treatment, the gentamicin protocol, outlined in Table 13-2, is recommended.

The duration of parenteral antibiotic therapy is determined by individual patient response to treatment but should be continued a minimum of 10 days. The patient may be maintained on an appropriate oral antibiotic if the clinical response to parenteral therapy was satisfactory. The duration of oral therapy varies depending on the type of infection and the patient's response; treatment periods of 4–8 weeks are not unreasonable.

Shock Therapy

Antibiotic therapy alone is of little benefit in treating septic patients. Realistically, the principal clinical challenge in the management of sepsis is maintaining an adequate plasma volume, cardiac output, and ventilation throughout antibiotic therapy.[5]

Because plasma protein losses may be extensive in septic shock, plasma and whole blood, given at a rate of 10 ml/kg/hr, are preferred for volume re-

Table 13-2. Antibiotic Therapy in Sepsis

Organism	Primary Drug	Alternate
Gram-positive *Staphylococcus aureus* *Streptococcus* spp. Anerobic bacteria (excluding *Bacillus fragilis*) *Corynebacterium* spp.	Na or K penicillin G 25,000 units/kg IV q 6 h	Cephalothin[a] 20–30 mg/kg IV q 6 h
Gram-negative E. coli Klebsiella spp. *Pseudomonas aeruginosa* *Proteus* spp. *Enterobacter* spp.	Gentamicin sulfate[b] 1–3 mg/kg IV q 8 h	Gentamicin 1–3 mg/kg IV q 8 h *coadministered with*[c] Carbenicillin 15 mg/kg IV q 8 h *or* Cephalothin[a] 20–30 mg/kg IV q 6 h

[a] May be given intramuscularly but injections are painful.

[b] Gentamicin nephrotoxicity is potentiated by dehydration and metabolic acidosis, both of which are common clinical findings in septic patients.

[c] Aminoglycoside antibiotics are often synergistic with β-lactam antibiotics.

placement. The total dose varies depending on individual circumstances; however, enough replacement fluid must be given to maintain the plasma oncotic pressure.[4] Alternately, 10% dextran solution can be administered intravenously at 0.5–1.0 ml/kg/hr to a maximum daily dose of 15 ml/kg.[4] Volume expansion may also be accomplished with lactated Ringer's solution given intravenously at 10–20 ml/kg/hr; in profound shock states, fluids may be given at a rate of 100 ml/kg/hr. A more detailed discussion of shock can be found in Chapter 2.

Other Considerations

Blood glucose levels may drop rapidly in septic shock. Monitoring glucose levels hourly determines when and if glucose administration is required. A 50% glucose solution, given intravenously at 0.25–0.5 g/kg/hr, is recommended. Metabolic acidosis is a characteristic clinical feature of septic shock. When blood gas (arterial or venous) monitoring is available, sodium bicarbonate can be administered intravenously to correct base deficits.*

The controversy over whether to use corticosteroids in septic shock continues with little relief in sight. Clearly, there is no indication for long-term corticosteroid therapy and little justification for short-term (more than 1 day) corticosteroid therapy in life-threatening sepsis. However, large, single doses of methylprednisolone sodium succinate (30 mg/kg IV) or dexamethasone sodium phosphate (3 mg/kg IV) given to dogs under experimental conditions

* Milliequivalents of sodium bicarbonate required = base deficit × 0.3 × kg body weight. (Give one-half the calculated dose in 20–30 min; the remainder is given over 3–5 hr).

suggests that these patients may benefit from single-dose corticosteroid therapy.

Recent studies into the role of nonsteroidal antiinflammatory drugs (indomethacin, aminopyrine, flufenamic acid, flunixin meglumine) in septic and endotoxin shock suggests that these drugs have an increasingly important role in the management of septic shock. Among these drugs, flunixin meglumine (2.2 mg/kg given twice daily at a single 12-hr interval) has been used in dogs with good results.[4] Nonsteroidal antiinflammatory drugs seem to prevent the development of hypotension by their ability to inhibit cyclooxygenase, thereby resulting in decreased levels of prostaglandins.

The principles of treatment for the disseminated intravascular coagulation that is sometimes precipitated by sepsis are described in Chapter 8.

PROGNOSIS

Although the prognosis of a patient with gram-positive sepsis is considered to be better than that of a patient with gram-negative sepsis accompanied by endotoxemia, the prognosis for both is poor. The mortality rate of sepsis in dogs, once shock ensues, is very high. Early recognition, although realistically difficult to accomplish in the clinical setting, and prompt specific intervention are critical factors in successful patient management. Another way of appraising the outcome of sepsis in veterinary medicine is to assume that patients treated with antimicrobials prior to the onset of clinical signs have significantly lower mortality rates than those treated after the onset of clinical signs. Although this statement has yet to be proved, it is logical to assume that risk management, i.e., treating those patients at risk of becoming septic at or before the time of exposure to potentially infectious bacteria, is prudent.

REFERENCES

1. Drazner FH: Bacterial endocarditis in the dog. Comp Contin Educ Pract Vet 1:918, 1979
2. Gilbert D: Endotoxemia and shock. In Sanford JP, Luby JP (eds): The Science and Practice Clinical Medicine. Vol. 8. p. 3. Grune & Stratton, New York, 1981
3. Hardie EM, Rawlings CA: Septic shock. I. Pathophysiology. Comp Contin Educ Pract Vet 5:369, 1983
4. Hardie EM, Rawlings CA: Septic shock. II. Prevention, recognition, and treatment. Comp Contin Educ Pract Vet 5:483, 1983
5. Haskins SC: Shock. In Kirk RW (ed): Current Veterinary Therapy VIII. p. 2. Saunders, Philadelphia, 1983
6. Rabinowitz SG: Bacterial sepsis and endotoxic shock. In Youmans GP, Paterson PY, Sommers HM (eds): The Biologic and Clinical Basis of Infectious Disease. p. 472. Saunders, Philadelphia, 1980
7. Reinhardt RA, Tussing GJ, Kalwarf KL: Endocarditis prophylaxis for patients with periodontal disease. AFP 27:129, 1983
8. Young LS: Gram negative sepsis. In Mandell GL, Douglas RG, Bennett JE (eds): Principles and Practice of Infectious Diseases. p. 571. Wiley, New York, 1979

Index

Page numbers followed by f represent figures; those followed by t represent tables.